For about a hundred years French medicine sheltered a highly influential intellectual tradition that was known as "the science of man." The medical science of man was holistic in character, encouraging physicians to focus – in medical theory and therapeutics – on the relation between the "physical and the moral." This study traces the history of this tradition from its roots in the medical vitalism of the University of Medicine in Montpellier, through its adaptation to the requirements of the Paris based "medical revolution," to its ideological and discursive fragmentation in the face of the heightened politicization of French medicine and the coming of medical modernity in the years from the Restoration to 1848. French physicians employed this tradition of linking the "physical and the moral" as their principal vehicle in seeking enhanced cultural authority throughout French society. Even after the vitalist underpinnings of the medical science of man were challenged, it exerted a powerful influence on the development of the human sciences – especially the conceptualization of degeneracy, hysteria, and racial inferiority – and undergirded the medicalization of French society.

The physical and the moral

Cambridge History of Medicine

Edited by

CHARLES WEBSTER, Reader in the History of Medicine, University of Oxford, and Fellow of All Souls College

CHARLES ROSENBERG, Professor of History and Sociology of Science, University of Pennsylvania

For a list of titles in the series, see end of book.

The physical and the moral

Anthropology, physiology, and philosophical medicine in France, 1750–1850

ELIZABETH A. WILLIAMS
Oklahoma State University

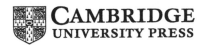
CAMBRIDGE
UNIVERSITY PRESS

CAMBRIDGE
UNIVERSITY PRESS

32 Avenue of the Americas, New York NY 10013-2473, USA

Cambridge University Press is part of the University of Cambridge.

It furthers the University's mission by disseminating knowledge in the pursuit of education, learning and research at the highest international levels of excellence.

www.cambridge.org
Information on this title: www.cambridge.org/9780521430678

© Cambridge University Press 1994

First published 1994
First paperback edition 2002

A catalogue record for this publication is available from the British Library

Library of Congress Cataloguing in Publication data
Williams, Elizabeth A. (Elizabeth Ann), 1950–
The physical and the moral: anthropology, physiology, and philosophical medicine in France, 1750–1850 / Elizabeth A. Williams.
      p.   cm. – (Cambridge history of medicine)
Includes index.
ISBN 0 521 43067 4 (hardback)
1. Medicine – France – History – 18th century.   2. Medicine – France – History – 19th century.   3. Medicine – France – Philosophy – 18th century.   4. Medicine – France – Philosophy – 19th century.
5. Université de médecine de Montpellier.   6. Ecole de santé de Montpellier.   7. Ecole de médecine de Montpellier.   8. Université de Montpellier. Faculté de médecine. I. Title. II. Series.
[DNLM: 1. Université de Montpellier. Faculté de médecine.
2. Université de médecine de Montpellier.   3. History of Medicine, 18th Cent. – France.   4. History of Medicine, 19th Cent. – France.
5. Vitalism. WZ 70 GF7 W7p 1994]
R504.W53   1994
610'.944'09033–dc20
DNLM/DLC
for Library of Congress
93-39511   CIP

ISBN 978-0-521-43067-8 Hardback
ISBN 978-0-521-52462-9 Paperback

To
Robert, Eleanor, and Susanna

CONTENTS

ILLUSTRATIONS

ACKNOWLEDGMENTS

For generous and efficient assistance in the research for this book, I wish to thank the librarians and staff of the Bibliothèque Nationale, the Archives Nationales, the Faculté de Médecine de Montpellier, the Faculté de Médecine de Paris, the Muséum national d'Histoire naturelle, the Musée de l'Homme, the Wellcome Institute for the History of Medicine, the History of Medicine Division of the National Library of Medicine, the Newberry Library, the Northwestern University Medical School, the library of the University of Georgia, and the Edmon Low Library at Oklahoma State University.

Financial support for the research for this book was provided by the National Science Foundation, the National Endowment for the Humanities, the Oklahoma Foundation for the Humanities, the Newberry Library, the College of Arts and Sciences of Oklahoma State University, and the Departments of History of the University of Georgia and of Oklahoma State University. I would like to express special thanks to Lester Stephens, former head of the History Department of the University of Georgia, for his generous support, at a crucial moment, of a young and very green scholar.

Scholarship has worth only insofar as it is a collective endeavor. I am thankful for this opportunity to express my gratitude to all those teachers, colleagues, and students who have shared with me the joys and vexations of the intellectual life: Roger Biles, Susan Blum, William B. Cohen, John Cornell, Maureen Flynn, the late Alf Heggoy, Ann Higginbotham, James Huston, Lionel Jensen, George Jewsbury, Ivan Karp, Tami Moore, Helen Nader, David Pace, Stanley Pierson, Bryant T. Ragan, Jr., Alain Saint-Saëns, Terry Shinn, Dale Sorenson, Gerald Strauss, Carol Summers, Greg Sutton, Rachel Webber, Kirk Willis, and Mary Victoria Wilson.

I wish to thank James Smith Allen, Joseph Byrnes, Robert Mayer, and Robert A. Nye, as well as Charles Rosenberg and the anonymous reviewer for Cambridge University Press, for their readings of the manuscript of this book. I greatly appreciate their labors on my behalf and regret those faults that persist despite their efforts.

Loving thanks go to Joe Lunn and Marsha Richmond, who have befriended me for virtually the whole of my life and whose generosity of spirit has always encouraged and strengthened me and my family.

It is not possible to repay, even to express, what I owe to Robert A. and Mary Jo Nye, whose friendship and intellectual companionship have been a source of joy for many years. I have a special debt to Bob Nye, without whose teaching my life as a scholar would have been impossible. Like so many others among his students, I will always be grateful for the privilege of having had, in him, a great teacher.

My mother and father, Grace Marie and the late Fred N. Williams, deserve more thanks than I can state in words. All the striving of my life is an attempt to return in some measure what they have given to me.

The help Robert Mayer gave me in the making of this book was immense, but it is trivial compared to everything else he has given me in our shared life. This book is dedicated to him and to our daughters.

ABBREVIATIONS

AGM	*Archives générales de médecine*
AHPML	*Annales d'hygiène publique et de médecine légale*
AN	Archives nationales
BHM	*Bulletin of the History of Medicine*
BSAP	*Bulletins de la Société d'anthropologie de Paris*
DBF	*Dictionnaire de biographie française*
Décade	*La décade philosophique, littéraire et politique*
DSB	*Dictionary of Scientific Biography*
DSM:BM	*Dictionaire des sciences médicales: Biographie médicale*
FHS	*French Historical Studies*
JHB	*Journal of the History of Biology*
JHMAS	*Journal of the History of Medicine and Allied Sciences*
MANM	*Mémoires de l'Académie nationale de médecine*
MAPB	*Mémoires d'anthropologie de Paul Broca*
MNHN	Muséum national d'histoire naturelle
MSME	*Mémoires de la Société médicale d'émulation*
RHS	*Revue d'histoire des sciences*

INTRODUCTION

For about a hundred years French medicine sheltered an intellectual tradition that contemporaries knew under the rubric "la science de l'homme," but that I have tried to capture in my title by referring serially to anthropology, physiology, and philosophical medicine. In devising a title for this study, I consciously avoided the English expression "the science of man" because it evokes a host of late eighteenth-century constructs, including "social science," "science of society," and "social art," that were connected only loosely to the specifically medical science of man that is examined here. I also wanted to avoid suggesting an exclusive focus on anthropology.[1] This book is certainly intended to contribute to the history of anthropology, but it also treats the history of physiology, before that discipline became what is now understood by the term, and, above all else, it is about medicine, from which both anthropology and physiology in large part derived.

Historians have been aware of the tradition of the medical science of man – or what I will interchangeably call "anthropological medicine" – for some time.[2] Excellent work has been undertaken on its development dur-

---

1 On the general science of man in the late eighteenth century, see Peter Gay, *The Enlightenment: An Interpretation*, vol. 2, *The Science of Freedom* (New York: W. W. Norton, 1969), 167–215; Keith Michael Baker, "The Early History of the Term 'Social Science,' " *Annals of Science* 20 (1964): 211–26; Henri Gouhier, *La jeunesse d'Auguste Comte et la formation du positivisme*, vol. 1, *Saint-Simon jusqu'à la Restauration* (Paris: J. Vrin, 1933), 42–48; Georges Gusdorf, *Les sciences humaines et la pensée occidentale*, vol. 8, *La conscience révolutionnaire: Les Idéologues* (Paris: Payot, 1978), 384–427.

2 I have used the term "anthropological medicine" in part simply for stylistic relief from the cumbersome and tiresomely sexist "science of man" but chiefly because numerous figures in this medical tradition conceived their work as constituting, or at the least contributing to, a new science of anthropology that was rooted in or subsumed by medicine. For usages of the term in medical works, see, for example, P. J. G. Cabanis, *Oeuvres philosophiques de Cabanis*, ed. Claude Lehec and Jean Cazeneuve, 2 vols. (Paris: Presses universitaires de France, 1956), 1:126, and 126, n. 1, 2:77; J.-L. Moreau de la Sarthe, "Pinel, Traité médico-philosophique sur l'aliénation mentale, ou la manie," *Décade* (20 pairial an IX [1801], 458–59n; Laurent Cerise, "Introduction," in *Rapports du physique et du moral de l'homme* by P. J. G. Cabanis (Paris: Fortin, 1843), xiii; Jacques Lordat, *Réponse à des objections faites contre le principe de la dualité du dynamisme humain* (Montpellier: Sevalle; Paris: J. B. Baillière, 1854), lxi–

ing the career of Pierre-Jean-Georges Cabanis and other physicians of the revolutionary era.[3] In this literature the science of man is generally seen as a product of the millenarian optimism of revolutionaries who hoped to transform the individual and society by medical therapeutics and social hygiene. This approach ties the medical science of man to monistic or materialistic philosophy and therefore to left-leaning politics. It explores the development of the medical science of man in the rapidly changing ideological environment of the revolutionary years. Finally, it traces the eclipse of the medical science of man to the political reaction that culminated in the rise to power of Bonaparte and brought disillusionment to the medical visionaries themselves.[4]

This conception of the origins, nature, and historical fate of the medical science of man is not, so far as it goes, inaccurate. The science of man *was* forcefully articulated during the Revolution. Its proponents in that era were mostly (although not always) linked to leftist politics. The science of man embraced during the Revolution was on the whole "optimistic" in its vision of humanity's future. This optimism did crumble amid the conflicts of an increasingly embittered politics.

These facts are but a small part, however, of a much larger and more complex history. The medical science of man originated well before the Revolution in the work of medical thinkers – the Montpellier vitalists – who were by no means millenarian visionaries. Although grounded in vitalist concepts, it was not a unitary medical doctrine or program linked to a particular political or social philosophy but a protean, often fragmented discourse. Furthermore, the medical science of man did not disappear with the end of the Revolution but instead, in the postrevolutionary era, underwent multiple terminological and ideological permutations. After the Revolution, the tradition of the science of man accreted conflicting meanings, repeatedly shifted institutional locus, and developed in company with a seemingly endless variety of theoretical and practical enterprises within the

---

lxii. On earlier usages of the term in France, see Georges Gusdorf, *Les sciences humaines et la pensée occidentale*, vol. 5, *Dieu, la nature, l'homme au siècle des lumières* (Paris: Payot, 1972), 405–08, 417–23, and for the revolutionary period, vol. 8, *La conscience révolutionnaire*, 384–92.

3 Gusdorf, *La conscience révolutionnaire*, esp. 305–427, 451–76; Martin Staum, *Cabanis: Enlightenment and Medical Philosophy in the French Revolution* (Princeton: Princeton University Press, 1980); Sergio Moravia, *Il tramonto dell'illuminismo: Filosofia e politica nella società francese (1770–1810)* (Bari: Laterza, 1968); idem, *Il pensiero degli Ideologues: Scienza e filosofia in Francia (1780–1815)* (Florence: La Nuova Italia, 1974); idem, "Philosophie et médecine en France à la fin du XVIIIe siècle," *Studies on Voltaire and the Eighteenth Century* 89 (1972): 1089–1151; Gouhier, *La jeunesse d'Auguste Comte*, vol. 1.

4 On monism and materialism, see Staum, *Cabanis*, 7–8, 205–6, 236–37, 263–65, 304–7; Moravia, *Il pensiero*, part 1; on the generally leftist associations of the science of man and its eclipse under Bonaparte, see Staum, *Cabanis*, chaps. 9 and 10; Gusdorf, *La conscience révolutionnaire*, esp. 305–30.

broad domain of medicine. It finally went into eclipse only after mid-century when its diverse elements gradually sedimented out into a range of emergent disciplinary constructs and medical specialties. And even then, forced into a subterranean and muffled existence, it continued to exert powerful influence in the human sciences.

Unlike the medical science of man of the revolutionary era, this larger tradition of anthropological medicine has generally escaped the attention of historians. The importance to the science of man of the work of the Montpellier vitalists, although by no means wholly ignored, has been underestimated because of the relative neglect of vitalism generally in the history of medicine and biology. The overemphasis on the labors and personality of Cabanis has resulted from the tendency to seek a univocal ideological register – leftism, materialism – for the medical science of man. Finally, the neglect of the medical science of man of the early to mid-nineteenth century has stemmed from two interrelated historiographical tendencies: to emphasize the development of forward-looking and progressive rather than traditional or archaic strains of French culture, and to reproduce and valorize ideological antinomies rather than to explore processes of adaptation, accommodation, and co-optation.

These various dispositions in turn reflected more fundamental methodological and ideological commitments that until recently undergirded general historiography and, most relevant to this work, the history of thought. In liberal historiography, individual historical actors who struggled for progressive change with exceptional clarity of vision or force of will figured prominently. In the historiography of the Left, social groups that mobilized for starkly delineated class and political conflicts dominated. In recent years, however, both these individuals and these social groups have tended to diminish in significance as the great contest of Left and Right that gave them meaning has lost its clarity. The minutely detailed examinations of ideological and class differentiation that preoccupied intellectual, social, and political historians into the 1960s (and especially historians of France, the motherlode of ideology) have come to seem strangely irrelevant.[5] At the same time, the various discursive, institutional, and administrative processes by which power is established and maintained in society, whatever the apparent or claimed ideological intentions of those who set them in motion, have commanded ever greater attention. Modes of manipulating lan-

5 This shift has taken place in historiographical contexts that have radically different implications. The contrast is perhaps best gauged by comparing the perspective of François Furet, who in his immensely influential *Interpreting the French Revolution* (Cambridge: Cambridge University Press, 1981), announced the end of ideological debate over the French Revolution, and Michel Foucault, who found ideology an impoverished framework for the analysis of power. On this feature of Foucault's thought, see the essays in *Foucault: A Critical Reader,* ed. David Couzens Hoy (New York: Basil Blackwell, 1986).

guage, of hiding behind professed ideology, of absorbing and co-opting discourses of challenge or resistance – these have assumed greater significance as the overtly articulated conflicts of Left and Right have come to have a hollow, even archaic ring.

The history of thought has not only shared in this general reevaluation of historical significances but has also become the terrain for a major campaign of methodological revisionism. This revisionism has undermined basic theoretical and procedural commitments, including the view that ideas originate and are conveyed in more or less readily definable units, that they circulate in a system of exchange whose principal value is reasoned choice, that ideas have natural or logical links to other ideas and to specific social practices, that when combined ideas form (or at least should form) rational doctrines, that coherence in intellectual traditions is achieved in a process of linear development, and that the focus of historical investigation should be those ideas that have proved the most fertile in influence on strains of thought that have remained recognizably and durably important.[6]

Such conceptions of how to study and evaluate the thought of the past have been forcefully contested both within and outside the world of working historians for some three decades, most compellingly by the diverse theorists of "discourse."[7] As conceived principally by Michel Foucault, discourses originate not as unit ideas but as socially engendered linguistic practices. They do not circulate in a system of rational exchange but rather accrete strata of sometimes wildly incompatible meaning. Discourses may be arbitrarily linked to other discourses by speakers who act to define and advance their specific social interests. They cohere not because of inner logic or empirical proof but because networks of conditions and practices hold them together. Finally, they exercise influence not as great ideas but as momentarily inescapable modes of thinking and talking about objects constituted by discourse itself.[8]

The concept of discourse has supplied a vehicle for rediscovering and reassessing patterns of thought – such as the fragmented, sometimes elusive

6 For reflections on the traditional practice of intellectual history and recent challenges to that practice, see the essays in *Modern European Intellectual History: Reappraisals and New Perspectives*, ed. Dominick Lacapra (Ithaca, N.Y.: Cornell University Press, 1982).

7 Allan Megill, "Foucault, Structuralism, and the Ends of History," *Journal of Modern History* 51 (1979): 451–503; Mark Poster, "The Future According to Foucault: The *Archaeology of Knowledge* and Intellectual History," in *Modern European Intellectual History;* Patrick H. Hutton, "The Foucault Phenomenon and Contemporary French Historiography," *Historical Reflections/Réflexions historiques* 17 (1991): 77–102. On the analysis of discourse in literary criticism, see Richard Terdiman, *Discourse/Counter-Discourse: The Theory and Practice of Symbolic Resistance in Nineteenth-Century France* (Ithaca, N.Y.: Cornell University Press, 1985).

8 Michel Foucault, *The Archaeology of Knowledge*, trans. A. M. Sheridan Smith (New York: Pantheon Books, 1972); *idem, Power/Knowledge: Selected Interviews and Other Writings, 1972–1977*, ed. Colin Gordon, trans. Colin Gordon et al. (New York: Pantheon Books, 1980). For a discussion of the evolution of Foucault's conception of discourse, see Ian Hacking, "The Archaeology of Foucault," in *Foucault: A Critical Reader*, 27–40.

tradition of the science of man – that earlier were neglected or simply lost from view since they failed to exhibit the characteristics demanded of "important" ideas. Discourse analysis legitimates inquiry into previously neglected realms of thought and speech by several means. At a fairly abstract level, it posits that whatever is said is significant by the very fact of its being said, thus delegitimizing the concept of an intellectual or scientific canon. More practically, it supplies a standard for judging the relative importance of ideas and intellectual traditions other than the criteria of clarity, rationality, and relevance to present thought. The standard it establishes is that of power, conceived not purely as the obvious power of the state apparatus and strategic institutions but also of those discursive practices that constitute social existence, identity, and relations. Thus discourses have power over those who speak within them – the architects of specific doctrines – and over those who are the objects of discourse, whether the discourse itself has any claim to truth, rationality, or transcendental meaning.[9]

This study is situated, then, within a new historiography conditioned by the insights and emphases of discourse analysis. It recovers for historical investigation a scientific discourse – the medical science of man – that always retained what Raymond Williams calls an "effective nucleus of meaning," but that was also marked by incoherence, fragmentation, unstable linguistic usages, methodological and logical evasions, and transparent political and ideological bias.[10] This discourse exerted intellectual and social power not in spite of these characteristics but precisely because it was friable, subject to apparently endless reformulation, extension, and adaptation to new circumstances. Yet these very qualities – the incoherence and adaptability of the medical science of man – have caused it to be lost from historical vision. Judged by traditional criteria, the history of the medical science of man appears to be one principally of failure, of an accumulation of statements subsequently thought unilluminating, wrongheaded, sometimes even vicious. Unlike familiar features on the intellectual landscape (such as the various "anticipations" of evolutionary theory), the discourse of the science of man could not be viewed as leading up to or generating any currently recognizable and valued scientific approach, theory, or paradigm. Indeed, one of the most telling features of this history is the way in which, after about 1850, the discourse of anthropological medicine was repudiated even in those domains where its influence was most compellingly registered. This process of repudiation then conditioned subsequent historiography. The single theorist of the medical science of man to remain widely known and in relatively good repute by the later nineteenth century was Cabanis, who was

9 Foucault, *Power/Knowledge*, esp. chaps. 3, 6, and 7.
10 Raymond Williams, *Marxism and Literature* (New York: Oxford University Press, 1977), 39.

claimed by physicians of that era as a forerunner of materialist neuroscience; it is unsurprising that the only conception of the science of man that we know very much about was his.[11]

Thus the perspective of discourse analysis has made it possible to see the larger science of man where earlier historiographical perspectives did not. All the same, I have sought to avoid what many historians have seen as serious problems presented to diachronic, genuinely historical analysis by the framework of discourse. These problems include the assumptions that discourse is autonomous and functions independently of the decisions and actions of individual speakers. This perspective has in turn seemed to imply that discourse is internally self-assured and untroubled, in short that discourse leaves no room for conflict. In some critiques these problems have been laid at Foucault's door; more recently the Foucauldian perspective has itself been plumbed for insights into the process by which "counter-discourses" emerge.[12] This study, which is an empirical investigation prompted by the insights of discourse analysis, does not address these problems at the level of theory. It does indicate, however, that in this case discourse was far from monolithic. Indeed I argue that the great power of the science of man derived from its supplying the basic but endlessly renegotiable terms of discussion of a problem – the relations of the physical and the moral – that had, from all ideological perspectives, become unavoidable.

A related but less tractable set of problems has to do with how discourses are formed and how they disintegrate. Foucault's own studies laid much greater stress on the power exerted by discourses in given synchronic settings than on how discourses are contested, undergo fragmentation, and ultimately suffer structural collapse. And at least one of his disciples has recently applauded historians who "frankly admit that they are incapable of explaining cultural mutations, and, even more, that they haven't the slightest idea what form a causal explanation might take."[13] If seen in this light, discourse analysis becomes a problematic tool for investigations, such as this one, that emphasize development and change. This study attempts not only to show the discursive power of the science of man at successive mo-

---

11 See the discussion in Chapter 2 and in the Epilogue.
12 For critiques by historians of the apparently monolithic character of discourse, see Dorinda Outram, *The Body and the French Revolution: Sex, Class and Political Culture* (New Haven: Yale University Press, 1989), 4–5, 19; Jan Goldstein, *Console and Classify: The French Psychiatric Profession in the Nineteenth Century* (Cambridge: Cambridge University Press, 1987), 3–4; Daniel Pick, *Faces of Degeneration: A European Disorder, c. 1848–c. 1918* (Cambridge: Cambridge University Press, 1989), 9–11. See also Terdiman, *Discourse/Counter-Discourse*, 18, 40, 72.
13 Paul Veyne, "The Roman Empire," in *A History of Private Life*, vol. 1, *From Pagan Rome to Byzantium*, ed. Philippe Ariès and Georges Duby, 4 vols. (Cambridge, Mass.: Harvard University Press, 1987), 43.

ments of French history but also to explore the dynamics of its history. It examines how the science of man accrued widespread support and then, having exercised dominance, collapsed into a substratum of principles and impulses no longer joined under one discursive rubric.

As a corrective to what I see as the excessively formalistic character of discourse analysis, I have also employed the framework of "tradition" to designate and analyze the medical science of man. To a much greater extent than discourse, tradition encourages attention to the way individual theorists deliberately positioned themselves in relation to the science of man. Tradition is seen here not as the "dead hand of the past," as Marx called it, or as an anonymous and inescapable framework for utterance, but as a body of transmitted texts, concepts, and linguistic usages that were available for conscious manipulation to diverse ends.[14] Some of the physicians working within the science of man deliberately embraced the tradition and trumpeted its value and authority. Others took up its thematics while avoiding identification with the tradition as a whole or noisily rejecting elements within it that they found objectionable. If discourse analysis enables us to perceive unintentionally registered effects and constraints, the framework of tradition reestablishes a context charged with immediacy and intentionality.

In any event some recognition of conscious contests – waged with and over tradition – is essential to understanding the fragmentation and collapse of the discourse of the science of man. Of the complex reasons for the demise of the science of man, the single most compelling was its identification with what came to be seen as discredited tradition in both the theory and organization of medicine. At one level of analysis, this rejection of the science of man may be seen as ineluctably determined since it resulted from the linked and powerful processes of the spread of scientism and the ever more complex division of intellectual and professional labor in medicine. Yet these social processes were themselves the work of myriad conscious and choosing individuals. The concept of tradition allows us to recover, as discourse analysis does not, the practical, often highly emotive, labor of devising and promoting intellectual constructs. It recognizes that in such labor the power of tradition, of what Raymond Williams calls the "practical continuities – families, places, institutions, a language" – is often great.[15] In so doing the framework of tradition supplies some sense of how conceptions and usages that are seemingly dispirited, discarded, even dead can continue to tug at the margins of a putatively unencumbered creative consciousness. Thus the history of the science of man is illuminated by viewing it alternately as an autonomous discourse of great and evident momentary

14 For a survey of concepts and uses of tradition, see Edward Shils, *Tradition* (Chicago: University of Chicago Press, 1981).
15 Williams, *Marxism and Literature*, 116.

power and as a tradition that, even after slipping from view, continued to exert real force.

The medical science of man cannot be precisely defined. As Nietzsche said of the concept of punishment, its history *is* its definition, and that history is the subject of this book.[16] But the science of man can be said to have four principal nodes of reference. First, it was holistic, both in its conception of the human persona as an integral, functionally interdependent whole and in its view of medicine as a science or art that must somehow embrace the myriad, interdependent phenomena of human experience. Seen in this light, medicine was not limited to a discrete set of physical phenomena but instead was extensive, to some theorists even comprehensive, in its purview.

A second defining feature derives from the first: the science of man postulated intimate relations (*rapports*) among separate domains of human experience that in the eighteenth century were usually conceived according to a tripartite scheme of the physical, the mental, and the passional but that later were reduced to what physicians of the revolutionary era called "the physical and the moral."[17] The science of man did not generally reduce the psychic domain to the physical, and thus was neither "monist" nor "materialist." Most physicians who worked within the tradition accepted some kind of distinction between mind and body and between willed and unwilled action. But they taught nevertheless that these realms of existence and experience were closely interdependent. "Rapport" meant, then, not control or determination of mind by body or vice versa but linkage, interrelation, reciprocity.[18]

16 "The concept 'punishment' possesses in fact not *one* meaning but a whole synthesis of 'meanings': the previous history of punishment in general, the history of its employment for the most various purposes, finally crystallizes into a kind of unity that is hard to disentangle, hard to analyze and, as must be emphasized especially, totally *indefinable*. . . . [A]ll concepts in which an entire process is semiotically concentrated elude definition; only that which has no history is definable." Friedrich Nietzsche, *On the Genealogy of Morals,* trans. Walter Kaufmann and R. J. Hollingdale (New York: Vintage Books, 1969), 80.
17 P. J. G. Cabanis, *Rapports du physique et du moral de l'homme,* 2 vols. (Paris: Crapart, Caille et Ravier, 1802). (All references here are to the 1956 edition of the *Oeuvres philosophiques* cited in note 2.) Cabanis's work gave this phrase its great currency, but it had been used for some time before. See, for example, the work of the Montpellier physician Louis de Lacaze (written in collaboration with Théophile de Bordeu), *Idée de l'homme physique et moral* (Paris: H. L. Guérin and L. F. Delatour, 1755). As we will see, the phrase had a firm place in medical discourse long into the nineteenth century. I have used the English "moral" for want of any more exact English equivalent. The French *moral* does not have so intense an ethical charge as the English, but as this work demonstrates, problems of morality were very close to the surface — and often fully there — for most of the physicians who employed the phrase "rapports du physique et du moral." See also L. S. Jacyna, "Medical Science and Moral Science: The Cultural Relations of Physiology in Restoration France," *History of Science* 25 (1987): 111–46.
18 For a discussion of this point, see Goldstein, *Console and Classify,* 49–55.

Third, the science of man pushed medicine into society, by its own internal logic as much as by any overt ideological or political intention, for it was a medical philosophy that regarded intellectual, passional, and social phenomena as intimately tied to the well-being of the body. In its earliest incarnations, the science of man owed this social construction of medicine largely to a certain reading of Hippocratism, which was construed as teaching that health was not individual but rather was dependent on social practices and milieux. Later these Hippocratic moorings were cut but anthropological medicine continued to insist on the importance to health of habit, occupation, climate, and similar influences.[19]

Lastly, the science of man privileged the problem of discerning human "types" amid the great variety of clinical and social detail gathered in the course of medical investigations. These types were generally articulated in terms of the variable distribution in individuals of vital energy and, more specifically, in terms of temperament, constitution, age, sex, climate, disease, and, ultimately, race. This disposition to typologize was rooted in the medical vitalism from which, as I argue, the science of man derived its original encouragement. Vitalism insisted by definition on the variability and diversity of human phenomena. It originally assumed coherence as a medical doctrine by attacking universals, in the form of the mechanical and physiochemical constants of iatromechanism and Cartesian conceptions of body physics. Rejecting mechanical constants, vitalist physicians looked instead for patterns, regularities, and generalities that would allow them to devise meaningful pathological, therapeutic, and physiological explanations. Thus the discernment of types showing regularities different from those found in the physical universe was one of the special contributions the science of man had to make to the larger scientific enterprise.[20]

It is the central argument of this book that from the late Enlightenment to around 1850 the medical science of man developed in the three principal discursive contexts of anthropology, physiology, and philosophical medicine. Of these three, only anthropology now seems naturally linked to some idea of a science of man. Indeed, one of the main tasks I hope to accomplish is to show how and why in France the medical science of man ultimately became detached from the "progressive" and mainstream development of the other two contextual fields, physiology and medicine. As early as the 1820s the dominant construction of physiology – the experimentalist, laboratory-based science of François Magendie and his associates – left little place for posing the sorts of broad sociomedical questions that only two de-

19 On Hippocratism in the science of man, see Moravia, "Philosophie et médecine."
20 On vitalism generally, see Jacques Roger, *Les sciences de la vie dans la pensée française du XVIIIᵉ siècle*, 2d ed. (Paris: A. Colin, 1971), 420–39.

cades before were commonly labeled "physiological."[21] Nor was the phrase science of man used much beyond 1850 to signify a conception of medicine itself, although before that date the interchangeability of the terms *médecine, art de guérir, science médicale,* and *science de l'homme* was an ordinary feature of the French medical vocabulary. From roughly the 1830s to the 1850s the complex of problems, concepts, and theoretical inclinations that had made up the science of man began to be shunted aside and marginalized as the concerns of "philosophical medicine," which, unlike "positive medicine," continued to address nonmedical, "metaphysical" problems with the antiquated procedures of philosophical argumentation. It was only after 1859 when a group of doctors clustered in the Société d'anthropologie de Paris proffered a new version of anthropology, one acknowledging its medical roots yet establishing independent claims to positivity, that mainstream medicine again lent support (and then somewhat grudgingly) to the development of a medically founded science of man.[22] But this new science of man – the consolidated discipline of anthropology – was only partially congruent with the earlier medical science of man whose history is examined here.

At the point where this book begins, medicine alone of these three was firmly constituted intellectually and socially, having existed for centuries as one of the chief divisions of learning and, with law and the clergy, forming one of the ancient professions.[23] Neither "anthropology" nor "physiology" enjoyed such status in the later eighteenth century, although both words were gaining currency. In this period the term anthropology began appearing in the writings of German physicians and philosophers and in France, too, was beginning to enter various scholarly lexicons. In the late eighteenth century, furthermore, scholarly projects that look something like modern anthropology were underway. Cabinets were filled with human skulls and pottery shards, and notebooks were crammed with measurements and descriptions of facial angles, cranial diameters, and shades of skin color.[24] Despite these endeavors, however, no distinct field of anthropology

21 John Lesch, *Science and Medicine in France: The Emergence of Experimental Physiology, 1790–1855* (Cambridge: Mass.: Harvard University Press, 1984), esp. 89–124; see also Joseph Schiller, "Physiology's Struggle for Independence in the First Half of the Nineteenth Century," *History of Science* 7 (1968): 64–89.

22 On the institutional support given Brocan anthropology by the medical establishment, see Elizabeth A. Williams, "Anthropological Institutions in Nineteenth-Century France," *Isis* 76 (1985): 331–48.

23 Eliot Freidson, *Profession of Medicine: A Study of the Sociology of Applied Knowledge* (New York: Dodd, Mead, 1970); see also the works cited in note 25.

24 On eighteenth-century anthropology, see Claude Blanckaert, ed. *Naissance de l'ethnologie? Anthropologie et missions en Amérique, XVIᵉ–XVIIIᵉ siècles* (Paris: Editions du Cerf, 1985); Michèle Duchet, *Anthropologie et histoire au siècle des lumières: Buffon, Voltaire, Rousseau, Helvétius, Diderot* (Paris: François Maspéro, 1971); Britta Rupp-Eisenreich, *Histoires de l'an-*

yet existed. There were no anthropologists as such and certainly no profession of anthropology.[25] Rather, there was a discourse of anthropology, just as there were discourses of aesthetics, economics, and ethics, without any of these constituting established disciplines or fields of learning. Anthropological discourse was created by philosophers, jurists, naturalists, and doctors, whose "anthropology" differed in keeping with the previously existing discourses of philosophy, law, natural history, and medicine and with the institutional and social structures supporting these endeavors. This book is not, then, about all of early "anthropology" or the early "science of man"; rather it is about the anthropology of the doctors, the medical science of man.

"Physiology" was a term more commonly used than "anthropology" in eighteenth-century France, but it too signified divergent types of investigation pursued by diverse inquirers. In general, physiology meant the study of living function rather than static structure, but the way in which such investigations should proceed, the specific problems physiological inquiry should encompass, and indeed the meaning of "function" itself were matters of dispute.[26] The first chapter of this book examines one crucially important conception of physiology that was developed by vitalist physicians at the University of Medicine in Montpellier in southern France and then adapted by Paris physicians in the context of the French "medical revolution."[27] To Montpellier doctors, physiology was the study of living organisms, as opposed to "dead objects" or "brute matter," and its central objective was to discover the unique "laws" governing the existence of organisms endowed with "life." The primordial law of organized beings was that they lived and functioned by virtue of the interconnected activities of the "animal economy," which was empowered by some kind of vital force or forces. Thus physiology was the study of the interrelated, systemic, harmonious operations that simultaneously manifested and sustained the life of bodies that enjoyed vitality.

thropologie, XVIe–XIXe siècles (Paris: Klincksieck, 1984); George W. Stocking, Jr., "French Anthropology in 1800," in *Race, Culture, and Evolution: Essays in the History of Anthropology* (1968; rpt. Chicago: University of Chicago Press, 1982), 13–41.

25 The diverse criteria used to define the outlines of a "profession" are surveyed and criticized in Andrew Abbott, *The System of Professions: An Essay on the Division of Expert Labor* (Chicago: University of Chicago Press, 1988); see also Magali S. Larson, *The Rise of Professionalism: A Sociological Analysis* (Berkeley: University of California Press, 1977); Eliot Freidson, *Professional Powers: A Study of the Institutionalization of Formal Knowledge* (Chicago: University of Chicago Press, 1986), esp. 20–62.

26 Lesch, *Science and Medicine in France*, 12–26; cf. Georges Canguilhem, "La constitution de la physiologie comme science," in *Etudes d'histoire et de philosophie des sciences* (Paris: J. Vrin, 1979), 226–73.

27 On different meanings attached to the phrase "medical revolution," see Elizabeth A. Williams, "The French Revolution, Anthropological Medicine, and the Creation of Medical Authority" in *Re-creating Authority in Revolutionary France,* ed. Bryant T. Ragan, Jr., and Elizabeth A. Williams (New Brunswick, N.J.: Rutgers University Press, 1992), 79–97.

As conceived by the Montpellier doctors, physiology ostensibly encompassed not only human beings but animals and plants as well. And indeed some Montpellier physicians undertook research on animals, arguing for the advantages of an approach that compared human to animal and vegetable phenomena.[28] In practice, however, the vitalist physiology of the Montpellier physicians focused almost exclusively on human beings. Because Montpellier vitalism was a product of medicine, and medicine itself was anthropological in the sense that it was human-centered, these inquirers were especially cognizant of problems specifically presented by human physiology. In Montpellier vitalism, then, there was an ineluctable connection between physiological and anthropological problematics. This link was compellingly reinforced by the Montpellier concept of "organization," which necessarily entailed investigation of any and all phenomena connected to the life of the organism – internal and external, physical and mental, healthy and pathological. *Nothing* could be justifiably excluded since any process or operation might constitute the key to explaining the activities of the interrelated whole. Physiologically based medicine had to take into account any influence, activity, or circumstance that affected general vitality and health. It had to be constituted as the science of *l'homme entier.*

Montpellier's conception of physiology and of the tasks proper to medicine had powerful resonance in late eighteenth-century medical and scientific circles in France. The paths along which its influence moved to Paris are considered in Chapter 2, which takes up the development of the medical science of man by the Paris medical revolutionaries of the 1790s. As adapted by Paris doctors in the context of the Revolution, vitalist physiology retained its focus on the human and indeed was conceived of as the fundamental framework for the larger science of man that was to claim authority in diverse regions of human life and experience. This science of man was to investigate not body, mind, or feeling in isolation but instead the "relations between the physical and the moral." Grounded in physiology, it promised to extract from the study of human "organization" fundamental principles for a science of human beings as individuals and in society.

In the course of the Revolution the program of forming a new anthropological medicine came to be associated particularly with a configuration of medical theory that some historians have identified as medical Ideology. Accordingly, anthropological medicine was for a time closely identified with the larger movement of Ideology and with the Ideologues' supposed embrace of a unitary eighteenth-century legacy of atheist materialism.[29] During the late Empire and Restoration this linkage between Ideology and

28 Réjane Bernier, "La notion de principe vital chez Barthez," *Archives de philosophie* 35 (1972): 423–41.
29 George Rosen, "The Philosophy of Ideology and the Emergence of Modern Medicine in France," *BHM* 20 (1946): 328–39.

anthropological medicine provoked a reaction, and, as is shown in Chapter 3, much angry debate then took place in medical circles between "materialists" and "spiritualists" over the nature of the mind-body relation.[30] Yet many medical theorists regarded the very existence of such debate within medicine as deleterious to the advance of medical science and to the interests of the medical profession. They began seeking in turn to cut medicine free from all ideological ties; their principal device for so doing was the construction, and simultaneously the marginalization, of "philosophical medicine."

Throughout the eighteenth century physicians had referred to their approach to medicine as "philosophical" merely as a way of saying that it was rigorous, genuinely scientific, and informed by sound method. Medicine was "philosophical" if it stood in contrast, on the one hand, to "routine" and blind obedience to tradition and, on the other, to hucksterism and superstition.[31] All of this changed after the Revolution, as the phrase "philosophical medicine" was given a pejorative connotation by those who sought to associate themselves with a new medicine that repudiated philosophy, and ideology along with it. As "positive" techniques of medicine – clinical observation, statistical inquiry, and especially pathological anatomy – gained more advocates, the old "philosophical" medicine of the erudite theoretician was dismissed as superannuated, speculative, and metaphysical. Just as eighteenth-century doctors had rejected seventeenth-century "systems," now nineteenth-century doctors renounced the "doctrines" of the eighteenth century.[32] At first "philosophical medicine" was condemned by detractors of both materialism and spiritualism, which were portrayed as metaphysical perspectives equally irrelevant to positive medicine. But when, in the late Restoration and especially in the 1830s, the scientistic values of the eighteenth century were rehabilitated, the process of cleansing medicine of ideology came particularly to mean eliminating its archaic, vitalist elements. Finally, by around 1850, "philosophical medicine" stabilized as a term of opprobrium used by forward-looking Parisian doctors to denigrate the vitalist medicine of the school of Montpellier and all those in Montpellier and elsewhere who continued to sympathize with it.

By the time this semantic development was accomplished, the science of man had fragmented into the diverse, often mutually antagonistic elements that are examined in Chapter 3. The intense struggles of the Revolution and

30 Jacyna, "Medical Science and Moral Science."
31 See, for example, Théophile de Bordeu, *Recherches sur l'histoire de la médecine* (1764; Paris: Auguste Ghio, 1882).
32 On the defects of "philosophical medicine," see, for example, "Introduction," *Annales médico-psychologiques* 1 (1843): viii; J. -B. Bouillaud, review of A. R. J. Lepelletier, *Physiologie médicale et philosophique*, in *Journal universel et hebdomadaire de médecine* 5 (1831): 26–28; obituary for J.-J. Virey, *Archives générales de la médecine*, 4th ser., 11 (1846): 117.

counterrevolution engendered an array of new formulations of the science of man developed by medical theorists across the ideological spectrum – erstwhile Ideologues, conservatives, "eclectics," Broussaisists, promoters of the new specialties of hygiene and mental medicine. All of them continued to use the phrase science of man to describe their efforts and orientation, but only the heirs of Montpellier remained content to accept the cognomen "philosophical medicine." For the self-styled progressives, this phrase has become a form of linguistic assault.

These developments – the devaluation of philosophical medicine, the advance of medical modernity, and the decline of vitalism – did not mean that medicine now abruptly eschewed questions posed by the science of man and still referred to even by fierce detractors of Cabanis as the "relations between the physical and the moral." Chapter 4 opens by examining theorists at either end of the vitalist-materialist divide who continued during the Orleanist era to argue that medicine must constitute itself as a comprehensive science of man. In these years vitalists in Montpellier persisted in the view that the only true medicine was one that recognized the uniqueness of human beings and grounded its investigations in a genuinely anthropological vision. At the opposite end of the spectrum, phrenologists insisted with full confidence that they held the key to the physical-moral relation, despite the judgment of its critics that phrenology itself was one last flight of philosophical medicine. The dominant trend of the 1830s and 1840s was, however, the attempt of diverse medical theoreticians who were still determined to address the problem of the physical and moral to develop new syntheses that would move the science of man beyond its old methodological and ideological polarities. The medical physiology and race science of the period attempted to maintain medicine's focus on the uniquely human while accommodating the comparativist perspective of general biological science. A new "social-Christian" medicine rejected all the old theoretical dichotomies of materialist and spiritualist, progressive and conservative, in favor of a socially engaged medicine focused on understanding and developing "faculties-in-action." Still other physicians gravitated toward the emergent disciplines of "ethnology" and "anthropology," which were grounded partly in medical inquiry and partly in pursuits – historical, geographical, linguistic – that, like the medical science of man itself, had gradually developed on the broad terrain of the human sciences charted in the eighteenth century.

In the 1840s and the 1850s none of these syntheses was successful in engendering a newly dominant discourse of the science of man. But their efforts did make clear the principal requirements that any successful reconfiguration of the science of man would have to meet. The enterprise had to be, by the standards of a rapidly evolving scientific community, genuinely "scientific," and it had to find some "positive" means by which to join the study of body and mind, the physical and the moral, without falling prey to the charges of metaphysical obscurity that had obstructed previous efforts. Beginning in the 1850s the vehicle increasingly used to achieve these ends was the view that human psychic characteristics were determined by physical heredity.[33] Hereditarian thinking was not altogether new by any means; it had played an ever more prominent role in the discourse of the science of man as well as in the larger domain of the biological sciences in the late 1830s and in the 1840s. But from the 1848 Revolution forward, the tendency of French medical and life scientists to ascribe to blood heritage the formation of physical and moral features was increasingly pronounced.

The complexly interwoven reasons for the heightened importance of heredity – theoretical, professional, institutional, and broadly cultural – can only be suggested in this study. The Epilogue indicates, by focusing on significant moments in the post-1850 development of the human sciences, how hereditarianism supplied a new ground of positivity to disciplines that gradually sedimented out of the old anthropological medicine. Medically grounded heredity theory was first formulated by alienists whose original theoretical orientation was supplied by anthropological medicine but who sought to give mental medicine new rigor by supplying it with an unambiguously physicalist explanatory mechanism. The ubiquity of hereditarian thinking in medicine was in turn linked to a shift in focus from individual to social pathology. Indeed the key development of the era was the emergence of the "degenerate," the individual whose inherited pathological proclivities worsened under the influence of a noxious environment and evil habits and were then passed on to a yet more enfeebled progeny. Hereditary, degenerative pathology then became the focus of work in a range of disciplines – psychiatry, neurology, criminology, and anthropology – that gradually displaced the medical science of man. In the Epilogue I argue that in all these fields claims were made to a new positivity on the basis of a putatively rigorous physicalism – a sense of determinism and law-bound behavior borrowed from the natural sciences – that was adopted in conscious opposition to the principles of the old anthropological medicine.

The chief emphasis of the Epilogue is on the emergent discipline of anthropology, whose appearance was encouraged by hereditarian discourse to which it in turn made a singular and powerful contribution by honing the concept of race. Where previous efforts to develop an independent science of anthropology had foundered for want of a clearly determinist and hence genuinely scientific paradigm, race provided a widely heralded device for linking the investigation of physical and psychic capacities. Racial analysis justified inquiry into subjects – human anatomy and physiology, speciation and tranformism, the historical development of language and civil society,

33 Robert A. Nye, *Crime, Madness, and Politics in Modern France: The Medical Concept of National Decline* (Princeton: Princeton University Press, 1984); Pick, *Faces of Degeneration.*

prehistory and archaeology – whose range and complexity had been only dimly perceived in the old anthropological medicine but that doctors seemed peculiarly well suited to approach precisely because of the medical tradition of the science of man.

The emergence of this new science of man did not mean that the old science of man was salvaged intact. Nor was it intended to be; the anthropology of the late nineteenth century at once borrowed from and worked to dismantle the constructs of anthropological medicine. Indeed the development of anthropology illustrates with particular clarity a process at work in all the disciplines in which anthropological medicine was reconfigured: the manifest rejection, yet simultaneously the unconscious reappropriation, of a tradition that was regarded as superannuated yet continued to command authority. This process unfolded most clearly on the very terrain – strict hereditarianism – where the newly positive human sciences sought to demonstrate their transcendence of the ambiguities of the old science of man. While the hereditarian constructs of the new human sciences ostensibly provided an austerely physicalist and determinist framework for the investigation of mental pathology, racial characteristics, and the like, these constructs in fact replicated the concept of physical-moral reciprocities that had always marked anthropological medicine. In important instances, furthermore, specifically vitalist features of the old science of man – its holistic approach to pathology, its emphasis on the husbanding and distribution of vital energy – returned in new guises. The cases traced in the Epilogue suggest that, although the human sciences of the later nineteenth century struggled to move beyond the archaic discourse of the physical and the moral, they were in profound ways still ensnarled in its problematics and language.

As these remarks will indicate, this book is in large part a history of the changing meaning of words. One of my central assumptions is that words stabilize or change in meaning depending on the specific contexts – strictly discursive, institutional, political, broadly social – in which they are employed by actual speakers in accordance with their peculiar interests.[34] These interests form too, then, a central theme of the book, and a word is in order about what kinds of interests I have investigated. This book is not conceived according to a rigorous theoretical scheme of the bond between thought and action, discourse and "real life." Thus I have not deliberately looked for a particular set of determinants – institutional antagonisms, religious influence, class or gender conflicts – although all of these appear at

34 My conception of these interests is derived in part from Foucault's idea of the power of discourse, but I also use the term "interests" in the more mundane fashion of the older sociology of science, with its concerns for patronage, funding, institutional clusters, and the like. See R. K. Merton, *The Sociology of Science: Theoretical and Empirical Investigations,* ed. Norman Storer (Chicago: University of Chicago Press, 1973); Robert Fox and George Weisz, eds. *The Organization of Science and Technology in France, 1808–1914* (Cambridge: Cambridge University Press, 1980).

various points in the history. Rather I have started from the words themselves and then, guided by certain fairly loose preconceptions about what constitutes the social grounding of words and thought, explored as much purely empirical information as I could gather about the speakers of the words.

When I began the book I was primarily concerned with institutional interests, such as the continuing rivalry between the Paris and Montpellier faculties of medicine. But the material itself began to demand being situated within a much more broadly political context, of which shifting institutional allegiances and objectives were but a part. As many historians have pointed out, French medicine was intensely politicized in the course of the French Revolution and thus, to a greater degree than one might find in the history of other cultural phenomena, there was often a more or less direct "fit" between medical and political developments.[35] The close links between medical and political culture in this era explain the structure of the book, which is divided into four parts corresponding to the great political divisions of the period covered: late Ancien Regime, Revolution and Empire, Restoration, and Orleanist monarchy. I do not present this viewpoint on the links between medicine and politics as a general truth about science or culture but rather attempt to demonstrate its accuracy and utility in this particular case by examining the political enmeshing of medicine at the successive stages of French history traversed here.

Aside from the institutional and political contexts of the medical science of man, this work also attempts to locate the individuals who elaborated the tradition of anthropological medicine within diverse social networks of exchange, hostility, reciprocity, and allegiance. The inadequacy of the kind of formal institutional history that operated only at the level of the university, the *grandes écoles,* and prestigious learned societies pressed itself upon me throughout the writing of this book. Some of the most important links, both cordial and antagonistic, among the theoreticians treated here operated not at the formal level of institutions but through small-scale or informal social networks of varying kinds – family, military service, sociopolitical movements like Saint-Simonism, and patronage clusters. If, as the Foucauldian perspective has taught us, discursive formations function with a high degree of autonomy, nonetheless the nuances and fine features of these discourses, those particularities that constitute the *événéments* of history, are produced in the diverse contexts in which individual lives unfold. These contexts are as important a part of this work, which is intended to be a close empirical history, as the autonomous discourse of the science of man itself.

---

35 On the political divisions among the French medical corps after the Revolution, see Jacques Léonard, *La médecine entre les pouvoirs et les savoirs: Histoire intellectuelle et politique de la médecine française au XIXe siècle* (Paris: Aubier Montaigne, 1981), 110–26.

A word is in order about exclusions. The reader might well expect that a book about early anthropology in France would include a good deal of information about the natural history tradition, in which the word "anthropology" also took root and which ultimately served as one of the principal sources for the concept of race. There is, however, little here on what was usually referred to in the nineteenth century as "the natural history of man." Although there were always theoretical congruences and institutional ties between the medical science of man and the natural history of man, this work emphasizes the differences between the two. Whereas the science of man claimed its medical origins and trumpeted its grounding in medicine, the natural history of man allied itself with general natural history and the emerging science of biology. With few exceptions, the medical science of man insisted on the sui generis character of its methods, whereas the natural history of man eagerly embraced those of the life sciences and even of the physical sciences where they seemed applicable. The science of man deliberately took up questions with philosophical and theological dimensions, whereas the natural history of man tended to eschew such problems, viewing them as beyond the purview of science.[36] I will have occasion throughout this work to venture into the domain of the natural history of man by touching on the work of Desmoulins, Lacépède, Cuvier, Lamarck, Geoffroy Saint-Hilaire, Flourens, and others. The overlap between medicine and natural history in the ethnological society and in the establishment of anthropological study at the Muséum d'histoire naturelle is also briefly considered. But the main line of development that this book follows is the evolution of the medical science of man. As that task alone seemed formidable enough for one book, the work of linking these two histories together in a unitary history of the development of anthropology in France remains to be accomplished.

The exclusions in respect to physiology will appear even more marked. There is nothing here on the development of physiology at the hands of Magendie and his followers after the 1820s. As my purpose is to explore not the general development of anthropology or physiology or medicine but those parts of each that intersected in the theoretical nexus of the science of man, I have not followed the history of experimental physiology beyond its hiving off from medicine and its establishment as a discipline that achieved self-definition in good part by repudiating the problem of the physical-moral relation that had engrossed physiologists of an earlier era. The physiology that *is* examined here is the one that by the 1830s and 1840s was coming to be perceived as a specifically medical physiology, focused still on

---

36 On natural history in France, see Pietro Corsi, *The Age of Lamarck: Evolutionary Theories in France, 1790–1830*, trans. Jonathan Mandelbaum (Berkeley: University of California Press, 1988), 1–39; Henri Daudin, *Les classes zoologiques et l'idée de série animale en France à l'époque de Lamarck et Cuvier (1790–1830)*, 2 vols. (Paris: Alcan, 1926); Paul Farber, "Discussion Paper: The Transformation of Natural History in the Nineteenth Century," *JHB* 15 (1982): 145–52.

problems of human organization, physical and mental. When the new physiology abandoned the focus on the human in favor of a comparativist perspective, this step created as salient a point of division with "medical" physiology as the experimental method itself, although the overt conflicts between physiological traditionalists and progressives were generally couched in strictly methodological terms.

The latter part of this book presents for the most part a story of decline. The medical science of man, despite the high ambitions of its early advocates, was not destined to march in step with dominant trends in either medical theory and methodology or the organization of medicine as a social enterprise. By 1850 it was evident that an omnibus, general, anthropological medicine rooted in vitalist holism would not flourish in an era dominated by positive philosophy, reductive and experimental methodology, and professional specialization. Accordingly, much of the discourse of anthropological medicine circa 1850 seems distinctly archaic. Nonetheless, although this story is about decline, it is not about nullity or insignificance. The discursive framework of the science of man may have disappeared but elements of the science of man survived in diverse and influential forms. By 1850 the root assumption of the medical science of man, that there existed an intimate link between the physical and the moral, was pervasive in French society. And although the human sciences of the later nineteenth century rejected medical conceptions of fluid, reciprocally flowing physical-moral *rapports* in favor of a putatively strict materialism, the immense prestige these sciences enjoyed nonetheless stemmed from the fact that they were able finally to explain in clear scientific terms what everyone already assumed to be true. This is not of course to say that the human sciences emerged solely from the tradition of anthropological medicine or that they would not have enjoyed acceptance in the absence of this tradition. It is to say that given the concatenation of historical circumstances that everywhere impelled human science toward a determinist, positivist, materialist posture in this era, the peculiar history of this process in France – the singular cast the human sciences took and the broad sociocultural approbation they enjoyed – cannot be explained without reference to the long-standing medical tradition of the linkage between the physical and the moral. Individual theorists believed they were transcending this medical past, or, at the very least, rigorously selecting from and reshaping its elements. They believed, in short, that they were dominating a tradition rather than being dominated by it. That this self-perception was in significant part illusory is the view developed in the Epilogue. At its most general level, then, this book concludes with an argument on behalf of the staying power of intellectual traditions, even those, or perhaps especially those, which like the medical science of man harbor ambiguities and inconsistencies, are particularly subject to the transformative power of external influences, and are finally reduced to a fugitive discursive existence.

1

Montpellier vitalism and the science of man

History has neglected the Montpellier vitalists. Even to specialists their work is little known, and their singular role in the eighteenth-century development of the biomedical sciences is only dimly perceived. This neglect of Montpellier is a consequence of two familiar patterns in the history of French science. One is the much-remarked tendency of historians both inside and outside France to stress developments in Paris at the expense of all other locales.[1] Given the long-standing dominance of Paris in French cultural life, this tendency is perhaps more justified than defenders of provincial science allow, but still it is a pattern that has helped to obscure important moments in French scientific life. In any event, although Paris-centrism can be easily enough overcome by further and deeper study of the scientific life of the provinces, the second familiar pattern, to which Montpellier long ago fell victim, is more problematic. That is the tendency in what we might call classical history of science to select for study only those figures, traditions, and schools that are judged to be significant forebears of modern science. This "presentist" bent, as G. W. Stocking, Jr., has termed it, has been much discussed, and I do not want to belabor the point or engage in hand wringing about the blinkered vision of an older historiography.[2] Still, it is important to recognize that Montpellier disappeared from historical view largely because for a long time medical historians in France have concentrated on the perspective of the so-called Paris clinical school, ignoring medical traditions and developments that seemed irrelevant to its history. In turn modern judgments about the medical past have depended to an extent not often enough realized on the Paris-centered perspective presented in classic nineteenth- and early twentieth-century texts by figures such as Louis Peisse, Charles Daremberg, Jules Rochard,

1 See Mary Jo Nye, *Science in the Provinces: Scientific Communities and Provincial Leadership in France, 1860–1930* (Berkeley: University of California Press, 1986); Terry Shinn, "The French Science Faculty System," *Historical Studies in the Physical Sciences* 10 (1979): 271–332.
2 G. W. Stocking, Jr., "On the Limits of 'Presentism' and 'Historicism' in the Historiography of the Behavioral Sciences," in *Race, Culture, and Evolution: Essays in the History of Anthropology* (1968; rpt. Chicago: University of Chicago Press, 1982), 1–12.

Table 1

Winners	Losers
Paris	Montpellier
positive method	philosophical method
statistics	prose
vivisection	antivivisection
use of the microscope	ordinary vision
reductionism	holism
autopsy	observation of the living
antivitalism	vitalism

Paul Delaunay, and others.[3] These older histories are rich, irreplaceable texts. But they are all embedded in particular ideologies of the medical enterprise and therefore function as actions in the great rhetorical battles that were waged within French medicine in the nineteenth century.

By about 1850 (which is not accidentally the end point of the story told in this book), a set of "victors" in these battles was beginning to emerge and medical history was coming to incorporate a set of dichotomies that clearly differentiated winner from loser (Table 1). Let me be clear: I am not saying that such "winners" and "losers" actually existed. Nor am I saying that these battles were over by 1850. Indeed this study is intended to undercut such views. Rather, I am saying that beginning early in the nineteenth century, partisans of Paris medicine used historical scholarship as part of an overall effort to undermine "philosophical medicine" in general and vitalism in particular, and that this perspective continued to inform medical history long thereafter. Nineteenth-century histories of medicine generally acknowledged the greatness of Montpellier "for its time," recounted how it was superseded by Paris clinical medicine, and denounced its nineteenth-century representatives and sympathizers as reactionary, retrograde, or, to use Laín Entralgo's phrase of 1947, "stupidly conservative."[4] All of this meant that sustained historical inquiry into the language, concepts, and doctrines of Montpellier was unnecessary since Montpellier lay outside the forward movement of medicine. In this literature, even Montpellier's eighteenth-century "greats" – Théophile de Bordeu and Paul-

3 Charles Daremberg, *Histoire des sciences médicales*, 2 vols. (Paris: J. B. Baillière, 1870); Paul Delaunay, *Le monde médical parisien au dix-huitième siècle* (Paris: J. Rousset, 1906); *idem, La vie médicale au XVIe, XVIIe et XVIIIe siècles* (Paris: Editions Hippocrate, 1935); Louis Peisse, *La médecine et les médecins*, 2 vols. (Paris: J. B. Baillière, 1857); Jules Rochard, *Histoire de la chirurgie française au XIXe siècle* (Paris: J. B. Baillière, 1875).
4 See, for example, Peisse, *La médecine et les médecins*, 1:238–97; Daremberg, *Histoire des sciences médicales*, 1157–97 (an especially severe treatment); Pedro Laín Entralgo, "Sensualism and Vitalism in Bichat's *Anatomie Générale*," *JHMAS* 5 (1948): 47–64.

Joseph Barthez – were ritually saluted rather than carefully studied, with the result that the intricate texture of Montpellier thought has been forgotten. In recent years the importance of Montpellier not only to the doctrinal and institutional history of medicine but to the larger history of sociomedical discourse in the crucial years between the late Enlightenment and early nineteenth century has been recognized.[5] Yet precisely what it is that has been lost to historical understanding by Montpellier's recession into shadow has not yet come clear.

The central argument of this chapter is that Montpellier medicine stands at the source of the long and important tradition in French medicine that contemporaries knew as "the science of man." The phrase "science of man" was first used in the title of a medical treatise by the Montpellier physician Paul-Joseph Barthez in 1778, although the idea that medicine constituted a science of man had been current in Montpellier for some time before.[6] A full explanation of why this tradition began and developed in Montpellier must await a later, comprehensive study of the scientific and cultural context of Montpellier medicine. My purpose here is rather to examine in detail the theoretical principles, concepts, and language of the vitalist science of man, and to situate Montpellier in the larger world of eighteenth-century medicine.[7] In so doing I will argue that the four principal "nodes of reference" of anthropological medicine – its holism, its insistence on an intimate

5 Like so many other developments in recent French historiography, this alteration of perception seems to have begun with Michel Foucault, who liberally cited Montpellier theorists in characterizing late eighteenth- and early nineteenth-century medicine; see *The Birth of the Clinic: An Archaeology of Medical Perception*, trans. A. M. Sheridan Smith (New York: Vintage Books, 1973). See also C. C. Gillispie, *Science and Polity in France at the End of the Old Regime* (Princeton: Princeton University Press, 1980), 217–18; John Lesch, *Science and Medicine in France: The Emergence of Experimental Physiology, 1790–1855* (Cambridge, Mass.: Harvard University Press, 1984), 19, 25–26; Sergio Moravia, "Philosophie et médecine en France à la fin du XVIIIe siècle," *Studies on Voltaire and the Eighteenth Century* 89 (1972): 1089–1151; Dorinda Outram, *The Body and the French Revolution: Sex, Class and Political Culture* (New Haven: Yale University Press, 1989), 53–56; Martin Staum, *Cabanis: Enlightenment and Medical Philosophy in the French Revolution* (Princeton: Princeton University Press, 1980), 86–90.

6 Paul-Joseph Barthez, *Nouveaux élémens de la science de l'homme*, 2 vols. (Montpellier: J. Martel, 1778). (All references here are to the 1806 edition published in Paris by Goujon; in it the two volumes are separately paginated although the chapter numbers are continuous. Citations to Barthez's notes supply page numbers in the separately paginated notes sections at the end of each volume.)

7 Most treatments of Montpellier medicine appear in works focusing on either Théophile de Bordeu or Paul-Joseph Barthez as individuals. See, for example, François Duchesneau, *La physiologie des Lumières: Empirisme, modèles et théories* (The Hague: Martinus Nijhoff, 1982), 361–404; Elizabeth Haigh, "Vitalism, the Soul and Sensibility: The Physiology of Théophile de Bordeu," *JHM* 31 (1976): 30–41; Louis Dulieu, "Paul-Joseph Barthez," *RHS* 24 (1971): 149–76. The only exception is Louis Dulieu, *La médecine à Montpellier*, 4 vols. (Avignon: Les presses universelles, 1975–90), which has invaluable detail but is essentially antiquarian in character and attempts little in the way of historical analysis of either the theoretical or institutional foundations of Montpellier medicine.

physical-moral relation, its construction of medicine as a necessarily social enterprise, and its disposition to typologize human beings according to categories discernible only to medical observers – were established in Montpellier thinking and were necessary implications of the vitalist doctrines that were Montpellier's singular contribution to eighteenth-century biomedical science.

THE CONTOURS OF EIGHTEENTH-CENTURY MEDICINE

All historians try to avoid anachronism, but historians of medicine, whose field of inquiry has been subject to dizzying change in the modern world, are particularly wary of it. The very word "medicine" evokes images and associations that have to be jettisoned before the professional, intellectual, and institutional contours of medicine in earlier eras come into relief. Medicine now is a skilled, prestigious, and highly remunerative profession. It rests on a corpus of exceedingly specialized scientific knowledge. It is, above all, a sophisticated body of techniques, often mechanical in nature, mobilized for the correction of discrete malfunctions in the human organism. Some of these features of modern medicine were in the making in the eighteenth century. Clearly, the medical "profession" was in the process of a fundamental restructuring that progressively entailed its exclusion of all but initiates as well as the elaboration of new procedures and standards of training.[8] In medical theory and doctrine, too, certain anticipations of the present may be discerned: by the mid-eighteenth century the mechanist conception of the body, which ultimately eventuated in experimental medicine and its concomitant technological instrumentalities, was triumphant virtually everywhere in Europe. The most widely read treatises and text-

8 The question of whether medicine did or did not constitute a "profession" in the eighteenth century has been much discussed. See especially Gerald L. Geison, ed. *Professions and the French State, 1700–1900* (Philadelphia: University of Pennsylvania Press, 1984), 1–12; Toby Gelfand, *Professionalizing Modern Medicine: Paris Surgeons and Medical Science and Institutions in the 18th Century* (Westport, Conn.: Greenwood Press, 1980); idem, "The Decline of the Ordinary Practitioner and the Rise of a Modern Medical Profession," in *Doctors, Patients, and Society: Power and Authority in Medical Care,* ed. Martin S. Staum and Donald E. Larsen (Waterloo, Ontario: Wilfrid Laurier University Press for Calgary Institute for the Humanities, 1981); Gillispie, *Science and Polity,* 84–92; Jan Goldstein, *Console and Classify: The French Psychiatric Profession in the Nineteenth Century* (Cambridge: Cambridge University Press, 1987), 8–40; idem, "Foucault among the Sociologists: The 'Disciplines' and the History of the Professions," *History and Theory* 23 (1984): 170–92; Caroline C. F. Hannaway, "Medicine, Public Welfare and the State in 18th-Century France: The Société Royale de Médecine of Paris (1776–1793)," (Ph.D. diss., Johns Hopkins University, 1974), 2–32; Matthew Ramsey, *Professional and Popular Medicine in France, 1770–1830: The Social World of Medical Practice* (Cambridge: Cambridge University Press, 1988), esp. 1–65. I have used the term "profession" as convenient shorthand for the domain of official medicine without intending to enter the debate on "professionalization" as such, which is not directly germane to my subject.

books were those of mechanist theoreticians, chief among them the Dutch teacher and practitioner Hermann Boerhaave who, as one observer insisted, "reigned supreme."[9]

Nevertheless, despite this incipient modernity, medicine of the late eighteenth century differed in essential ways from its modern counterpart. As an occupation, medicine was highly stratified, ranging from a tiny elite of doctors trained at the ancient faculties down to diverse popular practitioners (charlatans, midwives, itinerant healers) who worked in most cases wholly outside the official medical domain. For my purposes the most important distinction is that which divided "doctors" (*docteurs, médecins*), who took one or more of the official medical degrees and thereafter practiced "medicine" as such, from "surgeons," who earned a living not only by performing their own cutting operations but also by overseeing the various therapies – bloodletting, cupping, purging, bathing – prescribed by the doctors. This distinction between doctors and surgeons was also reflected in and reinforced by their separate corporate organization. Doctors belonged to the corporations formed either by the medical faculty from which they took their degrees or by the local *collèges* that conferred the right to practice in given locales. At the end of the Ancien Regime some nineteen faculties and fifteen colleges constituted the corporate base of doctors. Surgeons were attached to local *communautés*, of which there were about four hundred by the late eighteenth century; these were completely separate in organization, administration, and procedures from the corporate bodies of the doctors. These corporate forms corresponded to other realities of the social world of medicine: until the Revolution, the training, certification, clientele, habits of work, income, and social standing of doctors and surgeons were also markedly different. The only exception to this rule was the emergence of a surgical elite in the great medical capitals, that, throughout the century, pressed an ever more formidable challenge to the exclusivity of doctors.[10]

These social features of eighteenth-century medicine are important to this study because they indicate that elite physicians of the era were often accustomed by their own experience to viewing medicine primarily as a body of theory and to perceiving themselves as speculative thinkers in the honored style of the philosophe. Like students of other branches of learning, such doctors accepted only those limits established by "right method"; they rec-

<hr />

9 A.-B. Richerand, "Notice sur la vie et les ouvrages de Bordeu," in *Oeuvres complètes de Bordeu*, ed. A.-B. Richerand, 2 vols. (Paris: Caille et Ravier, 1818), i. On Boerhaave, see G. A. Lindeboom, *Herman Boerhaave: The Man and His Work* (London: Methuen, 1968); for mechanism generally, see Jacques Roger, *Les sciences de la vie dans la pensée française du XVIIIe siècle*, rev. ed. (Paris: A. Colin, 1971), esp. 161, 206–24, 731–61; Thomas S. Hall, *History of General Physiology, 600 B.C. to A.D. 1900*, vol. 1, *From Pre-Socratic Times to the Enlightenment* (Chicago: University of Chicago Press, 1969), 218–29, 352.

10 This discussion is based on Gelfand, *Professionalizing Modern Medicine*; Goldstein, *Console and Classify*, 8–40; Ramsey, *Professional and Popular Medicine*, 17–125.

ognized no a priori restrictions on their competence. Medical writers commonly asserted their authority on matters – social, cosmological – that to us have nothing of the medical about them. This tendency of eighteenth-century doctors to regard broad philosophical or social questions as their own was later repudiated by positivist-minded doctors in Paris medical circles who ridiculed the speculative bent of "philosophical medicine," with which they particularly identified the Medical University of Montpellier.[11] There is a certain irony in this fact since in the eighteenth century the Montpellier medical faculty embraced much more readily than its Paris counterpart those innovations in training and practice that ultimately transformed medicine. Well before the physicians of the Paris faculty, doctors in Montpellier took up dissection and autopsy, undertook investigations in the natural sciences, and worked to bridge the ancient distinction between the doctor's work of the mind and the surgeon's work of the hands.[12]

Nonetheless there are several senses, current in the eighteenth century, in which the term "philosophical medicine" does properly fit the Montpellier physicians. First, the Montpellier doctors defined aims for medicine that went beyond mere therapeutics and made of medicine a science that investigated the full range of circumstances determining or impinging on states of health and sickness. Second, the doctors of Montpellier were "philosophical" insofar as the word signified an embrace of the scientific spirit and method as opposed to what was called "routine" – medicine oppressed by the heavy weight of authority and age-old tradition. Thus the Montpellier doctors sought to place medicine firmly within the field of enlightened learning and to promote within medicine the use of methods that in other learned pursuits were encouraging breaks with the past. In brief, the Montpellier physicians endeavored to transform medicine into a broadly conceived science of man.

THE SCIENTIFIC WORLD OF MONTPELLIER

The Montpellier medical school was one of the earliest established in Europe (its first formal statutes date from 1220), and from the Renaissance forward, it was a highly prestigious center of medical training. Students from both western and eastern Europe traveled to Montpellier for their medical education. The reputation of the Montpellier medical school rested in good part on the fact that medical teaching there was well integrated with study of the other sciences. Throughout the sixteenth century the faculty had four standard chairs of medicine, to which were added chairs in anatomy and

11 See Chapter 3.
12 On Montpellier's receptivity to innovation in the eighteenth century, see Gillispie, *Science and Polity*, 217–18; Hannaway, "Medicine, Public Welfare," 18–20; Jacques Léonard, *Les médecins de l'Ouest au XIXème siècle*, 3 vols. (Lille: Atelier Reproduction des Thèses, Université de Lille III, 1978), 148–52.

botany in 1593, in pharmacy and surgery in 1597, and in chemistry in 1676. When the botanical chair was founded in 1593, the Jardin des plantes (the oldest one in France) was also established. From this point forward, botanical teaching in Montpellier was uninterrupted, and the *jardin* was much frequented by teachers and students.[13]

During the Renaissance Montpellier appears to have been an important point of interchange between the cultural centers of Italy and France. Montpellier scholars traveled across the Alps to the great north Italian medical schools and adopted from them novelties in both the theory and practical arts of medicine. It may have been the Italian contact that encouraged the founding in Montpellier of the first anatomical amphitheater in 1566. From that point on dissections were performed at Montpellier in the winter semester, though obtaining sufficient cadavers was a constant problem given hospital administrators' hostility to the practice of autopsy.[14] These dissections helped to foster a celebrated anatomical tradition that in turn encouraged Montpellier's early championing of the unity of medicine and surgery. The Montpellier master surgeon François de La Peyronie, who was First Surgeon to Louis XV, was instrumental in gaining the king's support for establishment of the Société royale de chirurgie in Paris in 1731. From the moment of its founding, the academy worked ceaselessly to enhance the status of surgery. In Montpellier La Peyronie helped to found the Collège de chirurgie, which by 1784 had eleven chairs of its own and an *école pratique*. Montpellier was the only medical school in France that accorded a mixed medical-surgical degree, known informally as the D.M.C. (*docteur, médecin, chirurgien*). For a long time there was only modest interest in this degree but as the century progressed it became increasingly popular and indeed tended to supersede the degree of *maître-chirurgien* given by the Collège de chirurgie. By 1794 the medical faculty had awarded over six hundred medical-surgical degrees. Thus long before the formal unity of medicine and surgery was achieved in France at large, the need to effect this union was recognized in Montpellier.[15]

By the opening of the eighteenth century there had long existed a special relationship between the Montpellier medical school and the crown. Constituted as an independent "University of Medicine," the school enjoyed an

13 "Introduction," *Cartulaire de l'Université de Montpellier*, 2 vols. (Montpellier: Ricard Frères, 1890); Montpellier: Maison Lauriol, 1912), 5; see also A. Germain, *L'Ecole de Médecine de Montpellier: Ses origines, sa constitution, son enseignement* (Montpellier: J. Martel ainé, 1880), 5–16. On the gardens, see Louis Dulieu, "Le mouvement scientifique montpelliérain au XVIIIe siècle," *RHS* 11 (1958): 227–49, esp. 229.
14 Dulieu, "Le mouvement scientifique," 228; François Granel, *Pages médico-historiques montpelliéraines* (Montpellier: Causse and Castelnau, 1964), 69–86.
15 Dulieu, "Le mouvement scientifique," 229; Granel, *Pages médico-historiques*, 78–79, 88; on the founding of the Académie de chirurgie, see Gelfand, *Professionalizing Modern Medicine*, chap. 5; Léonard, *Les médecins de l'Ouest*, 148; for the number of D.M.C. degrees awarded at Montpellier, see Dulieu, *Médecine à Montpellier*, 3:114.

institutional status not granted any other medical school in France, which gave the administrators and professors great freedom in internal governance, even in respect to local episcopal authority. The safeguarding of this status, as well as the establishment of the new chairs and the Jardin des plantes, seem to have formed part of a general royal effort to woo important institutions in Montpellier, which had been a major Huguenot center during the Wars of Religion, back to the royalist-centralizing camp. Throughout the seventeenth century the crown appointed celebrated Montpellier physicians to prestigious positions at court, a pattern that contributed not a little to the bitter resentment against Montpellier harbored by the Paris faculty in the eighteenth century.[16]

In the first decade of the eighteenth century, these marks of royal esteem were reinforced when the crown acceded to requests that Montpellier have its own scientific academy comparable to the Académie des sciences in Paris. In 1706 the Société royale des sciences de Montpellier was founded, modeled on the Paris academy in structure, organizational details, and plans for publication. According to the letters patent registered on its founding, the society was to give to Paris academicians full rights in its proceedings; in return Montpellier academicians were to be treated with special regard in Paris. The Montpellier society was originally divided into five classes for mathematics, astronomy, chemistry, botany, and physical science (*physique*). Like the Paris academy the Montpellier society consisted of full, adjunct, and honorary members. (In 1706 the honorary members included the archbishop of Narbonne, the bishop of Montpellier, the intendant of Languedoc, a *conseiller* of the Montpellier *Cour des Comptes, aides et finances,* and other notables.) Though at first plagued with money problems, the society eventually achieved a sure footing, in part by gaining the financial patronage of the archbishop and *président des Etats,* Arthur Dillon. The most striking physical proof of the society's financial prosperity was the building of an observatory in 1745.[17]

Professors at the University of Medicine participated fully in the activities of the Société royale des sciences, and in general there was a close interchange between medicine and the other sciences in the environment provided by Montpellier's learned institutions.[18] In his history of medicine

16 Gérard Cholvy, *Le diocèse de Montpellier* (Paris: Beauchesne, 1976); Delaunay, *Le monde médical parisien,* 94–165. See also Howard Solomon, *Public Welfare, Science, and Propaganda in Seventeenth Century France: The Innovations of Théophraste Renaudot* (Princeton: Princeton University Press, 1972), esp. 166–67.

17 *Histoire de la Société royale des sciences établie à Montpellier,* 2 vols. (Lyon: Benoît Duplain, 1766; Montpellier: Jean Martel, 1778), iii–xvi; Dulieu, "Le mouvement scientifique"; see also Dulieu, "La contribution montpelliéraine à l'Académie des Sciences," *RHS* 11 (1958): 255–62.

18 Of the two volumes of papers published by the society, roughly half the material was contributed by medical figures; see *Histoire de la Société royale.* Among the prominent medical figures who belonged to the Société des sciences in the eighteenth century were Jean

written in 1768, Bordeu associated himself and Montpellier generally with the larger development of science, asserting that Montpellier doctors had abandoned the sterile dialectic in which medicine of previous centuries had been trapped and had embraced in its place the methods of the "academy": experimentation, observation, and calculation. Bordeu traced Montpellier's respect for the other sciences to the influence of the Société royale and praised the king for the impetus its founding had given to modern methods of research.[19]

Yet there were limitations to Montpellier's receptivity to what were often called "the auxiliary sciences." Animals were studied with much less interest than plants; Montpellier had no menagerie and little in the way of animal collections.[20] Furthermore, although there was, from the early eighteenth century on, a frank and genial recognition that all the sciences were interrelated, many of the medical professors steadfastly asserted the fundamental autonomy of their own discipline. The reasons why doctors insisted on medicine's distinctiveness from the other sciences changed over time. In the seventeenth century Montpellier had been closely identified with Paracelsism, and thus physicians of the early eighteenth century who wanted to restore medicine's autonomy were especially determined to banish iatrochemistry from physiological and pathogenetic explanation. Bordeu noted in his history that his predecessors had regarded medical chemistry as "un amas de cornus, de poêlons, de fourneaux." For himself he denounced the old chemistry as "pernicious gibberish, which had filled all the writings and corrupted many heads" among the self-styled "Paracelsians." Although Bordeu had a high regard for the "purified" chemistry of his own day, he denied the applicability of chemical principles to medicine. He singled out for praise those chemists such as Georg-Ernst Stahl who recognized that the domains of chemistry and of medicine must be held separate:

The [chemistry] of our century is too wise to confound its object with the study of the living body; it distinguishes what belongs to it from what concerns the organism, the action of nerves, that of the passions, and that of the sensibility which is inherent in all parts [of the body].[21]

Astruc, Paul-Joseph Barthez, François Boissier de Sauvages, François, J. L. V., and P. M. A. Broussonnet, Pierre Chirac, Antoine Fizes, Antoine Gauteron, Etienne Gondange, Henri Haguenot, François de La Peyronie, Antoine Portal, and Gabriel Venel. On the relations between the medical corps and the society, see Dulieu, "Le mouvement scientifique," 236 and n. 1.

19 Théophile de Bordeu, *Recherches sur l'histoire de la médecine* (1764; rev. ed. Paris: Auguste Ghio, 1882), 255.

20 Dulieu, "Le mouvement scientifique," 244; Charles-Louis Dumas, *Principes de physiologie, ou introduction à la science expérimentale, philosophique et médicale de l'homme vivant*, 4 vols. (Paris: Crapelet, 1800–3), I:xxix.

21 Bordeu, *Recherches sur l'histoire de la médecine*, 251–52; see also Allen Debus, *The French Paracelsians: The Chemical Challenge to Medical and Scientific Tradition in Early Modern France* (Cambridge: Cambridge University Press, 1991), 199–201.

Bordeu was heartened that Stahl, who was better known for his theory of phlogiston than for his vitalism, denied the usefulness of chemistry to medicine. His praise for modern chemistry was, then, just another way of arguing against the invasion of medicine by outsiders.

The Montpellier doctors reserved their greatest disdain, however, for iatromechanists who extrapolated principles from physics, mechanics, and hydrodynamics. As a later apologist of the Montpellier doctors observed, they "succeeded in demolishing the mechanist doctrine, in habituating scholars to the empirical study of man considered as a whole . . . and in revealing as chimerical the project of reducing to chemistry and physics the phenomena of life."[22] Barthez reiterated ceaselessly his dismay that doctors could be content with explanations offered to medicine by mechanics and physics; these were valuable aids in comprehending "the perfection of [bodily] instruments" but could teach nothing about the fundamental processes of life.[23] Victor de Sèze, author of a 1768 treatise on sensibility, stated the matter this way:

Why should we not accord to living bodies a unique physics? Do not the faculties that one remarks in them, and that one remarks only in them, indicate that they form a class apart, which has its laws of action, its laws of movement independent of those which direct other bodies?[24]

If living bodies did not obey the same laws or exhibit the same phenomena as inert bodies, there could be no justification for or value in subsuming medicine within the physicochemical sciences. It was in the full elaboration of this sense of the uniqueness of life that Montpellier was to achieve its greatest renown.

THE SINGULARITY OF LIFE

Precisely how and why Montpellier became a privileged site for the development of vitalism is not presently known. C. C. Gillispie speculates in a recent work that the main currents that fed Montpellier's distinctive outlook were Sephardic and Arabic medicine, "botanical lore" from its superb gardens, and the Rabelaisian skeptical tradition.[25] In any event the vitalist

22 Jacques Lordat, *Exposition de la doctrine médicale de P.-J. Barthez, et mémoires sur la vie de ce médecin* (Paris: Gabon, 1818), 53–54.
23 Barthez, *Science de l'homme*, 1:34. As for chemistry, Barthez saw little value in it for medicine since chemistry studied only substances that had been evacuated or extracted from the body and were thus no longer "alive." In his view medicine had few points of contact with chemistry and its investigations of *la nature morte*. For this discussion, see *Science de l'homme*, 1:35–36.
24 Victor de Sèze, *Recherches physiologiques et philosophiques sur la sensibilité ou la vie animale* (Paris: Prault, 1786), quoted in Moravia, "Philosophie et médecine," 1093.
25 Gillispie, *Science and Polity*, 217–18; see also Germain, *L'Ecole de Médecine de Montpellier*, 5–9.

tradition in Montpellier began in the 1730s when the botanist and nosologist François Boissier de Sauvages introduced in his courses a version of the teachings of Stahl (1660–1734), the Halle physician, naturalist, and chemist whose medical doctrine constituted a fully elaborated challenge to all teachings that sought to base medicine on physicochemical principles. Stahl began teaching medicine at Halle when the university was established there in 1694. The medical world in which he functioned was marked by doctrinal contentiousness among Galenists, Paracelsians, Helmontians, and iatrophysicists.[26] Stahl's own doctrine was devised both to resolve the philosophical problems at issue among these schools and to propose a new therapeutics. Taking aim particularly at the mechanist teaching of Boerhaave, Stahl argued for an irresoluble distinction between the living and the nonliving. All living matter was characterized by purpose and striving directed by a principle Stahl called "anima." In Stahl's system anima was responsible both for voluntary, conscious activity and for involuntary, unconscious processes. His explanations of particular physiological functions sometimes made anima into a precise instrumentality – salivation occurred, for example, "when the soul judged it necessary."[27] In other cases Stahl's explanations owed a good deal to the apparatuses of mechanist models but always with the proviso that prior to the work of motion lay anima, the true cause and guide of any given functional activity.[28]

Why Stahl's teachings were sympathetically received in Montpellier will not be known until a general study of the vitalist tradition there is undertaken. Whatever the precise means by which Stahl was successfully introduced in Montpellier, Stahlian teaching helped to set Montpellier medicine on a new course.[29] Though Stahlianism was not universally embraced by the medical professors, it was enthusiastically taught by Boissier de Sauvages, and became a central subject of argument and commentary by critics through the 1730s and the 1740s.[30] By midcentury, however, Montpellier had its own doctrine of the singularity of life, developed principally by Théophile de Bordeu, propagated by Bordeu and his cousin Louis de Lacaze, and then given its fullest expression in the writings of Paul-Joseph Barthez.

26 On Stahl, see Duchesneau, *La physiologie des Lumières*, 1–31; Hall, *History of General Physiology*, 1:351–66; Lester S. King, "G. E. Stahl," *DSB* 12:599–606; *idem*, "Stahl and Hoffmann: A Study in Eighteenth-Century Animism," *JHMAS* 19 (1964): 118–30.
27 Théophile de Bordeu, "Recherches anatomiques sur la position des glandes, et sur leur action" (hereafter "Glandes"), in *Oeuvres complètes*, 203.
28 King, "G. E. Stahl."
29 The editor of Bordeu's history of medicine remarks that Bordeu's father, who was also a physician, corresponded with Stahl in the 1720s; see "Notice de M. Lefeuve sur Bordeu," in *Recherches sur l'histoire de la médecine*, 12.
30 On Boissier de Sauvages, see Hall, *History of General Physiology*, vol. 2, *From the Enlightenment to the End of the Nineteenth Century*, 73–76; L. S. King, "Boissier de Sauvages and Eighteenth-Century Nosology," *BHM* 11 (1966): 43–51. Bordeu discusses the disputes between the "Montpellier Stahlians" and their critics in "Glandes," 203–06.

Before examining the chief features of what came to be known as Montpellier doctrine, it must first be asked whether the vitalist teachings of Bordeu, Lacaze, Barthez, and other less famous representatives of Montpellier medicine (such as Gabriel Venel, de Sèze, Henri Fouquet, Charles-Louis Dumas) entailed the existence of a unified Montpellier "school." Claiming originality for his own work, Barthez angrily denied that he was the "leader of a vitalist sect."[31] And certainly to the end of the eighteenth century exponents of other medical doctrines – mechanists, Stahlians, and Hallerians – were still to be found on the Montpellier faculty.[32] Among the vitalists themselves, furthermore, there were important differences of opinion: Barthez emphasized, for example, his distance from Bordeu on the relative importance of fluids and solids. He also contested Bordeu's teaching on the separate "lives" of the individual organs of the body.[33] Other theoretical differences will become apparent in the subsequent discussion. If viewed in relation to the larger theoretical framework of late eighteenth-century medicine, however, Montpellier retains its unity despite such divergencies by virtue of its insistence on an empirically derived, noncorporeal and nonspiritual vital force that constituted the essential line of distinction between living and dead matter. A cluster of derivative concepts and principles – the primacy of sensibility, the harmony and integration of the living organism, the teleological character of physiological function – further unites the Montpellier theorists. If their definitions and arguments were not always precisely similar, they were nonetheless always articulated within the same terminological and conceptual universe. Despite their theoretical differences, moreover, all Montpellier doctors fostered the creation of a collective public image and encouraged a sense of institutional esprit de corps. Bordeu's encomium to Montpellier for its "liberty of thought" and its commitment to observation is typical of passages in which the Montpellier doctors praised the distinct and honored place occupied by the Montpellier medical school.[34] After 1800, finally, when vitalist doctrine came to hold full sway at Montpellier, institutional and theoretical solidarity merged, and the "école de Montpellier" came to have a unique identity in biomedical circles.[35]

31 Barthez, *Science de l'homme*, 1:"Notes," 98.   32 Lordat, *Exposition*, 42–44.
33 Perhaps thinking it more politic, Barthez specifically named Van Helmont rather than the much-heralded Bordeu as the originator of this view; see *Science de l'homme*, 1:21–22.
34 Bordeu, *Recherches sur l'histoire de la médecine*, 186, 248, 255.
35 Discussions of "the Montpellier school" appear, for example, in Philippe Pinel, *Nosographie philosophique, ou la méthode de l'analyse appliquée à la médecine* (Paris: Crapelet, an VI [1797]), xxviii–xxix; Daremberg, *Histoire des sciences médicales*, chap. 32; Peisse, *La médecine et les médecins*, 238–97. Cf. Duchesneau, *Physiologie des Lumières*, who argues that Barthez should not be seen as continuing or developing ideas of Bordeu; see also François Duchesneau, "Vitalism in Late Eighteenth-Century Physiology: The Cases of Barthez, Blumenbach, and John Hunter" in *William Hunter and the Eighteenth-Century Medical World*, ed. W. F. Bynum and Roy Porter (Cambridge: Cambridge University Press, 1985), 259–95.

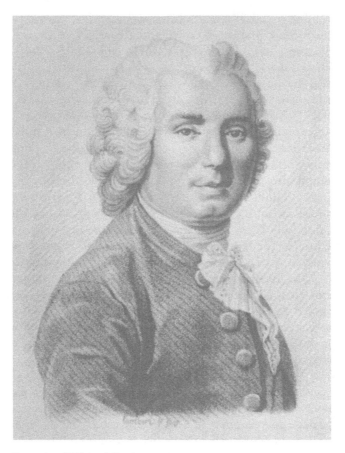

Portrait of Théophile de Bordeu (1722–76), by Ambroise Tardieu.

The core of Montpellier teaching was its doctrine of life, which held that among living beings there is at work a power or principle different in kind from other forces found in nature. In a series of works published in the 1740s and 1750s, Bordeu (1722–76) elaborated a medicophilosophical theory whose central precept was that "to live is only to feel, and to move in virtue of feeling."[36] Coming from a long-established family of doctors, Bordeu began his medical studies at Montpellier in the 1730s. He was an avid student of anatomy and also undertook a number of experiments, including some performed in collaboration with François Lamure (1717–87) that were published by the Société royale.[37] In the late 1730s and early 1740s Bordeu

36 Lordat, *Exposition*, 45.
37 Richerand, "Notice," i–iii; on Lamure, see *DSM:BM* 5:496–98. Lordat recounts that along with Tandon, Lamure was the main "Hallerian" on the Montpellier faculty in the 1760s; see Lordat, *Exposition*, 43.

was closely attentive to the controversies set off by the introduction of Stahlianism in Montpellier. As a result, he devoted his first student thesis, *Dissertatio physiologica de Sensu generice considerato* (Montpellier 1742) to the general nature of sentiment and movement.[38] This paper indicated the extent of his reading in van Helmont and Stahl and prefigured the attack on mechanism that he developed at length in *Recherches anatomiques sur la position des glandes et sur leur action* (1752).[39]

Although Bordeu's treatise on glandular function shows much evidence of the influence of Stahl, Bordeu opened the work by distancing himself from Stahl's controversial view that for doctors the study of anatomy was pointless. This position made sense in the context of Stahl's theoretical scheme, which attributed even the smallest details of bodily function to the direct intervention and guidance of the soul. Bordeu was wholly opposed to such a view, believing on the contrary that the contributions anatomy might make to medicine had scarcely yet been realized. Study of the glands was typical of the state of the anatomical art: everyone recognized the crucial importance of the "mechanism for excretion of the humors derived from the blood," but the precise nature of the excretory mechanisms and the "forces directing them" was unknown. Bordeu argued that this was a problem only anatomy – conceived not merely as "the simple history of parts" and "their structure" but rather as the investigation of "the uses of parts, their interplay, their links and relations with one another" – could solve.[40] According to Bordeu, nothing was more useless to medicine than the endless disquisitions of anatomists on such matters as the length and disposition of individual fibers in complete disregard for the role of organs and structures in health and sickness. Anatomy must be studied in conjunction with the practice of medicine; it must be learned at the sickbed as well as at the dissecting table.[41]

Unlike the Stahlians, then, Bordeu was not interested in posing a challenge to mechanist thought solely on the basis of philosophical and metaphysical arguments about the unassimilability of the living body to the "artificial machine."[42] Nor, as his explanation of glandular activity would make evident, was he ready to dispense wholly with the terminology or style of reasoning characteristic of iatromechanism. All the same, in surveying the history of opinion on glandular activity, Bordeu singled out as the principal teaching he hoped to combat the mechanist doctrine that the glands worked by means of compression of the glandular body by surrounding bones and muscles in the processes of mastication, digestion, the secretion of milk, and so on. The mechanist view was almost universally

38 In *Oeuvres complètes*, 1–13.   39 In *ibid.*, 45–208.
40 Bordeu, "Glandes," 45–46.   41 *Ibid.*, 46–47.
42 For use of this term, see *ibid.*, 205. The locution is revealing: Bordeu was not antagonistic to the idea of body as machine, only to that of body as *artificial* machine, that is, a machine lacking the initial vital force required to activate its properties and functions.

accepted, he noted, despite the fact that it had never been proved by investigations in fine anatomy. Nor could it be proved, he ventured to show, for the glands, instead of being "compressible" and acting in virtue of compression, were located in "pockets" where they were free to engage in their own activities.[43]

Bordeu first examined the location and functioning of the parotid glands, which did not function – as mechanists envisioned – as a kind of *pressoir* during chewing but in reality enjoyed augmented space created by the movement of the jawbone. This fact could be proved by a simple experiment involving a cadaver: when a wet sponge was placed in the cavity occupied by the gland and the jawbone was then worked as in chewing, the sponge was not compressed.[44] From the parotids Bordeu moved on to the other salivary glands, the glandular *couches* of mouth and throat, the brain, pituitary, thyroid, thymus, pancreas, liver, kidneys, and testicles, and ended with a discussion of the excretion of semen and milk, which together provided the model and explanation for all other secretions.[45]

It was in explaining excretion and secretion as generally similar processes that Bordeu elaborated his doctrine of the singularity of life and vital phenomena. Glandular action was not a mechanical process, dependent on the movement of parts surrounding the glands themselves. Rather glandular activity worked in essentially the same way as the erection and ejaculation that took place in the procreative act and in lactation. In all cases the process began with "a kind of convulsion" of feeling that brought on erection and ended with flowing (*découlement*) of semen, milk, tears, saliva, and the other humors in question. Of all the complicated circumstances and events involved in glandular activity, Bordeu isolated four as necessary conditions: a favorable disposition of the blood vessels (the humors being derived locally from the blood); a proper arrangement of the excretory canals themselves (for delivery of the humors); some kind of shaking, irritation, or friction (to assist in the erection); and, most important, the original "spasm" or "convulsion" that set the process in motion.[46]

Clearly, this representation of glandular function still owed a good deal to the mechanists' vessels, canals, and frictions, as Barthez later noted disapprovingly.[47] Yet the process ultimately rested on the primary phenomenon Bordeu called the spasm or convulsion, which in turn was the result of nervous action. Bordeu did not explain how or why the nerves in the region of the glands were first moved into action, although he noted the role of the passions in the salivation that came with the desire for food and in the "admiration" associated with acts of love. Nor was it clear what happened to

---

43 *Ibid.*, 50–58.   44 *Ibid.*, 57–58.
45 *Ibid.*, 64–130.
46 *Ibid.*, 117, 130–32; see the helpful discussion in Duchesneau, *Physiologie des Lumières*, 364–70.
47 Duchesneau, *Physiologie des Lumières*, 385.

the nerves or how precisely they performed their task: "Let us not be concerned with how these four conditions arise in the gland and with what the
change is that the nerves undergo; this is something we perhaps will never
know. It is sufficient to be convinced by experience that they [the condi-
tions] do exist."[48] Elsewhere Bordeu anticipates the objection that "one
cannot see" from his theory "what effect the action of the nerves has on the
glandular body" by asking "what does it matter, after all, if we understand
the use of nerve action so long as the action itself is demonstrated?"[49] The
most Bordeu could suggest was that the nerve action was "excited" by
some *force nouvelle* whose provenance we do not know but the existence of
which "is no less real."[50]

This is one of Bordeu's many references to the play of an unknown
"force," a term he often employed to signify the principle or principles that
guided and directed the activities of the body. In a similar usage elsewhere
he asked what "force" it might be that decided which humor would be separated in a particular gland – how the gland "knew," that is, not to separate
milk as opposed to bile or some other humor from among the constituents
of the blood.[51] Again the answer involved action of the nerves:

Secretion is reduced then to a kind of *sensation,* if one can so express it; the parts [of
the humor] that are appropriate to exciting such a sensation will pass [through the
orifices of the *vaisseau secrétoire*] and the others will be rejected; each gland, each or-
ifice thus has, so to speak, its individual taste [*goût particulier*]; everything that is foreign to it will in the ordinary course of things be rejected.[52]

This explanation, Bordeu recognized, removed the whole discussion to the
yet more difficult problem of what precisely was meant by sensation:

Those who closely examine these questions know how difficult it is to explain one-
self when one speaks of that force which directs with such fine judgment [*tant de
justesse*] the thousand individual movements of the body . . . and its parts; . . .
there are students of physics [*physiciens*] who, struck by these movements, have had
recourse to individual causes; and we will speak elsewhere of the hypothesis of
Stahl, who held that the soul directed everything in the animal body. Whatever the
case, one can say that all parts that live are directed by a *force conservatrice* that is
constantly on guard. Is . . . [this force] of the essence of . . . matter, or is it a necessary attribute of its combinations? Once again we pretend to nothing further than
a manner of conceiving these things, of metaphorical expressions, of comparisons.[53]

However obscure the operation of sensation might be, it nonetheless played
the determinative role in glandular activity. The special tasks of the particular glands were a result of the fact that each gland had a unique mode of

48 Bordeu, "Glandes," 133.   49 *Ibid.,* 147–48.
50 *Ibid.,* 145.
51 *Ibid.,* 162–63. This was a problem that vexed mechanists; see Lindeboom, *Boerhaave,* 278.
52 Bordeu, "Glandes," 163.   53 *Ibid.*

"tasting" or "touching," and in this respect the glands differed in no way from the other organs of the body. Completing his discussion of glandular activity proper, Bordeu moved to a series of comparisons between their mode of functioning and that of the throat and esophagus (which, following their own "taste," also knew what materials to keep and which to reject), the Fallopian tubes (which to do their work "became erect" and "seized" the material of the prepared egg), and so on.[54]

The glands further resembled other organs insofar as they exercised influence within what Bordeu called a "department" of action, a neighboring region in which the activities of the gland or organ had particularly marked effect, either positive (stimulating a related part to action) or negative (suppressing the activity of a neighboring part). He defined the "department" of the glands as "everything that enters into a sort of action when the gland acts."[55] Precisely how the gland exercised influence within its "department" Bordeu did not explain in this work, seemingly because he was more concerned at this point to explore the problem of periodicity and regularity in glandular action and in those functions influenced by it, matters with obvious medical applicability.

Bordeu did, however, return to the problem of how the glands and other organs influenced neighboring regions in the other of his two most celebrated works, the *Recherches sur le tissu muqueux* (1767), a study that earlier he had suggested would clarify many obscure questions about the animal economy.[56] In this work Bordeu defined the mucous or "cellular" tissue as that porous, spongy, irregular membranous material that spread throughout the whole body, in some cases forming for the viscera a kind of *poche* in which they lay sheltered, in others extending directly into and intertwining with the fibers of the visceral substance proper. This tissue was responsible for a host of essential body functions including, preeminently, that of providing passageways for movement of the humors. Ideally, humoral movement was free and unobstructed, but the ease with which the humors traveled depended on the condition of the connective tissue, "what one might call its penetrability, its spongy disposition."[57] The condition of the

---

54 *Ibid.*, 164–65.
55 *Ibid.*, 178–79; compare this discussion of the "department" of the glands to Bordeu's treatment of what he called the *cercle* of circulatory action, where he again envisioned a hierarchy of "general" and "particular" functional activity: "Il y a donc une circulation générale, et bien des circulations particulières. Ce sont, si nous osons le dire, comme de *petits cercles* qui viennent aboutir à un plus grand. Nous avons accoutumé de nous servir de cette dénomination de *cercle*, pour exprimer qu'une partie, quoiqu'elle reçoive le sang au moyen de la *circulation générale*, ou qui se fait dans les plus gros vaisseaux, a pourtant une *circulation particulière*, suivant qu'elle est en action ou qu'elle n'y est point: les autres parties qui se ressentent de cette action, sont du *département* de son *cercle*, etc."; *ibid.*, 187.
56 *Ibid.*, 208; "Recherches sur le tissu muqueux," in *Oeuvres complètes*, 735–96.
57 Bordeu, "Tissu muqueux," 752; another definition of the cellular tissue appears in "Recherches sur les maladies chroniques," in *Oeuvres complètes*, 829.

tissue depended in turn on how the organs embedded within it affected its character:

> The organs lodged [*nichés*] in the cellular substance . . . constrict, disturb, relax, and singularly modify it in its different portions; these modifications, which depend on the movement, even the simple presence of these organs, give a proper idea of what was called the *department* of the viscera and other parts in *Recherches sur les glandes;* the department of an organ is nothing other than its cellular atmosphere . . . or the portion of cellular tissue that is in relation to its [the organ's] action. When a part changes position or constitution, all the cellular tissue that is in its department is modified as well.[58]

This explanation seemed again to isolate a purely mechanical factor as the determinative element in a host of crucial activities: the movement or even the simple presence of a given organ disposed the cellular tissue in such a way as to define its local character. But once more, as in his account of glandular action, Bordeu was chiefly concerned not with mechanical action but with "the different degrees of force of this same cellular organ," whose ultimate cause was unknown.[59] Again, mechanical action – whether friction, obstruction, the exertion of pressure – was only a means for the expression or manifestation of the true empowering force that underlay it.

Given this emphasis on the force of the cellular tissue, Bordeu did not expect to find an invariable, mathematically expressible relation between the "departmental" influence of an organ and the character of the cellular tissue, the movement of the humors, or the other innumerable phenomena that the activities of organ and tissue together set in motion, sustained in activity, or otherwise determined. What he did expect to find was periodicity, regularity, coordination. The combined activities of all the "departments" of the body constituted its harmony, its "general life." Groping for an image to express his meaning, Bordeu hit upon one of the most famous metaphors ever devised for the independent yet harmonious functioning of the parts of the body, that of the beehive:

> We would compare the living body . . . to a swarm of bees who are massed in clusters [*pelotons*] and suspended from a tree like a bunch of grapes; . . . a celebrated Ancient said of one of the viscera of the lower abdomen that it was *animal in animali,* [and though] each part is . . . not of course an animal, it is a kind of separate machine that cooperates in its fashion in the general life of the body.[60]

This metaphor of the harmony of the body prompted Bordeu to a conclusive definition of the distinction between health and sickness:

> The organs of the body are linked one with another; they each have their own district and their own action; the relations among these actions, the harmony which

58 Bordeu, "Tissu muqueux," 752.   59 *Ibid.*
60 *Ibid.,* 187.

results from them, make for health. If this harmony is disturbed, either because a part flags [*se relache*] or because another overwhelms that which functions as its antagonist, or if the actions of the parts are reversed, or if they fail to follow one another in the natural order, these changes constitute maladies that are more or less grave.[61]

Life was not, then, a unitary phenomenon of the body but the end result of the activities and the interdependent properties of the individual organs. The "lives" of all the organs of the body functioned in constant reciprocal relations. The action of one organ necessarily entailed either diminution or augmentation of action in the others. If one acted too "vigorously" or if it "gave way," all the others, and the life of the whole, were disturbed. But so long as there was concourse, union, cooperation, there existed that state of harmony that doctors called health.

As this discussion of Bordeu's theory of glandular activity indicates, there was a fair component of mechanism still to be found in his vitalism. He employed diverse mechanical images to describe the process of secretion. His lingering mechanism is evident too in his concept of the body's "antagonisms," reciprocal actions and reactions operating between organs that had special affinities and relations. Finally, this mechanist tendency is fully evident in Bordeu's conception of the connective tissue, which provided a multipurpose apparatus for the execution of diverse moments and functions.[62] Yet, if there are elements in Bordeu's work that remain mechanistic, there are others that surpass even Stahl in affirming the autonomy and sui generis character of vital functions. Bordeu cast back beyond Stahl to van Helmont, for example, in postulating the existence of three vital "centers" – the brain, chest (*poitrine*), and lower abdomen – that enjoyed "supremacy" in the body and acted as a "triumvirate" in coordinating its activities.[63] Each of these centers had special kinships with other parts of the body, kinships that Bordeu sought to explain with the help of specific anatomical apparatuses. Thus the brain exercised influence over its subordinate parts with the aid of the nervous pathways, and the chest over its by the movement of blood to the tiniest vessels of the body. He could not account in such terms, however, for the work of "the central organ which departs from the lower abdomen and which has certain relations with all the other parts."[64] And even where the apparatus of "influence" seemed clear, as in the case of the nervous structures, the primary activating force was still to be found in the nerves' peculiar "virtue" of sensation. Though the nerves

61 *Ibid.*
62 On Bordeu's concern with mechanisms and structures, see Duchesneau, *Physiologie des Lumières*, 363–84.
63 Bordeu, "Glandes," 193n. The reference to a "triumvirate" is in Lordat, *Exposition*, 45.
64 Bordeu, "Glandes," 193n.

seemed to be especially important in the operations of sensibility, there was nothing to indicate that they were essential to the functioning of the vital forces, which were diffused throughout the body.[65]

In treating the general character of the brain and nervous system, Bordeu took up the much-argued question of whether the brain had its own independent movements or, in its pulsations, was merely responding to the diastolic-systolic action of the underlying arteries.[66] Unable to answer the question, Bordeu nonetheless strongly emphasized the fact of the brain's movement, suggesting that in so doing it imparted a series of "tremors" (*secousses*) and "irritations" along the nervous apparatus that were important in innumerable particularized activities of the different organs. It appeared to be the case, he argued, that the nerves in the individual parts of the body had two sources of movement: one set originating in the brain, and another originating in the organ itself. Whichever was the case (Bordeu did not himself decide the matter), it was clear that the tiny fibrillations of the nerves were instrumental in a great host of corporal activities. The mechanist cast of all this is striking, but again Bordeu moved beyond exploration of the mechanics of nervous action to consider the general nature of this force of "sensation" to which he attributed so much importance:

As the nerves are the depositories of sentiment, we must repeat what we said earlier in respect to this kind of sentiment that is proper to each part. What is this "virtue" in the nerves? It is their life, [it is] an action that is the necessary result of their constitution and their position. Why try to go further with this? It is enough to know that the nerves have an action that increases the more they are irritated; the action of the brain on the nerves is but a species of irritation which has its effect because the nerves are disposed to receive it. If [the nerves] were like those of a cadaver, or if they lost the force which is of their essence in living [beings] . . . , it is clear that all these tremors would be fruitless. One can conclude, following this idea, that the nerves of a cadaver lack – in respect of having action of their own – only *d'être mis au ton qui fait la vie.*[67]

This "ton qui fait la vie" Bordeu then compared to the "the heat of the sun without which all nature would languish," and to the fire which when applied to *verre métallique* lent it "a thousand new properties." "Why and how does all this happen?" Bordeu asked, "This is what we do not know."[68]

65 For a fuller discussion, see Michael Gross, "The Lessened Locus of Feelings: A Transformation in French Physiology in the Early Nineteenth Century," *JHB* 12 (1979): 231–71.
66 On eighteenth-century models of brain action, see Max Neuburger, *The Historical Development of Experimental Brain and Spinal Cord Physiology before Flourens,* trans. Edwin Clarke (Baltimore: Johns Hopkins University Press, 1981); and Jules Soury, *Le système nerveux central, Structures et fonctions: Histoire critique des théories et des doctrines,* 2 vols. (Paris: Georges Carré and C. Naud, 1899), 1:458–76.
67 Bordeu, "Glandes," 200n. 68 *Ibid.*

Given the extraordinary degree of interest in the general problem of sensation and sensibility not only in medical but also in larger intellectual and literary quarters in the eighteenth century, it would be wrong to argue that Bordeu stands alone as the source of what was to be an increasingly intense preoccupation with the operations and effects of sensibility.[69] Yet his importance in establishing a language and context for subsequent discussion of sensitive force is undeniable. He made his most famous appearance as a theorist of sensibility in Diderot's *Rêve de d'Alembert,* where Diderot used Bordeu's persona to represent advanced medical opinion on the problem of the origin and causation of life in a godless universe.[70] François Duchesneau has argued that Diderot's commentary destroyed the coherence of Bordeu's theory; he points out that Bordeu never embraced a genuine hylozoism but sought only to answer the limited question of how anatomical apparatuses were set in motion for the performance of the functional tasks.[71] Duchesneau's emphasis on the self-imposed limitations of Bordeu's theory is apt. Bordeu treated the problem of the origin of vitality in various terms, speaking at times of a generalized *force nouvelle,* at others of the role of "organization" in producing the individualized "lives" of the diverse anatomical apparatuses. But he never extrapolated a general theory of the origin or motive force of life in matter from these specific and delimited physiological considerations. Yet if Diderot's construction of Bordeu's thought was partly fictive, it nonetheless helped to give currency to Bordeu's name and to establish Montpellier as a source of original and provocative thinking on the origins of animal vitality. But in any event this fixing of Bordeu's reputation as the interlocutor of d'Alembert did not occur until the nineteenth century. Like all of Diderot's most daring works, the *Rêve* remained unpublished until long after its composition in 1769.[72] It is properly viewed then as sign rather than as cause of Bordeu's celebrity.

The extent of Bordeu's larger literary and philosophical reputation cannot be charted here, but his importance in medical circles in the later eighteenth and early nineteenth centuries will become apparent in subsequent chapters.[73] For now it may be noted that the elements of Bordeu's work that had the greatest significance for medical theorists were his doctrines of the natural harmony of the operations of the body (his beehive metaphor was to

---

69 See Gross, "The Lessened Locus of Feelings"; G. S. Rousseau, "Nerves, Spirits, and Fibres: Towards Defining the Origins of Sensibility," *Blue Guitar* 2 (December 1976): 125–53; for literary usages, see Northrop Frye, "Towards Defining an Age of Sensibility," *English Literary History* 23 (1956): 144–52, and R. F. Brissenden, *Virtue in Distress: Studies in the Novel of Sentiment from Richardson to Sade* (New York: Barnes and Noble, 1974), esp. 11–55.

70 Denis Diderot, *Le Rêve de d'Alembert,* ed. Jean Varloot (Paris: Editions sociales, 1962).

71 Duchesneau, *Physiologie des Lumières,* 362–63.

72 The work was circulated in paraphrase by Naigeon in 1821 and then published in an 1830–31 collection of Diderot's manuscripts. See Arthur M. Wilson, *Diderot* (New York: Oxford University Press, 1972), 829, n. 6.

73 See esp. Chapter 2.

reappear in diverse contexts) and of the separate but interrelated "lives" that together constituted its general life. The former conception was one that came to be identified with Montpellier generally; all the major Montpellier theorists drew important physiological and therapeutic implications from this view of the body's natural harmony. But the idea of the separate "lives" of the body was associated particularly with Bordeu and, as will shortly be seen, with his relative and sometime coauthor Louis de Lacaze. The "Bordeu-Lacaze school" was often criticized for the mechanist, materialist, and "solidist" implications of the separate-lives doctrine. Barthez and his followers decried Bordeu's readiness to see the diverse systems of the body operating on their own without direction by some generalized vital principle; others were to lament the opening to "materialism" Bordeu putatively made by positing independent "lives" without ascribing them to specific vital forces.[74] Modern medical historians have tended to see Bordeu's importance principally in his theory of the connective tissue, which was significant not only in itself (many and diverse functions were to be attributed to this newly described anatomical element) but for the encouragement it gave to the development of larger histological thinking, especially Bichat's theory of the body's elemental "tissues."[75] The last of these matters will be examined in Chapter 2, but at this juncture it will be useful to examine a variation on Bordeu's theme of sensibility that was developed in the work of the Montpellier physician Louis de Lacaze and that drew out the implications of Bordeu's ideas for both physical and moral therapeutics.

"THE WELL-ORDERED LIFE"

In his early years Bordeu worked for a time in close association with his cousin Louis de Lacaze (1703–65), who had received his medical degree at Montpellier in 1723 and then moved to Paris to take up a position as *médecin ordinaire* to Louis XV. (He later served as *médecin* to the duc d'Orléans.) Though Lacaze held these prestigious posts, he never established the kind of medical reputation other Montpellier practitioners (Senac, La Peyronie, Chicoyneau) had built in the capital. By 1751, when Bordeu arrived in Paris, Lacaze had not yet published a major theoretical work and was eager to go into editorial collaboration with Bordeu, whose *Recherches sur les glandes* had been well received several years earlier. In many respects the Lacaze-

---

74 Lordat, *Exposition*, 44–49; Frédéric Bérard, *Doctrine médicale de l'Ecole de Montpellier, et comparaison de ses principes avec ceux des autres écoles d'Europe* (Montpellier: Jean Martel, 1819), 56–57.

75 Russell C. Maulitz, *Morbid Appearances: The Anatomy of Pathology in the Early Nineteenth Century* (Cambridge: Cambridge University Press, 1987), 15–17; Maulitz sees Bordeu as an important precursor to Bichat but emphasizes the Hippocratist, holistic context of Bordeu's tissue theory. For a treatment that seeks to place Bordeu in line with modern histology, see Granel, *Pages médico-historiques*, 94–95.

Bordeu relationship was typical of the extended family and patronage relationships that were an important part of Montpellier's collective identity: Lacaze was wealthy and well established in the capital, and when Bordeu set out to build his own reputation there, he naturally turned for professional sponsorship and financial assistance to his cousin.[76] Lacaze took Bordeu and Bordeu's friend, the Montpellier graduate Gabriel Venel, into his household, exacting in return for his hospitality the collaboration of the two younger men on a book with which he had been struggling for some time.[77] Personally this venture did not prove a happy one – Bordeu ended by denouncing Lacaze's "impudent and lying character" – but it did yield one of the Montpellier school's most famous titles: *Idée de l'homme physique et moral,* which appeared in 1755.[78] Bordeu wrote his mother that the book "was not worth much," but, for better or worse, he came to be widely identified with it.[79] No less an authority than the celebrated *Dictionaire des sciences médicales* (published by the Panckoucke house in the 1820s) attributes the book to Bordeu, and though Lacaze's biographer thinks it the "unintelligible" work of a lunatic, it was subsequently cited by many physiologists as an illuminating and useful source.[80]

This work continued the attack that Bordeu had initiated on medical mechanism, calling for an end to the "subjection of medicine to the laws of experimental physics."[81] Medicine could not aspire to a degree of certitude comparable to that achieved by such sciences; it could hope only to establish "rules" that were sometimes "vague, indeterminate, and almost arbitrary."[82] Similarly, experimental techniques imported from the physical sciences and intended only for investigations of *le corps mort,* were altogether inappropriate to medicine. Boerhaave's experiments on the blood, for example, were pointless since "blood in the living body" had different properties from blood manipulated in the laboratory.[83] In place of such an approach, Lacaze advocated observation of the living in health and sickness, a procedure that, in spite of its difficulties and complexities, would eventually yield "the laws of the animal economy."[84]

---

76 Lucien Cornet, "Un protecteur de Théophile de Bordeu: Le médecin Louis de Lacaze (1703–1765)," *Bulletin de la Société des sciences, lettres et arts de Pau,* 3d ser., 26 (1966): 55–63. On the importance of patronage relationships generally in "the Mediterranean south," see André Jardin and André-Jean Tudesq, *Restoration and Reaction, 1815–1848,* trans. Elborg Forster (Cambridge: Cambridge University Press, 1983), 233–40.

77 On Venel, see *DSM:BM* 7:407–11.

78 Bordeu's remark is quoted by Cornet, "Un protecteur," 60; Louis de Lacaze, *Idée de l'homme physique et moral* (Paris: H. L. Guérin and L. F. Delatour, 1755).

79 Quoted in Cornet, "Un protecteur," 61.

80 *DSM:BM* 2:388, 402; see, for example, the references to Lacaze in Bérard, *Doctrine médicale,* 56–57.

81 Lacaze, *Idée de l'homme,* 11.   82 *Ibid.,* 306.

83 *Ibid.,* 9, 43–45; on Boerhaave's blood doctrine, see Lindeboom, *Boerhaave,* 276–78.

84 Lacaze, *Idée de l'homme,* 66–67; this phrase is the title of the work's second chapter.

Lacaze's remarks on the nature of "observation" are of some interest in light of the attention later paid to Montpellier teaching on method. In Lacaze's usage, observation was not the simple fact gathering of the *empirique* who would use any treatment if it seemed efficacious on one or two occasions. Nor was it the repetition of innumerable pointless experiments (again Boerhaave was the target). Indeed no procedure was of any use unless based on a "solid theory" of "natural and easily recognized genres" of maladies.[85] As was increasingly common among doctors, Lacaze invoked the authority of Hippocrates to support his notions of method and theory. Contrary to a widespread misunderstanding, Lacaze argued, Hippocratism was not antitheoretical. Genuine Hippocratic medicine was "undogmatic" but it was also "theoretical" insofar as it sought "general principles." Lacaze denounced those *empiriques* who claimed the authority of Hippocrates without in fact knowing anything of Hippocratic procedures. No approach, "Hippocratic" or otherwise, was of any value unless it attempted to show the relations between cause and effect.[86]

Medicine was, then, not merely a collection of more or less haphazard therapeutic techniques but also a theoretical enterprise. It was the science of living, organized beings characterized by the fundamental properties of movement and sentiment, whose "union and concourse" were responsible for the maintenance of life in the face of challenges to it.[87] Lacaze attributed great significance to the role of movement or, more precisely, to "the ensemble of movements that are linked in mutual dependence" in the "general life" of the organism.[88] Unlike Bordeu, who avoided speculation on the nature of vital forces, Lacaze did hazard a hypothesis about the character of the general motive force of the body, suggesting that "electrical fluid, a universal agent" was the underlying "physical principle of all movement."[89] Yet simple recognition of this agent meant little; what remained to be explained was "the natural order of its actions," something that experimentation of the sort undertaken in the auxiliary sciences could never discern because experiments necessarily interrupted and disturbed the functioning of nature.[90] Despite this fashionable interest in electricity, Lacaze seldom used electrical action to explain the specific "movements" responsible for vital functions. For the particulars of his system he relied much more on Bordeu's concept of the "antagonistic" motions of action and reaction working between the individual organs of the body and especially among the three vital centers of brain, "phrenic region," and the "exterior organ," whose interconnections formed the "principal *ressort* of the play of the body economy."[91] Of these, the "phrenic region" was the most important for it

85 *Ibid.*, 47–48.   86 *Ibid.*, 66.
87 *Ibid.*, 12–13.   88 *Ibid.*, 74.
89 *Ibid.*, 76.   90 *Ibid.*
91 *Ibid.*, 329–30.

operated as a "center of reaction for all other parts" of the body. The proper resolution of these "antagonisms," the integrated "unfolding" (*enchaine-ment*) of actions and reactions, assured the general harmony of the body that was fundamental not only to physical well-being but to "moral" health as well.[92]

In his own writings Bordeu had not been much concerned to develop the psychological and moral implications of vitalist doctrine, nor was he ever to take up such matters except in passing in the works that were unambiguously and exclusively his. Even his occasional references to the play of the "passions" were intended to explicate organic functions rather than to consider the nature or operations of the passions themselves. Lacaze, on the other hand – desiring perhaps to be seen in company with Montesquieu and the other philosophes to whose work on similar matters he alluded – sought to encompass both the "physical" and the "moral" dimensions of physiology. That he did so is one reason that *Idée de l'homme*, despite its peculiarities and shortcomings, was a text that survived; the inextricability of the physical-moral relation was to become one of the cardinal elements of the vitalist legacy.[93]

Lacaze's work was organized using the framework of the ancient doctrine of the "non-naturals," the six primary influences – air, ingesta, movement and repose, sleep and waking, secretion and excretion, and the "affections of the soul" – that most directly affected the state of the body and determined its conditions of health or illness.[94] Keeping the promise of the title to treat the physical and the moral, Lacaze discussed at length the last of these influences, the "affections of the soul." His overall purpose was to explain the "necessary relations of the play of the animal economy with the state of men in society" as well as the "principal advantages and disadvantages that necessarily result from a good or bad disposition of the organs."[95]

Throughout this section of the work, Lacaze gave special attention to sensation and sensibility, the nervous apparatus, and the mechanisms of nervous action. Like Bordeu he held to an idea of diffuse sensibility, distributed throughout the body and not exclusively dependent on the presence of nerve endings. Sensibility was conveyed not only along the nervous apparatus but reciprocally among the three spheres of vital action. The esophagus and trachea, for example, as organs of "phrenic force," conveyed to the head the sensible movements of the entrails and diaphragm.[96] In this view, sensation was a general, universally dispersed "force" that was linked not only to nerve action but also to a multitude of diverse vital phenomena. All sensa-

---

92 *Ibid.*, 344–45, 351–56.   93 See Chapter 2.
94 On the doctrine of the "non-naturals," see William Coleman, "Health and Hygiene in the *Encyclopédie*: A Medical Doctrine for the Bourgeoisie," *JHMAS* 29 (1974): 399–421.
95 Lacaze, *Idée de l'homme*, 308.   96 *Ibid.*, 316–30.

tions were either pleasurable or painful, depending on the extent to which they satisfied or obstructed the fundamental "needs" of the animal economy; pleasurable sensations "augment the feeling of our existence" and encourage the development of physical and moral "habits" (*habitudes*).[97] Everywhere and at all times, then, fundamental *moeurs* are established not by society but by pleasure and pain as experienced by the animal economy. Yet, since the "complexions" of men differ in varying circumstances, "usages" differed too, a fact demonstrated by the long-recognized distinction between "men of the North" (robust, violent, strong in body) and "men of the Midi" (weaker, "livelier in sentiment").[98] If the "constitution" of the body was reflected in the "constitution" of society, however, it was reciprocally true that a particular constitution of society entailed changes in the animal economy. Social organization created a certain *manière d'exister* that apportioned tasks, encouraged the use of different "talents," and motivated the habitual use and development of particular organs. Thus men in the "savage state" were accustomed to muscular action requiring cooperation between the head and the phrenic center, whereas "civilized men" used only their heads. Too much headwork, at the expense of muscular action, caused the ill effects (timidity, fearfulness) characteristic of overrefinement.[99] In this construction of reciprocal physical-moral influence, the crucial concept was that of habit. Habits served to develop talents and faculties but were also responsible for vice: "Virtually every physical and moral ill is the effect of decisions taken unknowingly, and hasty judgments result not so much from lack of enlightenment but from a habitual evil disposition."[100]

This line of argument culminated in an extension of Bordeu's definition of health as harmony and balance to social practice: moderation was the key to health because any kind of excess disturbed bodily harmony, promoted "disorder," and put the all-important connective tissue into a state of "vicious sensibility." An individual characterized by excessive sensibility was dependent on the "objects" that satisfy heightened needs, governed by habit rather than reflection, and made prey to "the empire of the passions."[101] Disorder of this kind disrupted that "natural state of the body" that best fitted us to "acquit our duties toward society and enjoy rightful pleasures." "By habits of sobriety, suitable exercise for the body, and, especially by worthy occupations, one is happily distanced from the manner of life and disposition that lead almost inevitably to excessive passions."[102] In this classic Montpellier text, then, the moral and physical domains were conflated: only the "well-ordered life" could assure the health of both body and spirit.

97 *Ibid.*, 340–42, 363.   98 *Ibid.*, 365–66.
99 *Ibid.*, 363, 367, 384–85.   100 *Ibid.*, 406–7.
101 *Ibid.*, 426.   102 *Ibid.*, 423–24, 428.

THE VITAL PRINCIPLE

By the time Bordeu ended his collaboration with Lacaze he was well established in his medical practice and in learned circles in Paris. He was friendly with d'Alembert, Diderot, and others among the encyclopedists and had wealthy and powerful clients. Despite all his connections, however, Bordeu failed to attain the professional heights he had expected to reach; he never became the First Physician, for example, though he had been widely thought the likeliest successor to Jean Senac. On several occasions Bordeu was the victim of gossip and of false charges about his competence and honesty made by his Paris competitors. His innocence in these matters seems clear and the scandals themselves would appear to be nothing more than effects of the Paris-Montpellier rivalry. By the early 1770s, however, an exhausted and embittered Bordeu retreated from Paris to the south.[103]

Bordeu's place as Montpellier's most illustrious representative in the capital was eventually taken by Paul-Joseph Barthez, who was to produce the most influential synthesis of vitalist thought. Barthez first came to Paris in 1754 as a protégé of Camille Falconet, the powerful court physician. He too moved in d'Alembert's circle and wrote for the *Encyclopédie*.[104] In the mid 1750s Barthez served as an army physician and then in 1761, having triumphed in a competition for a chair, returned to Montpellier. For twenty years Barthez taught at the Montpellier faculty, served as adjunct chancellor, and built a large practice among the local nobility. In 1781 he returned to the capital, where he too was the victim of public charges made by Paris rivals, who claimed that he had killed, or at best neglected, his patient d'Alembert, who died in 1783. These scandals did not prevent Barthez from building a great reputation both in medical and wider learned circles, however, or from accumulating many honors and positions.[105] When the Revolution came, Barthez declared himself opposed to the joining of the nobility with the clergy and Third Estate and then fled the capital. From

103 Details on Bordeu's career appear in Louis Dulieu, "Théophile de Bordeu," *DSB* 2:301–2. Bordeu's contributions to the *Encyclopédie* are described in Pierre Astruc, "Les sciences médicales et leurs représentants dans l'*Encyclopédie*," *RHS* 4 (1951): 359–68. Much personal information is available in *Théophile de Bordeu: Correspondance,* ed. Martha Fletcher, 4 vols. (Montpellier: CNRS, Université Paul Valery, n.d.). The "scandals" in which Bordeu was caught up, and the antagonisms between Montpellier and Paris doctors, are described in Delaunay, *Le monde médical parisien,* 135–40, and in the article "Bordeu," *DSM:BM* 2:387–402. The view that the king passed over Bordeu for appointment as First Physician for fear of further antagonizing the Paris faculty is stated in the article "Lorry," *DSM:BM* 6:102–9.
104 Barthez's biography is recounted briefly in Louis Dulieu, "Paul-Joseph Barthez," *RHS* 24 (1971): 149–76; *idem,* "Paul-Joseph Barthez," *DSB* 1:478–79; see also Dulieu, *La médecine à Montpellier,* 3:183–89. The *Encyclopédie* articles are discussed in Henri Zeiler, "Les collaborateurs médicaux de l'*Encyclopédie* de Diderot et de d'Alembert" (Thèse, Faculté de Médecine de Paris, 1934).
105 "Barthez," *DBF* 5:689–90.

1789 to 1802 he lived in the south, where he published his second most famous book, *Nouvelle mécanique des mouvemens de l'homme et des animaux*
(1798). When Montpellier's Ecole de santé was created in 1794, Barthez was
passed over for appointment, but in 1802 he was rehabilitated by the Montpellier graduate and minister to Napoleon, Jean-Antoine Chaptal. That
same year Barthez also became *médecin consultant* to Napoleon, a post he
held until he died in 1806.[106]

Barthez's reputation, both contemporary and posthumous, rested chiefly
on his treatise *Nouveaux élémens de la science de l'homme,* first published in
1778, revised and "greatly augmented" in 1806, and reprinted in 1858. Barthez had already published several Latin works (including his *Principio vitali
humanis* [1773]) that made an impression in Montpellier, but his treatise on
the science of man secured for him a national, and even international, reputation as the preeminent expositor of vitalist doctrine.[107] In this work Barthez argued that there was but one "cause that produces all the phenomena
of life in the human body," a cause he elected to call the "principle of life"
or "vital principle."[108] The vital principle was not a metaphysical or occult
force used to "explain" the "functions of corporal life." Indeed "explaining" – in the sense of tracing phenomena to their ultimate cause or causes –
was no part of Barthez's task:

I never used the term vital principle to *explain* any of the phenomena of life but [em-
ployed it] only to make comprehensible and certain new conclusions in respect to
the effects of these phenomena, which I attempted to combine in a simpler, more
general, and consequently more useful manner than anyone had done before me.[109]

The essential nature of the vital principle was completely unknown. It was
pointless, for example, to ask whether the vital principle was a "substance"
because this term had been rendered meaningless and obscure by metaphysical dispute. The vital principle was not "a being existing of itself, distinct
from the soul and body of man," but rather a "necessary abstraction," the
use of which was required to make possible statements about the observed
phenomena of experience. He did not hold that the vital principle "orders
and regulates its acts" but suggested only that it existed in the fashion of
"a faculty attached to the combinations of movement and matter of which
a living body is formed."[110]

106 "Barthez," *DSM:BM* 1:572–88.
107 *Oratio academica de principio vitali hominis* (Montpellier: Rochard, 1773); *Nova doctrina de
   functionibus naturae humanae* (Montpellier: A.-F. Rochard, 1774). The third edition of *Nouveaux éléments de la science de l'homme,* edited by Barthez's grandnephew and published in
   1858 by J. B. Baillière, was prompted by a general debate on vitalism at the Académie
   impériale de médecine; the publisher called the book the "most important work of medical philosophy published in France in the eighteenth century" (editor's front note, n.p.).
108 Barthez, *Science de l'homme,* 1:20. 109 *Ibid.,* 1:"Notes," 4.
110 *Ibid.,* 1:97, 1:"Notes," 97–100.

Barthez was at pains to distinguish his vital principle from formulations with which it might be confused or conflated, especially the "thinking soul" of the Stahlians. Though he praised Stahl for combating the iatro-mechanists, Barthez distanced himself from the "animists" for whom "the influence of the thinking soul" was "the exclusive cause of spontaneous action in all parts of the body."[111] To Barthez such a conclusion was insupportable: although the thinking soul undeniably influenced voluntary movements, it clearly had no directing power over spontaneous and wholly unconscious activities like circulation. The existence of two different controlling principles, one guiding voluntary movements and the other involuntary processes, was inadmissible: "Good philosophical method in the science of man requires that one attribute to a single principle of life in the human body the living forces that reside in each organ and that are responsible for its functions."[112] The same principle sufficed to discredit the system of van Helmont, which multiplied "occult forces" to explain the "separate lives" of the independent organs, and the teachings of modern physiologists like Johann Blumenbach, who classified a range of "vital forces." Against all such views, Barthez asserted that it was "more natural and philosophical" to postulate one vital principle, with modifications.[113]

Barthez was scarcely less critical of the "solidist" view that he identified with the Italian physician Baglivi as well as Lacaze, a doctrine that attributed all vital phenomena to "an innate force of elasticity in the fibers" (*une force innée de ressort de fibres*). The solidists' hypothetical "antagonisms," "ensembles of movements," and "centers of effort" could not be demonstrated and were no more valuable than the bizarre explanations proposed by iatromechanists.[114]

It is ironic that Barthez was so critical of the hypotheses and "metaphysical entities" of his opponents for he himself was frequently viewed, both by his contemporaries and by later critics, as the expositor of an occult or mysterious force at work in the body.[115] Yet Barthez was careful to refer to the vital principle as an abstraction employed only to facilitate discussion of activities whose inner dynamics were not understood but whose effects were accessible to observation. This procedure enabled him to treat the "forces of the human vital principle, their communications or sympathies, their joining in one system, their distinctive modifications according to

---

111 *Ibid.*, 1:19.   112 *Ibid.*, 1:20.
113 *Ibid.*, 1:21, 78–79; 1:"Notes," 22–23. On Van Helmont, see Walter Pagel, *Joan Baptista Van Helmont: Reformer of Science and Medicine* (Cambridge: Cambridge University Press, 1982); Blumenbach's physiology is examined in Timothy Lenoir, *The Strategy of Life: Teleology and Mechanics in Nineteenth-Century German Biology* (Boston: D. Reidel, 1982).
114 Barthez, *Science de l'homme*, 1:22–25.
115 See, for example, Daremberg, *Histoire des sciences médicales*, 1175–77.

temperament and age, and their extinction at death."[116] To him such a procedure was the essence of Baconian induction, and it was within the tradition of Bacon that he sought firmly to lodge his own inquiry.

Barthez saw Bacon as the first philosopher clearly to differentiate between the soul of the theologians and the principle of life.[117] More important, it was Bacon who diagnosed the worst "vices" of the philosophy of his time and taught the method of induction, the only sure and reliable guide for inquiry in the "natural sciences." To Barthez the Baconian system entailed both the definition of correct scientific procedure (amassing data through observation and experience) and the establishment of the inquirer's proper objective (seeking to understand cause and effect relations only in the limited, skeptical, and prudent manner possible on the basis of such data). Investigators working in the spirit of Bacon, Barthez insisted, must abandon that search for "essences" or "final causes" that stimulated metaphysical inquiry: "Natural philosophy has for its object research into the causes of the phenomena of nature but only insofar as these can be known from experience. . . . Experience cannot teach what any of these [causes] are in essence."[118] Barthez supplemented the authority of Bacon by referring to Hume's *Treatise*, agreeing with Hume that to impute "cause did not imply any real understanding of cause and effect but only a recognition that certain phenomena succeed one another in a regular, and apparently constant, way. He agreed with Hume that we imagine succession to mean cause, and that such imagining or belief is all we can hope to attain in the way of certainty.[119] Thus it was under the aegis of the inductive method that Barthez defended the use of an abstraction such as the vital principle. Inductively derived "causes" could be called by various names – "principles, powers, forces, faculties"; whatever they were called, their ultimate nature could not be known. Newton's gravitation was one such "force"; Barthez's own vital principle was another. If the origin and fundamental nature of the vital principle would be forever unknown, its operations could nonetheless be demonstrated by observed facts.[120]

The title chosen by Barthez for his treatise of 1778 – the "new elements of the science of man" – indicated not only his Baconian posture but also his sense that medicine enjoyed privileged access to the most crucial phenomena of human experience and thus offered a unique approach to investigation of the human subject. "Hippocrates in his genius saw that human nature cannot be fully understood by anyone who does not possess the en-

116 Barthez, *Science de l'homme*, 1:33.
117 *Ibid.*, 1:76–77.   118 *Ibid.*, 1:5; see also 1:"Notes," 10–11.
119 *Ibid.*, 1:"Notes," 11–13; on Hume's treatment of cause, see Keith Michael Baker, *Condorcet: From Natural Philosophy to Social Mathematics* (Chicago: University of Chicago Press, 1975), 136–55.
120 Barthez, *Science de l'homme*, 1:7–8.

tire system of knowledge of the healing art."[121] But not all doctors were equally good observers. Medicine that denied or obscured the exercise of vitality – reducing what was protean, variable, and unpredictable to laws that in reality extended only to brute nature – lacked any means to explore phenomena that were peculiarly human. The only physicians who could hope to pierce the mysteries of human existence were those who recognized the role of the vital principle.[122]

VITALITY AND VARIABILITY: AGE, SEX, TEMPERAMENT, CLIMATE

The concept of variability was essential to Barthez's formulation of the science of man, so much so that the terms "variable" and "vital" occasionally function almost synonymously. The very idea of vital action or force was necessitated by the fact that "life-phenomena" failed to exhibit constancy and uniformity in the fashion of inert bodies. Barthez's "life-phenomena" encompassed a wide range of bodily functions and experiential activities, including the general forces of sensibility and movement; the special functions of particular organs; the "sympathies" and "synergies" that linked parts of the body economy; the multitudinous signs and symptoms of the body in sickness; the capacities and qualities of the body ("modifications of the vital principle") as it varied with age, sex, and temperament; the influence on the body of external factors such as Hippocrates's "airs, waters, and places"; and the mental states that corresponded to all of these. In short the "life-phenomena" embraced everything experienced by the "whole person," in whom "corporal instrument," vital force, and thinking soul were united. All these phenomena showed great variability and could not be reduced to determinative laws.[123]

The variability and spontaneity of vital phenomena were manifest in the operation of sensibility. Barthez found fantastic the doctrine of "animal spirits" upheld by Cartesians and other mechanists, and he also rejected any

---

121 *Ibid.*, 1:28. Cf. Bordeu, *Recherches sur l'histoire de la médecine*, 261, where he wrote: "La médecine a les droits très-légitimes sur la connaissance des passions des hommes et sur celle de leurs moeurs, qui tiennent plus ou moins de leurs passions naturelles, ou de leurs différents tempéraments."

122 Cf. Réjane Bernier who sees Barthez evolving away from preoccupation with the human toward considerations of how his vitalism might be extended to the plant and animal domains; see "La notion de principe vital chez Barthez," *Archives de philosophie* 35 (1972): 432–41. Although this argument introduces a valuable nuance into our understanding of Barthez, the textual changes noted between the 1778 and 1806 editions do not, to my mind, demonstrate any fundamental alteration in Barthez's system.

123 For discussions of the variability of vital phenomena, see Barthez, *Science de l'homme*, 1:123–24 (on muscle force); 1:182–98 (on sensitive force); 1:198–99, 221 (on the relation between irritants and movement); 1:232–34 (on the vital qualities of blood); 2:2–3 (on sympathies); 2:"Notes," 48–50 (on intelligence and brain size); 2:153–62 (on sleep); 2:177–81, 201–02 (on remedies and poisons); 2:289–99 (on age).

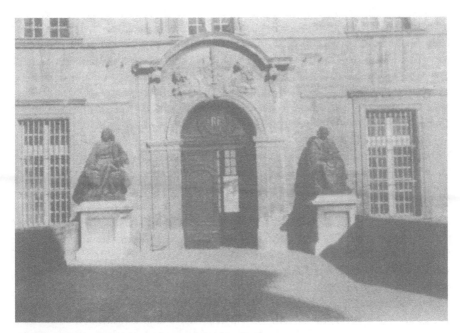

Facade of the Faculté de Médecine de Montpellier.

model of sensibility that made it dependent on mechanical "impulsion." He dismissed the distinction drawn by the Swiss physiologist Albrecht von Haller (1708–77) between "sensibility" (conscious feeling conveyed by the nerves) and "irritability" (unconscious reactive movement without feeling). To Barthez sentience was an independent "force" subsidiary to and governed by the general force of the vital principle. It was "an active force, not a passive state of the vital principle."[124] It did not depend on nerve action: anatomical investigation proved that parts and regions of the body that were sparsely supplied with nerves were still highly sensitive, while experiments by Haller himself had proved that sensibility operated in creatures like the polyp, which had essentially no nervous apparatus at all.[125] Barthez acknowledged that there was often some correlation between the degree of sensibility exhibited by a body part or region and either the number of nerve endings that supplied it or its proximity to major nerve centers such as the dispersed ganglia (which Barthez referred to as "miniature brains" distributed throughout the body).[126] Intense sensibility could also reflect, however, an intimate relation between a given organ and the "epigastric center" – the conjuncture of heart, diaphragm, and stomach – which, be-

124 Barthez, *Science de l'homme*, 1:177; on Haller, see 1:192–97.
125 *Ibid.*, 1:192–93, 182.   126 *Ibid.*, 2:60–63 (this is specifically on sympathies).

cause of its clustering of the vital forces of these critical organs, was the body's most sensitive region. Barthez referred to the concentrated, location-bound, or special types of sensibility observed in the particular organs or regions as "local sensibility." But he argued that general sensibility operated independently of the mechanical apparatus of the nerves and partook in some fashion of the general vital force: "All organs of the living animal body are doubtless susceptible to that general sensibility which is common to them all."[127]

Barthez attached great significance to the fact that sensibility varied, sometimes extremely, depending on diverse internal and environmental influences, including internal anatomical dispositions (such as the degree of "integrity" of the nervous system in cases of poisoning, paralysis, and nervous disease), temperament, climate, the volume and type of ingestibles, age, sex, and so on. With its high degree of variability, sensibility was the paradigmatic vital phenomenon. Its workings could not be attributed to clear-cut mechanical operations nor could its intensity be predicted, individual to individual, because it was influenced by apparently infinite internal and external circumstances.[128]

Barthez was not alone in identifying vitality with variability; the significance attached to variability in vital phenomena was a hallmark of Montpellier medicine. One of Bordeu's most widely cited works was an article he wrote for the *Encyclopédie* entitled "Crise" in which he took issue even with the revered Hippocrates on the supposed regularity to be found in the appearance of symptoms, duration, and moments of crisis in disease. He disputed the special significance of the "critical days," those days (the seventh, fourteenth, and twentieth from onset) when an illness supposedly underwent some kind of crucial metamorphosis. Pointing out the frequent difficulty of determining the "day of onset" and exploring the ambiguities of the doctrine when considered in relation to chronic disease, he concluded that the ancient teaching on "crises" was "obscure, vague, and subject to errors." All this proved that nature itself was "irregular" and that those who tried to capture it with calculations were bound to fail:

It is not by scrupulous calculations that one learns to judge an illness or how to use remedies; in calculating, one becomes timid, temporizing, indecisive, and as a result less useful to society; nature has its laws, but one can neither count nor classify them.[129]

"Rational medicine" made the constant mistake of attempting to harness the facts of illness to unvarying principles. Bordeu criticized those who

---

127 *Ibid.*, 1:182, 197.   128 *Ibid.*, 1:177–254.
129 Bordeu, "Crise," in *Encyclopédie ou dictionnaire raisonné des sciences, des arts et des métiers* (Paris: Briasson, 1751–65), 3:471–89; the quotation is on p. 488.

"sacrificed to this idol [the theory of crisis] . . . their own observations," and he intended his essay as a lesson in proper observational technique.[130] For Bordeu and Barthez, the value of "observational medicine" was that it alone properly recognized the unpredictability of the human organism in sickness.

This acceptance, indeed valorization, of the variability of "life-phenomena" encouraged Montpellier theorists to take up problems surrounding growth and aging that were necessarily slighted in mechanist analyses of body function. If the body was in fact a clocklike machine as Descartes had insisted, its slow and subtle transformations throughout life were difficult to explain.[131] Vitalist medicine gave special attention to growth and aging, tracing for each of the four "stages of life" (childhood, youth, maturity, old age) the relative proportions and "influence" of the various regions of the body, the varying condition of the vital forces, and the peculiar conditions and diseases characteristic of that stage. Barthez argued, for example, that in youth the upper region of the body exercised "dominance," a fact reflected in the large size of the head in relation to the body, the high degree of sensibility among the young (resulting from the importance of the head and the epigastric center), and the intense and rapid effects of external irritants such as poisons, bites, and noise. In old age all these factors were reversed: the lower part of the body dominated (a fact proved by the chronic digestive woes of the old), sensibility was dulled, and irritants were slow to exercise effect.[132]

Physicians were not the only eighteenth-century theorists interested in the question of human diversity according to age; Buffon too devoted separate sections of his *Natural History* to the human "stages of life." Nevertheless, medicine had a privileged role in this area, as Bordeu reminded readers of his history of medicine when he remarked on Buffon's many borrowings from medical teaching.[133] Montpellier's special importance in this connection stemmed from the fact that vitalism established a theoretical basis for the study of age variation. In accenting variability in the "life-phenomena," it made investigation of age-related differences significant rather than epiphenomenal. Age variations were not oddities or exceptional departures from the body's normative modes of operation but rather were manifestations of "modifications" in the vital principle naturally occasioned by the varying circumstances of the life of the organism.

130 *Ibid.*, 474–75.
131 Boerhaave attributed old age to the stiffening of the fibers but otherwise had little to say on growth or aging; see Hall, *History of General Physiology*, 1:384, and see 1:395–96 for Haller's "Boerhaavian" explanation of aging.
132 Barthez, *Science de l'homme*, 2:291–95.
133 Georges Louis Leclerc de Buffon, *De l'homme*, ed. Michèle Duchet (Paris: François Maspéro, 1971), chaps. 2–5; Bordeu, *Recherches sur l'histoire de la médecine*, 256. A detailed study of Buffon's relation to Montpellier vitalism is needed.

In considering particular age variations, Barthez brought into play one of his most important theoretical tools, the distinction between what he called "active" and "radical" force, the former signifying force currently or "actively" engaged and the latter meaning the potential or untapped force of the economy.[134] Reflecting on why hemorrhaging took the form of nosebleeds in children but was expressed as uterine or "hemorrhoidal" blood-loss in the old, Barthez argued that all such phenomena were linked to the way in which the "various ages effect changes" in the "constitutional intensity of the radical forces" at the same time as they work "general modifications in the active forces" of the vital principle. In the young the "active forces" are "precipitous, rapid, and irregular," whereas in the old they are slow, regular, tending toward dissipation. In the young, diseases are "impetuous and effervescent," whereas in the old they are sluggish. In the young sensation, appetite, and passion are at a high pitch; in the old they show "but feeble activity."[135]

Sexual differences were linked to age differences since "the feminine sex generally shows marked similarities to youth."[136] Such a view was a commonplace among medical theoreticians of the female sex and of femininity. But here too Barthez developed his treatment of specifically female characteristics within the context of his larger theory. Women shared with children "vivacity" in the "exercise of the forces," such vivacity finding expression in heightened sensibility, a lively play of the passions, and rapid alterations of mood. This "vivacity of force" rendered women's constitution "feeble and delicate" in comparison to the "active and supple" constitution of men. Consequently men were able to undertake enterprises of a sort women never could, but they also suffered from a greater tendency to those "faults in regimen" (such as excess in food, drink, and sex) that women, who had more reason to fear the effects of such habits, took care to avoid.[137]

Although the Montpellier doctors taught that sex determined important differences in the constitution, diseases, and mortality of women and men, they stopped short of certain extreme conclusions about the feebleness of women that earlier doctors had drawn. Bordeu criticized as "completely outmoded," for example, the Renaissance physician Juan Huarte's view that the constitution and faculties of women rendered them incapable of intellectual labor.[138] In other respects, however, vitalist medicine reinforced conventional views that women differed inherently from men, and taught that women had but limited capacity for any activities other than those for

---

134 Barthez, *Science de l'homme*, 2:163–65, 290–95.   135 *Ibid.*, 2:291–95.
136 *Ibid.*, 2:295.
137 *Ibid.*, 2:295–99; this section closely follows Pierre Roussel, *Système physique et moral de la femme* (Paris: Vincent, 1775).
138 Bordeu, *Recherches sur l'histoire de la médecine*, 269.

which nature had intended them – gestation, birthing, nursing, and the care of children. The Montpellier-trained physician Pierre Roussel published in 1775 one of the eighteenth century's most famous treatises on women, the *Système physique et moral de la femme,* which was devoted to "the constitution, organic state, temperament, *moeurs* and peculiar functions of the sex."[139] This work was a classic vitalist text. It took issue with medical teaching that treated women as if they were men except for certain special functions. Women were not women "in one place only" but from "every perspective." Only if one considered the whole – physiology, *moeurs,* character, inclinations – could one get at the truth of women. And only in studying the relations between the body and the "affections of the soul" could medicine accomplish its full task, which – beyond healing the sick – was to teach a way of life based on *bonne morale.* Finally, only that medicine which ceased trying to reduce the human to the mechanical could aspire to these ends. Roussel paid his respects to Stahl, attacked Boerhaave, and praised other Montpellier doctors – Venel, Lamure, Barthez, Fouquet, and especially Bordeu – who had initiated the "revolution" in medicine.[140]

The study of sensibility was as important in Roussel's treatise as it was in other vitalist analyses: sensibility, he argued, "provides the basis" for all knowledge of the interrelations of the physical and the moral. Like children, women exhibited high sensibility; their "existence consists more in sensations than in ideas or in corporal movements."[141] Dominated by rapidly changing sensations, women were capricious and inconstant; they lacked interest in politics, ethics, or science; their lives were characterized by those "sweet and affectionate sentiments" so necessary to the happiness and well-being of society.[142] Education and training could not alter the basic character of women: "Doubtless education, social *moeurs,* and an infinity of circumstances can alter in a thousand ways, and almost efface, the original character that nature has given to women; it is no less true that in general women are and must naturally be sweet and timid."[143] No matter what their education or circumstances, the "occupations" of women would never vary much; from the physiological point of view once the work of gestation, birth, and nursing were completed, woman's work was over and "the plan of nature fulfilled."[144]

Roussel was deeply impressed by Bordeu's theory of the mucous tissue and embraced the latter's view that variation in its character explained differences not only between the sexes but among people of varying climate,

139 Roussel, *Système;* this phrase is the book's subtitle.
140 *Ibid.,* xvi–xxiii, 2; Roussel wrote of Bordeu's book on the glands that "of all the books on physiology that we know, [it is] that which offers the most exact ideas on some of the most interesting particulars of the animal system"; see *Système,* 195. The reference to *bonne morale* is on p. xi.
141 *Ibid.,* 28–36.   142 *Ibid.*
143 *Ibid.,* 36.   144 *Ibid.,* xxxv.

occupation, and the like. Thus the development of women began in child-hood when the "mucous tissue" began to harden and to occasion changes in complexion, voice, height, movements, tastes, and ideas. Along with the state of the "soft parts," vessels, nerves, and fibers, the condition of the cellular tissue established that "passive state to which nature destines women."[145] External factors might modify the organization and constitu-tion of women, but between women and men there remained "an innate, radical difference that has been found in all countries and among all peoples."[146] Women were naturally characterized by the "sanguine temper-ament," which was the most conducive to a gentle, untroubled state of health. Their economy was characterized by equilibrium and "a pleasant balance." As women did not practice the "arts" that "modify the constitu-tion [of men] in a thousand ways," their economy was little subject to change.[147] The regime of women properly consisted of moderate exercise, restraint in eating and drinking, and avoidance of both indolence and ex-cessive passion.[148] Roussel disputed claims that organization and climate counted for little in establishing the physical-moral character. It was not so: "A Frenchman has more wit than a Samoyed; an old man is less active than a young one; women differ from men," all because "different instruments must produce different effects."[149]

These very ordinary statements about women are not of much interest in themselves; what is interesting is the vitalist imperative that informs Roussel's general approach to women – the demand for a holistic perspec-tive, the stress on sensibility, the insistence that variability is fundamental. Most important of all, however, is the fact that the vitalist perspective sup-plied a coherent and adaptable rationale for the construction of more or less stable physiological types, whose fundamental organization could not be al-tered by "external circumstances." Women were perhaps the most easily discerned of such types but others too – formed by age, temperament, cli-mate, and similar factors – were evident to the careful observer. In this re-spect vitalist medicine embodied a paradox that would be found in all subsequent anthropological enterprises: the very perspective that insisted most forcefully on the importance (and by implication, value) of diversity came to emphasize its own power to discern patterns and regularities amid such diversity and, yet more crucial, to insist on the "natural" stability and hence endlessly ramifying significance of those patterns.

145 *Ibid.*, 15.   146 *Ibid.*, 16.
147 *Ibid.*, 64–69, 91.   148 *Ibid.*, 93–132.
149 *Ibid.*, 22–23, note (a). This passage, disputing the claims of a "writer of this century," was probably directed at Helvétius, whom the Montpellier doctors frequently criticized for denying the influence of "physical causes" on character and intellect; on Helvétius, see Michèle Duchet, *L'anthropologie et histoire au siècle des lumières: Buffon, Voltaire, Rousseau, Helvétius, Diderot* (Paris: François Maspéro, 1971), 377–406; see also D. W. Smith, *Hel-vétius: A Study in Persecution* (Oxford: Clarendon Press, 1965).

These basic tenets of Montpellier medicine were to be found in discussions not only of age and sex but also of temperament and climate. The treatment of these latter topics was of course rooted in one of the most influential and long-lived elements of ancient medicine, the doctrine of the humors – blood, phlegm, bile, and atrabile – which, according to the Hippocratic text *The Nature of Man,* were the most important determinants of the body's "constitution" and "its pains and health." Health itself was defined in this text as "that state in which these constituent substances are in the correct proportion to each other, both in strength and quantity," and pain was described as that condition produced "when one of the substances presents either a deficiency or an excess, or is separated in the body and not mixed with the others."[150]

The humors not only determined health or sickness, moreover, but also provided the central point of reference in the ancient doctrine of "temperament," the ensemble of features, habits, and tendencies that characterized each individual. In Galen's system there were four simple temperaments corresponding to the primary qualities (warm, cold, dry, and wet); four mixed temperaments – sanguine (warm and moist), phlegmatic (cold and moist), bilious (warm and dry), and melancholic (cold and dry); and one ideal "temperate state." Later versions of temperament theory often simplified these systems into a one-to-one correspondence between the four humors and the four basic temperaments, the latter being attributed to the predominance of a given humor within the body economy. These versions yielded the correspondences sanguine-blood, pituitary-phlegm, bilious-bile, melancholic-atrabile, with the humor in question presumed to be "dominant" in the body system.[151]

In the eighteenth century humoral medicine was still widely resorted to, though it was frequently regarded as theoretically nugatory.[152] Montpellier medicine, however, revived and placed new emphasis on the doctrine of temperament in keeping with its close attention to the fact and causes of human variability. Indeed the controlling "influence of temperament," which could not be defined with exactitude but whose effects could be charted in more or less regular patterns, was a perfect instance of what Barthez saw as generalizations that were significant and meaningful although lacking in lawlike rigor.[153]

150 "The Nature of Man," in *Hippocratic Writings,* ed. G. E. R. Lloyd, trans. J. Chadwick et al. (New York: Penguin, 1978), 26.
151 On ancient temperament theory, see E. D. Phillips, *Greek Medicine* (London: Thames and Hudson, 1973), who argues that the "constitutions" of Hippocratic medicine "are always directly linked to the doctrine of physical humours, and do not yet take on an almost separate life as psychological expressions" (pp. 51–52); see also Raymond Klibansky et al. *Saturn and Melancholy* (New York: Basic Books, 1964); Staum, *Cabanis,* 49–55.
152 For a discussion of the predominantly "humoralist" cast of popular medicine in eighteenth-century France, see Ramsey, *Professional and Popular Medicine,* 145–46.
153 Barthez, *Science de l'homme,* 1:222.

Barthez disavowed popular doctrines that construed temperament solely as the product of an "overabundance" of one or another of the humors. Even recent works in physiology, he complained, described the sanguine temperament as that in which blood was dominant, the "pituitary" as that in which phlegm was excessive, and so on. This conception was erroneous, Barthez argued, both because "overabundance" of any humor was pathological and produced disease, and because humoral excess was only one of the "constant affections whose joint operation determines temperament."[154] There is a significant ambiguity in this formulation. Barthez was reluctant to accept that there could be humoral excess without illness since according to Montpellier teaching on pathology, humoral imbalance was a leading, if not always primary, cause of disease. Yet temperamental variation did exist, and the quantity and relative balance of the humors was critically important in explaining it. Embedded in Barthez's doctrine was the suggestion that the temperaments were all inherently pathological because they indicated humoral imbalance and represented divergence from an ideal or norm of "equilibrium" that therapeutic medicine was supposed to be able to restore. Yet he seemed to imply too that medicine was powerless against inherent imbalances in the body economy. His own version of temperament doctrine was based not simply on the humors but on a kind of dynamic interplay among the character of the vital forces, the proportions of the humors, the "physical state" (*physique*) of humors and solids, and the effects on the economy of "natural and political causes."[155] This conception of fundamental imbalance – the dominance of one principle and weakness of others – was later to play an important role in establishing a specifically physiological conception of social and racial types.[156]

Barthez argued that temperament could be investigated by both "direct" and "indirect" means. The "direct" method involved observation of what he called the "constitutional intensity or permanent energy of the radical forces" as well as study of the influence of the "non-naturals" on the "active forces." "Indirect" investigation entailed observation of people in society, a procedure that was less exact than the former but still reliable since "in general, *moeurs* . . . are in harmonious relation with the permanent affections of the system of [vital] forces."[157]

Barthez believed temperament to be directly linked to the weakness or strength of the "radical forces," the generalized potentialities of the economy for vital action of whatever sort. The strength or weakness of the radical forces could in turn be known in various ways. One sure indicator was the degree of sensibility, which was evident from such signs as the "vivacity

<hr />

154 *Ibid.*, 2:229.
155 *Ibid.*, 2:229–51; on the "inherent vices" of the body, see also Dumas, *Principes de physiologie*, 1:45.
156 See Chapter 4, "Seeking Middle Ground," and the Epilogue.
157 Barthez, *Science de l'homme*, 2:233, 251–52.

of sensations and spontaneous appetites" and from the extent of "anxiety or discomfort" attendant on body functions. An excess of sensibility indicated not powerful but "weakened" radical force; the expenditure of excessive energy in fulfillment of the appetites as in the performance of ordinary functions was a sign, then, of systemic debilitation. The play of sympathies, both those operating organ to organ and those that spread the influence of one organ throughout the body, was also a direct sign of the strength or attenuation of "radical force." Sympathies were most active in people who lived in a chronic state of heightened sensibility (women, children) or who were under attack by some affection of the sensible system.[158]

This equation between temperament and the degree of "radical force" was linked by Barthez and in vitalist theory generally to what may be termed a principle of limited energy that set inalterable boundaries on the human potential for exercising emotional, intellectual, sexual, procreative, and varied other functions. Barthez held that, in every individual, "radical force" was concentrated in one or more "organs" of the body and that, reciprocally, there was always at least one organ in the body that was deficient in vital energy. The temperament of each individual thus corresponded to the fashion in which his or her "radical force" was concentrated.[159] Barthez did not attempt any general typology of temperaments corresponding to the dominance or feebleness of specific regions of the body. Although he hinted at such a typology in ascribing special strengths and weaknesses to peoples across the globe, he devised no systematic classification. Barthez's silence in this regard suited both his epistemological modesty and his sense of the spontaneity of vital phenomena. It was left to his successors in the vitalist tradition to draw out the implications of this theory, as we will see in the next chapter when we look at Xavier Bichat's tripartite model of sensory, motor, and rational man, a doctrine based on the principle of limited energy and the notion that each individual had a particular center of vital force.[160]

In looking at the effect of the non-naturals on temperament, Barthez also approached matters that were to have great resonance with later theorists. He limited his consideration to three of the non-naturals – air, nutriments, and exercise – whose effects were readily established by reference to medical tradition. The effects of air on the vital forces were recognized by all doctors: "a change of air" was a remedy frequently resorted to in therapeutics. The consequences of "exercise" (not general exercise but the use of particular parts such as hand or eye in special tasks) were also well documented. It was well known, for example, that manual workers were incapable of fine writing because of the intensive, gross use made of their hands

158 *Ibid.*, 2:235; for Barthez's general doctrine of sympathies, see 2:1–104.
159 *Ibid.*, 2:237–39, and see 2:188, where Barthez remarks that the vital principle is weakened when forced by an "error of regimen" to work at two functions simultaneously; such efforts "caused a pernicious distraction of forces in the principal organs" (p. 18).
160 See Chapter 2, "Doctrine of Human Types."

in labor. This case illustrated further the chief theoretical principle that Barthez believed must guide observation in this sphere: the non-naturals did not act on the body in the fashion of "mechanical agents" but merely showed "nature somehow subject to a sort of necessity."[161] Although there seemed to be clear patterns in the effects nature exerted through means such as repetitive body movements, there was no precise mechanical relation of cause and effect. If a particular agent such as handwork had a strict mechanical effect, Barthez argued, that effect would be manifest only so long as the agent itself was still operating. But such was not the case. The worker whose hands lost their capacity for fine movement suffered the effects of "habit," not of repeated mechanical action whose effects ceased when his work ended. Barthez stated the general principle thus:

Such effects cannot be attributed to any mechanical cause but must be conceived in relation to the primordial laws which cause the vital principle to repeat spontaneously movements that were first caused by agents foreign to it [i.e., the non-naturals] whose action is repeated for a greater or lesser amount of time.[162]

To Barthez the extent to which habitual use could alter parts of the body or improve their functions was an open question. On one highly controversial point he asserted the great significance of "exercise" when he denied the German physician Samuel Soemmering's claim that there was an absolute relation between "intelligence" and the size of the nerves in relation to the size of the brain. In Barthez's view, Soemmering's argument failed to account for the "marked development that the intelligence can undergo as a result of training," even in animals with very small brains, such as the crocodile or the lizard.[163]

But although in this case "exercise" was seen to have an improving effect, Barthez did not think habitual use of an organ always had beneficial results. The instance of the manual workers whose hands lost the capacity for fine movement by overwork merely illustrated the general vitalist principle that overuse of any organ was potentially hazardous. Lacaze had considered at some length the harm potentially caused by excessive activity of any sort, arguing that "civilized man" was made timid and fearful by excessive thinking and the "savage" rendered heedless of the future by doing only brutish manual work.[164] Thus to the Montpellier doctors "exercise," like all the non-naturals, was beneficial only in moderation. Montpellier medicine lacked utterly any general teleological progressivism, such as that pervading Lamarck's thought, which saw individuals "improving" by means of habitual activity, and nature as a whole impelled to progress by virtue of

161 Barthez, *Science de l'homme*, 2:244.   162 *Ibid.*, 2:245.
163 *Ibid.*, 2:"Notes," 48–50.   164 Lacaze, *Idée de l'homme*, 378–80, 387, 395–96.

Table 2

Temperament	Dominant fluid	Character of fibers
Sanguine	Blood	Spongy/flexible
Bilious	Bile	Dry/elastic
Pituitary	Phleghm	Loose/soft
Melancholic	Black bile	Tenacious

the movement of species up a scale of perfection.[165] The Montpellier ideal of the organism was not one of ever greater adaptiveness to the exigencies of environment but of moderation, balance, and harmony both within the internal world of the body, and between the body and the external world of natural and social circumstance. The Barthezian formulation of the centrality of habit in forming temperament was enormously important to the medical science of man, but neither Barthez himself – nor any other Montpellier theorist – sought to penetrate that "hidden necessity" of nature that produced more or less constant states of the animal economy out of repetitive actions.

Barthez held that such "direct" investigation of temperament, through observation of the vital forces in action and of the effects of the non-naturals, could be supplemented by inquiry into "moral and physical causes," even though the role of such causes in establishing temperament could only be approximated. Indirect observation revealed "manifest analogies" between "*moeurs,* the physical state of the body, and the most regular and constant *manière d'être* of its principle of life."[166] To suggest correspondences between temperament and the "physical state of the body," Barthez reproduced a classification devised by the English physician John Huxham showing the apparent relation between temperament, humoral dominance, and the condition of body "solids" (Table 2).

Once again, Barthez questioned whether these peculiar states were natural or pathological. He noted that Stahl had regarded the state of the fibers as either the mark of an "original constitution" or of a "style of life too far removed from nature," that is, in some respect unbalanced or excessive.[167] Whatever the case, it was clear that all temperaments interacted with the "general causes" acting on "man and his *moeurs,*" causes that fell into the

165 J. B. de Lamarck, *Zoological Philosophy: An Exposition with Regard to the Natural History of Animals,* trans. Hugh Elliot (Chicago: University of Chicago Press, 1984), 349–54; see also the introduction to this volume by Richard W. Burkhardt, Jr. "The Zoological Philosophy of J. B. Lamarck," esp. xxviii–xxxiii.
166 Barthez, *Science de l'homme,* 2:247.   167 *Ibid.,* 2:249–51.

two broad categories of the natural ("climate" and "terrain") and the "political" ("way of life" and "form of government").[168] Reduced to "methodical" form, this last section of his discussion of temperament had the following shape:

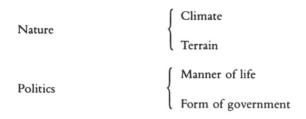

Nature
{
Climate

Terrain

Politics
{
Manner of life

Form of government

Under the rubric of natural causes, Barthez considered heat and cold, "terrain," and the quality of "exhalations" from the interior of the earth, all of which seemed to exercise profound influence both on human physical character (height, facial form, skin color, state of the vital forces) and on moral constitution (degrees of timidity, fierceness, courage).[169] Barthez cited standard authorities on these matters (Blumenbach, Camper, Montesquieu) but, in respect to climate in particular, he was not finally convinced by any of the explanatory mechanisms such authors had proposed and concluded that the precise character of climatic influence was unknown:

Nature has determined by primordial laws whose causes are unknown to us to create – either at the origin of the human genus or in the sweep of time in places of the earth subjected to four or five principal climates – diverse races of men, each of which is suited to his own climate.[170]

The effects of climate could be "changed or overcome," moreover, by the actions of government or by a settled way of life, a fact "the great Montesquieu" had neglected in deferring "overmuch to the role of climate."[171] For a permanent "race" to be formed, therefore, the character of both natural and political circumstances must endure; once a race was formed it could travel anywhere and remain unchanged so long as it did not intermarry with other peoples.[172] On the inevitable subject of whether "political causes" could assure the "perfectibility of the human intelligence," Barthez was doubtful. He denied that certain races – Africans, Americans – had "imperfections of the intelligence" as profound as some authors claimed. Yet he wondered how, given the extreme diversity and inequality in the existing state of things, anyone could believe in "a perfectibility unlimited in its progress."[173]

168 *Ibid.*, 2:252–53.   169 *Ibid.*, 2:262–70.
170 *Ibid.*, 2:260–61.   171 *Ibid.*, 2:273.
172 *Ibid.*, 2:275.   173 *Ibid.*, 2:280.

THE IMPACT OF MONTPELLIER VITALISM

Montpellier was by no means the sole locus for the development of vitalist thought in mid-eighteenth-century France. Other variants of vitalism – found in the work of Maupertuis, Needham, Buffon, and others – were in the process of formation around 1750. All rejected the mechanist models of nature, both Cartesian and anti-Cartesian, that had been dominant from the mid-seventeenth century.[174] The genetic and structural relationship between what we might call "general vitalism" and "medical vitalism" as found in the work of the Montpellier doctors remains to be charted.[175] Clearly, however, it was the emergence of Montpellier vitalism that marked a decisive departure away from mechanism within medical circles. As we will see in the next chapter, Montpellier doctrine had far-reaching implications for the medical innovators of the 1780s and the revolutionary era. Given the present state of research, one can only speculate on the question of why French medicine allowed vitalism an entry from Montpellier when it had neglected developments stemming from more general work in the life sciences. Two points might be ventured: one, the obvious observation that doctors were more likely to encounter and accept theoretical revisions that stemmed from within their own institutional domain. This was especially true since medical theorists, though accustomed by 1750 to importing doctrines from mechanics or chemistry, tended to be hostile to anatomical or physiological speculations that were not medical in origin.[176]

Another reason that Montpellier vitalism found acceptance in medical quarters where other "vitalisms" did not is that Montpellier teaching was politically and ideologically innocuous. When Abbé Needham taught that life was a force of its own, critics had responded that such a doctrine implied that no creator of life was required.[177] Montpellier doctrine did not appear to carry any such implications. Although Montpellier writings on the vital principle were determinedly secular in tone, never resorting to divine action or intervention to explain the workings of nature or the body, they were also determinedly respectful of orthodoxy, religious feeling, and the church. Vitalism of this sort was a welcome development to medical reformers who had grown increasingly dissatisfied with Christian-mechanist orthodoxy but who were wary – at a moment when they sought not only the theoretical but also the institutional rejuvenation of medicine – of embracing what royal authorities might construe as dangerous teachings. Barthez's doctrine of the vital principle could easily have lent itself to the view that since life was a force sui generis, God was dispensable. But no

174 Roger, *Sciences de la vie*, 458–584.
175 I hope to accomplish this task in a projected work on the place of Montpellier doctrine in eighteenth- and nineteenth-century biological and social thought.
176 Roger, *Sciences de la vie*, 7–19, 48, 160.   177 *Ibid.*, 494–520.

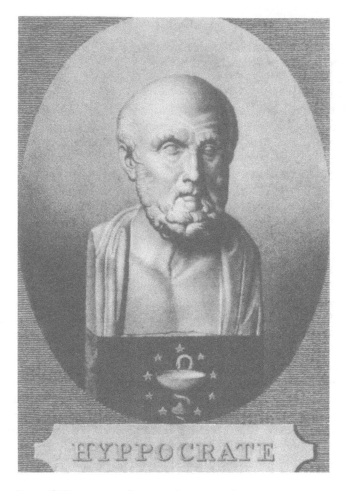

Bust of Hippocrates, by an unknown sculptor.

Montpellier theorist ever argued in such a fashion against the *Dieu-Artisan* or *Dieu-Législateur* of Christian naturalists. Indeed Barthez went to considerable lengths to shield himself from criticism of this sort after he had several close calls with religious and legal authorities, once with a church tribunal in Rome and, on another occasion, with the parlement of Toulouse. Barthez extricated himself without great difficulty from these imbroglios but he retained afterward a horror of judicial proceedings. "Above all else," he is supposed to have said, "I want to live a tranquil life."[178]

178 "Barthez," *DSM:BM* 1:576.

Whether these observations on why Montpellier teaching was more acceptable to physicians than other versions of vitalism are fully justified, it is true that Montpellier teaching was embraced in Paris by elements who were bent on effecting major changes in both the theory and practice of French medicine. Sergio Moravia has isolated what he regards as the major elements of Montpellier doctrine that exerted appeal among Paris medical innovators: the attempt to restore the autonomy of medicine after its long subjection to the physicochemical sciences; the search for methods that would restore medicine's "scientific dignity" in the face of criticism by "empiricists" and skeptics; and finally, the desire to give medicine an anthropological cast, to make of it a "science of man."[179] To these may be added the fact that the Paris reformers played Montpellier as an institutional counterweight to the Paris Faculty of Medicine, which by the late eighteenth century was a decaying institution remarkable chiefly for its hostile and defensive attitude toward all competitors in the medical domain and for its undisguised antagonism toward the increasingly prestigious natural sciences and their sponsoring institutions.[180] For a number of reasons, the Montpellier doctors did not share with the Paris faculty this sense of institutional and professional defensiveness. The medical school's ties with the Société royale des sciences de Montpellier encouraged cooperation between medical and scientific investigators and – in contrast to Paris – the school's reputation ran high in larger intellectual circles. Montpellier's reputation meant, furthermore, that its doctors were much sought after by the rich and the titled, a fact that may seem relatively trivial but which in a profoundly hierarchized "society of orders" was in fact crucial in determining the social prestige of competing elements of the service professions. Not having the institutional motivation of Paris doctors to resist encroachment from outside, the Montpellier physicians adopted the attitude that medicine must be open to the other sciences, the better to encourage its own development as an autonomous domain enjoying full scientific legitimacy.

Yet the Montpellier doctors were not ready to ascribe medicine's "new methods" solely or even chiefly to the example provided by other sciences. Instead they discovered a medical exemplar in Hippocrates, to whom Barthez referred as "the greatest genius who has ever written on human nature."[181] In Montpellier teaching, Hippocratism represented genuine "empirical" medicine as opposed to the false "empiricism" of the tradition-bound medicine still taught in most medical schools. Where traditional "empirics" followed "blind routine," true "empirical" Hippocratists were dedicated to genuine observation that employed careful techniques and was informed by larger principles. They developed and used "hypotheses," which were invaluable in guiding observation, rather than "systems" or

179 Moravia, "Philosophie et médecine," 1091.
180 Delaunay, *Le monde médical parisien*, 21–27.   181 Barthez, *Science de l'homme*, 2:87.

"dogmas," which rendered observation pointless. Hippocrates had taught these lessons; medicine, to its shame, had ignored them. In becoming "scientific," then, medicine was really doing no more than returning to its origins.[182] The "cult of Hippocrates" was a valuable rhetorical device allowing late eighteenth-century doctors to embrace scientific ideals and methods without betraying the autonomy or "dignity" of medicine. That the Montpellier doctors and their disciples employed such a device is important not only because they thus gave medicine a line of defense against the other sciences, but also because, in privileging medicine in this way, they supported the claim that medicine was the only branch of science that could engender a full-blown "science of man." "Man," it was universally agreed, stood alone in nature; the science that studied him must itself be unique and independent.

182 For a general explanation of the rhetorical uses made of Hippocrates by eighteenth- and nineteenth-century doctors, see Wesley D. Smith, *The Hippocratic Tradition* (Ithaca, N.Y.: Cornell University Press, 1979).

2

Anthropological medicine and the medical revolution

If Montpellier was the principal source of the medical science of man, it was nonetheless in Paris that the idea of an embracive, anthropological medicine was to be more fully developed. In the late eighteenth century, Montpellier and Paris were keenly, sometimes bitterly, competitive. Each center was aware that the other was its most potent rival, and much was made in both places of the special virtues of the native tradition.[1] Despite such rivalry, however, there was a good deal of intellectual and social exchange between Montpellier and Paris into the revolutionary period. Montpellier students moved back and forth between the two faculties. Montpellier professors were highly visible in the capital, thanks to posts they held at court. Montpellier theoreticians reached a Paris audience through the *Encyclopédie*, in books produced by Paris publishers, and in learned periodicals including the *Journal des sçavans*, the *Journal des beaux-arts*, and the *Mercure de France*. And although it was unusual for Parisian medical men to venture toward Montpellier, this fact was more a reflection of the general cultural dominance of Paris than of Montpellier's subsidiary position in the world of medicine.[2]

Many critics of medicine used Montpellier's reputation as a weapon against the Paris faculty, which was widely seen as the chief enemy of medical reformers. At first glance, it might seem anomalous that the Montpellier doctors functioned both as court physicians and as exemplars of medical reform. No such contradiction really existed, however. The Montpellier

---

1 C. C. Gillispie, *Science and Polity in France at the End of the Old Regime* (Princeton: Princeton University Press, 1980), 215–18; Caroline C. F. Hannaway, "Medicine, Public Welfare, and the State in 18th-Century France: The Société Royale de Médecine of Paris (1776–1793)," (Ph.D. diss., Johns Hopkins University, 1974), 18–28.

2 On the contributions of Montpellier doctors to the *Encyclopédie*, see Pierre Astruc, "Les sciences médicales et leurs représentants dans l'*Encyclopédie*," *RHS* 4 (1951): 359–68; Henri Zeiler, "Les collaborateurs médicaux de l'*Encyclopédie* de Diderot et de d'Alembert" (Thèse, Faculté de Médecine de Paris, 1934); on Barthez at the *Journal des Sçavans*, see Louis Dulieu, "Paul-Joseph Barthez," *RHS* 24 (1971): 149–76, at 155–56. Pierre Roussel wrote for the *Journal des beaux-arts* and the *Mercure de France*; see "Pierre Roussel," in *Biographie médicale par ordre chronologique d'après Daniel Eloy, etc.*, ed. A. L. J. Bayle and Thillaye, 2 vols. (Paris: Adolphe Delahays, 1855), 2:668–69.

doctors refrained from explicit political or social commentary and consciously avoided controversy.[3] And even if they had staked out positions in political and social debates, they would not in all likelihood have alienated their highborn clients. In medical circles the contest between established authority and reforming critics found the court, and by extension its physicians, in a progressive rather than a conservative position. On repeated occasions throughout the century, the court had given support to movements that challenged the power of the Paris Faculty of Medicine, especially in the assistance it lent to the institutional and social enhancement of surgery and to the founding of the Société royale de médecine.[4] Thus the prominent position of Montpellier doctors at court in no way precluded their association with progressive trends in French medicine.

Whether Montpellier could ever have used this favorable situation to develop precedence over Paris medicine seems unlikely, given the long-standing cultural supremacy of the capital. In any event, from the late 1770s onward reform elements in Paris medicine came to function as the undisputed center of a movement to rejuvenate French medicine, and a process was set in motion by which Montpellier was eventually eclipsed by Paris. As part of their larger effort, Paris reformers appropriated and turned to their own account the idea of transforming medicine into a general science of man. Key features of what historians have come to call the "medical revolution" – the renovation of medical education, the new significance given to clinical observation, the mapping of social and political ambitions for medicine – reveal the power the idea of a science of man held in the revolutionary setting. Indeed it may be argued that the most important and long-lasting result of the medical revolution – the creation of a new species of medical authority – stemmed in large part from the anthropologizing of medicine that occurred in the political context of the revolutionary years.[5] As the sacral authority of monarch and church was shaken, physicians sought to establish their own authority in diverse intellectual and social domains. They did so by arguing that medicine alone could comprehend the intricate relations among physical, mental, and passional phenomena, and that it was therefore uniquely capable of guiding society to new certitudes amid revolutionary upheavals.

The claims of doctors to augmented authority met with a checkered response through the years from 1789 to 1815. The prospect of a medical sci-

3 On Montpellier's reputation in larger learned circles, see Chapter 1.
4 Gillispie, *Science and Polity*, 203–5, 217–18. On the institutional reform of surgery, see Toby Gelfand, *Professionalizing Modern Medicine: Paris Surgeons and Medical Science and Institutions in the Eighteenth Century* (Westport, Conn.: Greenwood Press, 1980).
5 Elizabeth A. Williams, "The French Revolution, Anthropological Medicine, and the Creation of Medical Authority," in *Re-creating Authority in Revolutionary France*, ed. Bryant T. Ragan, Jr., and Elizabeth A. Williams (New Brunswick, N.J.: Rutgers University Press, 1992), 79–97.

ence of man was greeted warmly by the critical and reforming circles of the early Revolution, rebuffed by the Jacobins, and then selectively endorsed by the Directory, Consulate, and Empire. The science of man developed in turn in relation to the exigencies of a complex and rapidly changing political environment, so that eventually it became a rhetorical rubric for varied, even contradictory, formulations of the capabilities of medicine. By 1815 the science of man had been irrevocably lodged within the larger ideological conflicts – between clericals and anticlericals, spiritualists and materialists, conservatives and liberals – whose language and framework were largely created by the Revolution itself.[6] Thus the fate of the medical science of man ultimately had less to do with institutional struggles in the world of medicine than with the general transformation of French culture and society worked by the Revolution.

THE INSTITUTIONAL FRAMEWORK OF THE MEDICAL REVOLUTION

In the years just before the Revolution, official French medicine was intensely criticized by observers who found fault with medical education, with the therapeutic capabilities of most practitioners, and with the greed and pomposity of elite doctors to whom, as one critic wrote, nothing mattered but "ostentatious show" and an "elegant situation."[7] Yet for some time vigorous efforts at reform had been underway. If the critical articles in Diderot's *Encyclopédie* are taken as a benchmark, the movement for medical reform antedated the Revolution by some three decades. The date can be set even earlier if emphasis is placed on the surgeons' campaign to break the physicians' monopoly on medical practice.[8] In the late 1770s these reform efforts coalesced in the work of the Société royale de médecine, a crown-sponsored medical society that was founded in 1776 as a royal commission charged with investigating epidemics. This society was subsequently transformed into an academy of medicine in all but name by a group of reforming doctors led by Félix Vicq d'Azyr, who served as the society's permanent

6 On the Revolution's creation of new political vocabularies, see Keith Michael Baker, *Inventing the French Revolution: Essays on French Political Culture in the Eighteenth Century* (Cambridge: Cambridge University Press, 1990), esp. 203–305.
7 René-Nicolas Desgenettes, "Antoine Fizes," *DSM:BM* 4:161. The intellectual, moral, and physical decay of official medicine in the late eighteenth century is described in Erwin Ackerknecht, *Medicine at the Paris Hospital, 1794–1848* (Baltimore: Johns Hopkins University Press, 1967), 31–32; Paul Delaunay, *Le monde médical parisien au dix-huitième siècle* (Paris: Jules Rousset, 1906); Paul Triaire, *Récamier et ses contemporains, 1774–1852: Etudes d'histoire de la médecine aux XVIIIe et XIXe siècles* (Paris: J.-B. Baillière, 1899), 60–62 (but see pp. 89–90 for a defense of the Paris faculty). A useful corrective appears in Matthew Ramsey, *Professional and Popular Medicine in France, 1770–1830: The Social World of Medical Practice* (Cambridge: Cambridge University Press, 1988), 46–48.
8 Astruc, "Les sciences médicales"; Gelfand, *Professionalizing Modern Medicine;* Richard Schwab, "The History of Medicine in Diderot's *Encyclopédie*," *BHM* 32 (1958): 216–23.

secretary from 1778 to 1790.[9] Although the Société royale was originally charged with inquiry into only a limited range of questions connected to epidemics, Vicq d'Azyr and the other leaders of the society considerably broadened its scope to include investigation of climatic and meteorological conditions, the quality of waters (especially mineral waters), topography, fauna, and the "manner of life" of local populations. The society established an extensive system of correspondents throughout the country and, in the short period of its existence, amassed voluminous information on local conditions. Its principal focus, as Caroline Hannaway has argued, was "the health needs of the nation at large" rather than individual doctor-patient relationships.[10]

Although the Société royale de médecine was very much an Ancien Regime institution, when the Revolution came it attempted to transform itself into a body that would find favor with the revolutionary leaders and that would guide the transformation of medical institutions. Vicq d'Azyr developed a reform plan that was widely hailed in moderate circles, but as the Revolution radicalized in the harrowing circumstances of 1792–93, the society and its leaders came under attack for elitism and royalism. In August 1793 the Société royale de médecine was suppressed along with all other corporations.[11]

In this and in other ways the coming of the Revolution had momentous consequences for the organization and practice of medicine. By 1793 the Ancien Regime medical structure – with its three independent corps of doctors, surgeons, and apothecaries; its corporatist organization and system of regional licensing; its clerically dominated hospitals – had been abolished. A decade was to pass before a new organization of medicine was devised. After the old medical faculties were closed, there was virtually no formal medical schooling for a time, and the state exercised no supervision over medical practice. Finally, under the pressures of war, the Thermidorian Convention passed legislation calling for the establishment of three *écoles de santé* in 1794, but until the establishment of the Consulate these schools were left very much to their own devices. Hospitals too functioned with a high degree of autonomy and developed distinctive personalities without direction from any larger umbrella organization. For those interested in the future of medicine the ten years between 1793 and the passage of the law of Ventôse, an XI (March 1803) were marked by intense controversy. Countless proposals for the future of medicine were put forward, both in medical circles themselves and by political groups and bodies

9 Hannaway, "Medicine, Public Welfare," 81–95; on Vicq d'Azyr, see *DSM:BM* 7:429–32; Jacques-Louis Moreau de la Sarthe, *Eloge historique de Vicq d'Azyr* (Paris: n.p., an VI/1798).
10 Moreau de la Sarthe, *Eloge historique*, 19; Hannaway, "Medicine, Public Welfare," 147.
11 [Félix Vicq d'Azyr], *Nouveau plan de Constitution pour la médecine en France, présenté à l'Assemblée nationale par la Société royale de médecine* (Paris, 1790); Delaunay, *Le monde médical parisien*, 158–60.

who saw the reconstitution of medicine as fundamental to the ordering of the new society.[12]

Much has been written recently about practical medical politics in the revolutionary period, especially hospital reform, the revamping of the legal basis for the practice of medicine, and the restructuring of medical training and education.[13] Rather less attention has been given to the reworking of medical theory and therapeutic doctrine, although many physicians were as convinced of the necessity to transform the theoretical basis of medicine as they were of the need for new medical institutions and practices. These doctors presented their principles and proposals in varied forums. The new *écoles de santé* that opened early in 1795 in Paris, Montpellier, and Strasbourg provided an important site for theoretical discussion, especially since their personnel was considerably altered from that of the old faculties. The Paris school had an influx of new professors including Philippe Pinel, François Chaussier, and P. J. G. Cabanis, figures who either had never been considered for appointment or had been deliberately excluded from the old faculty.[14] Outside the official institutions of teaching, "free" medical education flourished. Private courses and institutes were initiated, some of them using facilities and building on organizational structures already present in the 1780s but many others making a new beginning in the era of medical laisser-faire opened by the Revolution. Of these the most important were the Ecole polymathique, the Lycée des arts, and the Lycée républicain, where medical theorists including Jacques-Louis Moreau de la Sarthe, Vicq d'Azyr, Jean-Noël Hallé, Fourcroy, and others taught courses emphasizing the new character and mission of medicine.[15] Some of these figures continued to stress, in the style of the Société royale de

12 Jacques Léonard, *Les médecins de l'Ouest au XIXème siècle*, 3 vols. (Lille: Atelier Reproduction des Thèses, Université de Lille III, 1971), 197–252; Ramsey, *Professional and Popular Medicine*, 71–84. Biographical details on doctors who served in the successive assemblies or figured in some way in revolutionary politics are found in Constant Saucerotte, *Les médecins pendant la Revolution, 1789–1799* (Paris: Perrin, 1887).

13 For hospital reform, see Louis Greenbaum, " 'Measure of Civilization': The Hospital Thought of Jacques Tenon on the Eve of the French Revolution," *BHM* 49 (1975): 43–56; Colin Jones, "Picking Up the Pieces: The Politics and the Personnel of Social Welfare from the Convention to the Consulate," in *Beyond the Terror: Essays in French Regional and Social History, 1794–1815*, ed. Gwynne Lewis and Colin Lucas (Cambridge: Cambridge University Press, 1983). On the legal restructuring, see Jean Imbert, *Le droit hospitalier de la Révolution et de l'Empire* (Paris: Recueil Sirey, 1954); Ramsey, *Professional and Popular Medicine*, 77–84. On medical training and education, see Charles Coury, "The Teaching of Medicine in France from the Beginning of the Seventeenth Century," in *The History of Medical Education*, ed. C. D. O'Malley (Berkeley: University of California Press, 1970); Gelfand, *Professionalizing Modern Medicine*, 165–70; David M. Vess, *Medical Revolution in France, 1789–1796* (Gainesville: University of Florida Press, 1975), chaps. 9–10.

14 On the changes in the Paris faculty, see Triaire, *Récamier et ses contemporains*, 96–100.

15 M. Berthelot, "Sur les publications de la Société philomathique et sur ses origines," *Journal des savants* (1888): 477–93; Charles DeJob, "De l'établissement connu sous le nom de Lycée et d'Athénée et de quelques établissements analogues," *Revue internationale de l'enseignement* 18 (1889): 4–38; Paul Delaunay, "La médecine et les Idéologues: L. J. Moreau de la Sarthe," *Bulletin de la Société française d'histoire de la médecine* 14 (1920): 24–70, at 33–35.

72   *Anthropological medicine*

médecine, the possibilities for collaboration between doctors and a self-aggrandizing state apparatus. Others, like Fourcroy, emphasized the benefits to medicine of closer links to the natural sciences. Yet increasingly doctors articulated the ambitions of medicine in the expansive rhetoric of the science of man.

In this period medical societies proliferated; some of them were independent while others were linked to larger institutions or to political organizations. In 1796 a group of doctors who were associated with the Paris Ecole de santé in various capacities founded the Société de santé de Paris (renamed Société de médecine de Paris in 1797). This society proclaimed its intention to function as "a center and meeting-place for all men dedicated to the enrichment of a science intimately tied to the well-being of humanity."[16] This group was made up largely (although not exclusively) of the older and more conservative elements of the Ecole de santé; it included six men who were later to serve on the Paris Health Council, which was to be established under the Empire to further the Bonapartist conception of public health. A few months later, a younger group of doctors led by Xavier Bichat, Dominique-Jean Larrey, and J.-L. Alibert established the Société médicale d'émulation, a group that did as much as any other institution to encourage the development of the medical science of man. From its founding until the moment when imperial censors began to repress free-ranging medicomoral discussion, the society encouraged consideration of manifold topics within the problematic of the physical and the moral. Finally, under the Consulate the Société de l'école de médecine de Paris was founded under the sponsorship of Lucien Bonaparte; it too included doctors who were eager to pursue the statist and bureaucratizing ambitions of medicine.[17]

In the 1790s the membership of these specifically medical societies frequently overlapped with those of more general learned societies such as the Société philomathique (founded in 1788), which was intended to function as an organization for mutual instruction of young scholars, and the Société des observateurs de l'homme, which during its brief existence (1799–ca. 1805) brought together investigators interested in gaining knowledge of distant peoples. Doctors were not especially prominent in this society, which from a twentieth-century perspective seems more clearly "anthropological" in scope and intention than any learned organization of the period. But some physicians did join in the society's attempt to forge links between the natural sciences and the investigations of historians, geogra-

16 Pierre Astruc, "Les sociétés médicales françaises de 1796 à 1850," *Le Progrès médical* (January 10, 1950): 29.
17 Dora B. Weiner, "Public Health under Napoleon: The Conseil de Salubrité de Paris, 1802–1815," *Clio Medica* 9 (1974): 283–84, n. 46; other societies included the Société anatomique, founded in 1803, and the Société de médecine pratique; see Astruc, "Sociétés médicales françaises," 28–29.

phers, legal scholars, and the like.[18] The medical societies also overlapped with political organizations, the most important of which was the Société de 1789, a political society of moderate constitutionalists (Sieyès, Condorcet, Talleyrand, Cabanis) who sought, among other objectives, to develop a "social art."[19]

Particularly gratifying to doctors was the welcome given physiological investigation by the Institute, which on its founding in 1796 included physiology within the Class of Moral and Political Sciences in the section devoted to the "Analysis of Sensations and Ideas." It was there that Cabanis delivered the famous addresses that were to be collected and published in 1802 as the *Rapports du physique et du moral de l'homme*. On the occasion of one of his presentations, Cabanis praised the Institute's founders for recognizing that the philosophical and moral investigations of this Second Class must begin with "the physical knowledge of man, [which] is their common foundation."[20] As these diverse institutional linkages indicate, then, the medical revolution unfolded within the larger movement of social criticism and transformation that characterized the revolutionary era. We turn now to examine the role that Montpellier doctrine played in this movement and to consider in detail the changing contours of the science of man.

THEORY AND THERAPEUTICS: THE MONTPELLIER-PARIS CONNECTION

The revamping of medical theory and therapeutics proposed in these years had many dimensions. A number of doctors argued, for example, that the old medicine had become dangerously interventionist, relying on drastic remedies such as copious bloodletting, violent purges, and great doses of questionable medicaments. Such procedures were challenged not only because they seemed practically inefficacious but also because drastic intervention violated the whole spirit of "Hippocratic" medicine, which, as noted earlier, enjoyed a steadily accelerating reputation in the late eighteenth century.[21] A fundamental teaching of Hippocratism, as it was con-

18 Delaunay, "La médecine et les Idéologues"; Benjamin Kilborne, "Anthropological Thought in the Wake of the French Revolution: The 'Société des Observateurs de l'Homme,'" *European Journal of Sociology* 23 (1982): 73–91; George W. Stocking, Jr., "French Anthropology in 1800," in *Race, Culture, and Evolution: Essays in the History of Anthropology* (1968; rpt. Chicago: University of Chicago Press, 1982); Ernest Wickersheimer, "Bichat à la Société philomathique," *La France médicale* (October 25, 1909), 380–82.

19 Keith Baker, *Condorcet: From Natural Philosophy to Social Mathematics* (Chicago: University of Chicago Press, 1975), 272–85; Sergio Moravia, *Il tramonto dell'Illuminismo: Filosofia e politica nella società francese (1770–1810)* (Bari: Laterza, 1986), 152–61.

20 Martin Staum, "The Class of Moral and Political Sciences, 1795–1803," *FHS* 11 (1980): 371–97; P. J. G. Cabanis, "Rapports du physique et du moral de l'homme," in *Oeuvres philosophiques de Cabanis*, ed. Claude Lehec and Jean Cazeneuve, 2 vols. (Paris: Presses universitaires de France, 1956), 1:126.

21 See Chapter 1.

structed by the medical revolutionaries, was that cures were effected not by physicians but by nature. Doctors merely assisted nature in its healing processes, and their most important function was to teach patients how best to receive nature's ministrations. Monitoring and control of diet, air, movement, and surroundings were significant tasks, and good doctors performed them with care. But the actual physiological labor of healing was nature's work, and the role of doctors in this respect was to show restraint and patience. "Remedies that interrupt nature," as Philippe Pinel termed them, were not only useless but actively harmful; bleedings, purges, and medicines altered the body's functions and "stood in the path of healing."[22]

Amid general adulation of "the divine Hippocrates," it was increasingly Montpellier medicine that was most clearly identified with Hippocratism. Thus when doctors of the revolutionary era sought to put Hippocratism into practice they did so in the shadow of Montpellier. Yet the influence exercised by Montpellier over the Paris medical revolution was much more profound than vague references to Hippocratism suggest. Instead, Montpellier's influence was chiefly at work in the insistence of the medical revolutionaries that medicine expand beyond the narrow terrain of practical therapeutics and establish its claims to the larger field of the science of man. The opening *discours* to the *Mémoires* of the Société médicale d'émulation stated that medicine must reform itself on the "reasoned and philosophical basis of method." It paid tribute to "the illustrious professor Barthez, the glory and pride of the old school of Montpellier," and insisted that medicine must establish ties with all the "human sciences." "Medical theory will be all the wiser and more firmly established the more fully it identifies with the general science of relations, of which practical medicine is only the corollary or application."[23]

The pedagogical, intellectual, and institutional connections tying the Montpellier theorists to Paris are apparent in the biographies of individuals who figured prominently in the medical revolution. One important case of a Montpellier-Paris tie is that of Philippe Pinel, whose role in hospital reform and in treatment of the mad has attracted much attention in recent scholarship.[24] After a stint at the medical faculty of Toulouse, Pinel studied

22 Philippe Pinel, "Recherches et observations sur le traitement moral des aliénés," *MSME* 2 (an VII/1798): 255. See also Moreau de la Sarthe's review of Alibert, *Nouveaux Elémens de thérapeutique* in *Décade*, no. 32 (20 thermidor, an XII/1804), 392, where he supports Alibert's contention that "the goal of the doctor must be analogous to that of nature." For another treatment of this theme, see Sergio Moravia, "Philosophie et médecine en France à la fin du XVIIIe siècle," *Studies on Voltaire and the Eighteenth Century* 89 (1972): 1089–1151, esp. 1098–1105.

23 "Discours préliminaire," *MSME* 1 (an VI/1797): i–xiii.

24 Michel Foucault, *Madness and Civilization: A History of Insanity in the Age of Reason* (New York: Vintage Books, 1965), esp. chap. 5; Jan Goldstein, *Console and Classify: The French Psychiatric Profession in the Nineteenth Century* (Cambridge: Cambridge University Press, 1987), esp. 67–105; Dora B. Weiner, "Introductory Essay," in *The Clinical Training of Doctors: An Essay of 1793*, by Philippe Pinel (Baltimore: Johns Hopkins University Press, 1980), 3–22.

at Montpellier from 1774 to 1778. Although he did not take his degree there, Pinel nonetheless becomes a great admirer of "the famous school of Montpellier," to which he wrote tributes in his celebrated treatise, the *Nosographie philosophique* (1797), and from which he said he derived the "principles" of his own work.[25] Many elements of Pinel's work – his denunciation of excessive intervention, his classificatory enterprise undertaken in the fashion of Boissier de Sauvages, his insistence that nervous ailments were not purely physical in origin but engaged the whole person – indicate the extent to which his medical perspective was shaped in Montpellier.[26]

Another Parisian medical reformer with strong ties to Montpellier was J.-L. Alibert (1768–1837), who was the secretary of the Société médicale d'émulation from 1796 to 1802. Alibert did not attend school in Montpellier, but he was closely tied both to Pierre Roussel (who by the late 1780s had established himself in Paris) and to Barthez, whose portrait (along with Bordeu's) hung on his walls.[27] One of Alibert's more important theoretical contributions was his article "Discours sur les rapports de la médecine avec les sciences physiques et morales," published by the Société médicale d'émulation in 1798. In this piece Alibert upheld a position on the relation between medicine and the other sciences that was fully in keeping with Montpellier teaching. Like the Montpellier doctors, he contended that medicine must be at once autonomous and receptive to the other sciences. He rejected both the obscurantism of medical traditionalists and the thirsting after novelty of enthusiasts who were ready to harness medicine to the carriage of chemistry, physics, or mechanics.[28]

Diverse other connections tied Parisian reformers to Montpellier. One of the chief figures in Cabanis's intellectual training was J. B. L. Dubreuil (1748–83), whose own mentor was Bordeu's comrade Gabriel Venel. Cabanis's biographer Martin Staum observes that in the company of Dubreuil, Cabanis "undoubtedly received a thorough introduction to the Montpellier clinical school."[29] Xavier Bichat was linked to Montpellier through his father, who studied with Barthez in the 1760s and took his medical degree

25 Although Pinel admired the great figures of Montpellier, he was one physician who believed that instruction in Paris was "much superior." See Goldstein, *Console and Classify*, 67; see also Pierre Chabbert, "Les années d'étude de Philippe Pinel: Lavaur, Toulouse, Montpellier," *Monspeliensis Hippocrates* (Spring 1960): 15–23; Philippe Pinel, *Nosographie philosophique, ou la méthode d'analyse appliquée à la médecine* (Paris: Crapelet, an VI/1797), xxvii–xxix.
26 On Pinel's debt to Montpellier, see Moravia, "Philosophie et médecine," 1095–1100.
27 L. Brodier, *J.-L. Alibert, médecin de l'Hôpital Saint-Louis* (Paris: A. Maloine, 1923), 297, 317–18.
28 J.-L. Alibert, "Discours sur les rapports de la médecine avec les sciences physiques et morales," *MSME* 2 (an VII/1798): i–cxii.
29 Martin Staum, *Cabanis: Enlightenment and Medical Philosophy in the French Revolution* (Princeton: Princeton University Press, 1980), 16. On Dubreuil's regard for Barthez, see Jacques Lordat, *Exposition de la doctrine médicale de P.-J. Barthez, et mémoires sur la vie de ce médecin* (Paris: Gabon, 1818), 277.

from Montpellier in 1769.[30] In still other cases the exchange between Montpellier and Paris developed during the Revolution itself. One of the principal forums in which the movement for medicosocial reform unfolded was the salon maintained first by Anne-Catherine Helvétius and later by Sophie de Grouchy Condorcet. At the "salon d'Auteuil" there was contact and interchange between Parisian medical leaders and Montpellier physicians such as Pierre Roussel, Victor de Sèze, Barthez, and others.[31]

Although these instances in no way constitute a definitive adumbration of the Paris–Montpellier link, they do suggest bonds of considerable importance. Cabanis assessed the significance of Montpellier to medicine in these terms:

> Bordeu, Venel, Lamurre – one might say the whole school of Montpellier – have given a new doctrine great force and many partisans. Developed since the [days of] these celebrated masters by the vast labors of Barthez; strengthened by his students and successors . . . ; perfected by the application of philosophical methods . . . it draws closer and closer to truth. Soon it will no longer constitute a particular doctrine: by profiting from genuine discoveries . . . and jettisoning that sense of exclusivity that hinders true collaboration, it will become the sole incontestable theory in medicine. It will serve as the natural and necessary meeting-ground for all the knowledge amassed by our art to this day.[32]

With this statement Cabanis situated himself and the medical revolution generally on the broad terrain of vitalism. In Cabanis's view Montpellier teaching would eventually constitute not the doctrine of a particular medical sect but simply a new way of looking at nature, one that focused with special keenness on the phenomena of life. To Cabanis the key element of the Montpellier approach to medicine was what he saw as its accent on the operations and multiple functional tasks of sensibility. Yet paradoxically it was precisely at that point in the structure of Montpellier's influence that the Paris medical revolutionaries in fact found Montpellier teaching least satisfying. To complement and extend Montpellier thinking on sensibility, they looked beyond strictly medical doctrines to larger philosophical currents in which the complex epistemological problems associated with the terms sensation and sensibility had for some time received sustained attention.

THE MEDICAL REVOLUTION AND IDEOLOGY

In their efforts to reformulate medicine as a broadly gauged human science, the medical revolutionaries of the 1790s frequently took their lead not from

---

30 Elizabeth Haigh, "The Roots of the Vitalism of Xavier Bichat," *BHM* 49 (1975): 77.
31 For a portrait of life at the salon d'Auteuil, see Antoine Guillois, *Le salon de Mme. Helvétius: Cabanis et les Idéologues* (Paris: Calmann-Lévy, 1894). See also Brodier, *Alibert*, 296–99; Delaunay, "La médecine et les Idéologues," 38–39.
32 Cabanis, "Coup d'oeil sur les révolutions et réformes de la médecine" in *Oeuvres*, 2:143–44.

medicine proper but from the general intellectual movement of Ideology, whose importance in the larger history of the medical science of man can hardly be exaggerated. The tradition of the Ideologues comes into play at crucial junctures – epistemological and theoretical, institutional and political – throughout this work. Ideology established the sensationalist epistemological orientation that was subjected to intense scrutiny by all subsequent proponents of the medical science of man. Ideologues honed for use in the human sciences those methods of observation, analysis, and classification that eighteenth-century figures had promoted for the general advancement of learning. They were prominent in the attempt to organize and perpetuate investigation in the human sciences within learned societies, the educational establishments created by the Revolution, and the Institute. By these means Ideology set its stamp on all later efforts to make human beings into objects of scientific inquiry. In later years proponents of alternative approaches to the human sciences often denied their connection to Ideology because of its identification with a "materialist" and antireligious heritage. But the very fact that such denial was necessary bespoke links between Ideology and the science of man that were recognized by its sympathizers and detractors alike.

The question of who exactly was an Ideologue has been variously approached by historians. François Picavet, in his classic study *Les Idéologues* (1896), included any figure who accepted the general philosophical stance implied by the term and he identified three successive generations of Ideologues.[33] Recently scholars of Ideology have been more restrictive in their coverage, applying highly specific criteria such as attendance at the salon d'Auteuil or contribution to the review *Décade philosophique* in gauging the extent of the Ideologues' network.[34]

Both Picavet's broad definition and the narrower ones of recent literature have merit: Picavet's shows the breadth and sweep of Ideology and, more important, demonstrates that many self-declared enemies of Ideology (such as Maine de Biran) used its categories, language, and concepts.[35] Recent definitions provide, on the other hand, a useful reminder that there was a specific small group of thinkers, at a precise historical locus, who called themselves *idéologistes,* shared a common program of reform, and were perceived by their contemporaries as constituting a political and intellectual

---

33 François Picavet, *Les Idéologues* (Paris: Alcan, 1896), esp. 24.
34 Emmet Kennedy, *A Philosophe in the Age of Revolution: Destutt de Tracy and the Origins of Ideology* (Philadelphia: American Philosophical Society, 1978); Joanna Kitchin, *Un journal "philosophique": La Décade philosophique (1794–1807)* (Paris: M. J. Minard, 1965), 117–20; Staum, *Cabanis,* 4–5. Sergio Moravia has emphasized the broad range of their work in *La scienza dell'uomo nel settecento* (Bari: Laterza, 1970). A useful summary of the question is found in Brian Head, *Politics and Philosophy in the Thought of Destutt de Tracy* (New York: Garland, 1987), 15–18 and notes 43–50, p. 60.
35 Picavet, *Les Idéologues,* 418–19.

Table 3. *Physicians associated with Ideology during the revolutionary era*

J.-L. Alibert	C.-L. Dumas
Xavier Bichat	J. N. Hallé
Jean-Baptiste Bory de Saint-Vincent	J.-L. Moreau de la Sarthe
F. J. V. Broussais	Etienne Pariset
Jean Burdin	Philippe Pinel
P. J. G. Cabanis	A.-B. Richerand
François Chaussier	Pierre Roussel
J. P. R. Draparnaud	Pierre Sue

coterie.[36] Still, for the purposes of this chapter, which seeks not to define Ideology as such but to show how the medical revolution was affected by its broad objectives and undertakings, the grand sweep is best. Taking the revolutionary era as the chronological frame of reference and considering for inclusion all individuals whom historians have categorized as Ideologues, we can devise a list of sixteen figures who were both associated with Ideology in some fashion and connected to medicine by medical education, practice, authorship, or membership in medical societies (see Table 3).[37] In varying degrees and with differing emphases, the efforts and labors of all these figures were linked to the framework of Ideology, whose epistemological program, methods of investigation, and sociopolitical objectives were incorporated into the medical science of man.

EPISTEMOLOGY AND METHOD: OBSERVATION, ANALYSIS,
AND THE PRIMACY OF SENSATION

The creation of a medical science of man entailed above all else a commitment to the view that medicine must be based on proper method. Thus methodological and epistemological concerns occupied a central place in projects for medical renovation, and a favored vehicle for approaching these concerns was the rewriting of medical history. Cabanis's treatise *Coup d'oeil sur les révolutions et sur la réforme de la médecine* exemplifies this preoccupation.[38] In this work Cabanis sought to be both comprehensive (tracing the development of medicine from its appearance among "the most primitive of peoples") and critical (drawing from each "revolution" in medicine conclu-

36 Head, *Politics and Philosophy.*
37 The table is based on Brodier, *Alibert,* 297; Delaunay, "La médecine et les Idéologues"; Picavet, *Les Idéologues,* 184–85, 218, 435–37, 450–52; George Rosen, "The Philosophy of Ideology and the Emergence of Modern Medicine in France," *BHM* 20 (1946): 328–39; Triaire, *Récamier et ses contemporains,* 237.
38 The original title of this work was *Considérations générales sur les révolutions de l'art de guérir;* it was revised and published with the title *Coup d'oeil sur les révolutions et les réformes de la médecine* in 1804; Cabanis, "Coup d'oeil," in *Oeuvres,* 2:65–254.

sions pertinent to contemporary concerns). One of the most prominent themes Cabanis addressed was the millennia-old antagonism between priests and physicians. Egyptian medicine was wholly captive to sacerdotal despotism; priests used the medical art to dupe the ignorant and credulous mass of people. The priest-doctors enjoyed their privileges solely by virtue of heredity; they nurtured an exclusivist "esprit de corps"; they encouraged superstitions and "popular prejudices."[39] In Greece too medicine was first "cultivated in the temples" by "lying and avaricious priests."[40] The stranglehold of malevolent clerics was broken definitively only by Hippocrates whose "genius" for observation and analysis opened a new era:

This new spirit imbuing the healing art was like a sudden light that dissipated the phantoms of night and lent objects their true form and natural color. Repudiating the errors of past centuries, . . . Hippocrates saw, with a clarity until then unknown, the connections and interdependence of observed facts and the results legitimately to be drawn from their comparison. . . . From that point a sure means was available, to any who would grasp it, for judging precisely those new ideas that time in its fullness would now bring. If the disciples of Hippocrates had only understood his teaching, they would have proceeded to lay the foundations of that analytic philosophy with whose aid the human spirit would now, day by day . . . devise new and ever more perfect instruments.[41]

The *parti pris* in this passage was probably as transparent to Cabanis's own audience as it is to us today. Written in 1795 in response to urging by the Ideologue Dominique-Joseph Garat, who had been charged by the Thermidorian Convention with rewriting the public education laws, this work sought to establish the teaching of medicine on the immovable foundation of "certain method."[42] Once this undertaking was assured, all else – the selection of particular subjects, the fostering of proper pedagogical spirit, the choice of means to cultivate students' minds – would follow naturally.[43]

Historical precedent is similarly invoked in the introduction to Pinel's *Nosographie philosophique*. Again Hippocrates was the object of high praise; his methods of rigorous observation had been "preserved for twenty centuries in their unalterable purity."[44] Yet in the spirit of all medical "moderns" who rejected authority for its own sake, Pinel counseled against unthinking imitation of particular Hippocratic dicta. Hippocrates was to be admired, he urged, as much for providing methods of self-criticism as for his substantive observations.[45] All this was used, in Pinel's hands, to debunk what he called "popular and humoral medicine" – both the medicine

39 *Ibid.*, 84–88. 40 *Ibid.*, 91. 41 *Ibid.*, 100.
42 On Garat and the education laws, see Georges Gusdorf, *Les sciences humaines et la pensée occidentale*, vol. 8, *La conscience révolutionnaire: Les Idéologues* (Paris: Payot, 1978), 310–14.
43 Staum, *Cabanis*, 151–64.
44 Pinel, *Nosographie*, ii, vii–viii. See also Philippe Pinel, *Traité médico-philosophique sur l'aliénation mentale* (Paris: Richard, Caille et Ravier, 1801), ix.
45 Pinel, *Nosographie*, vii–viii.

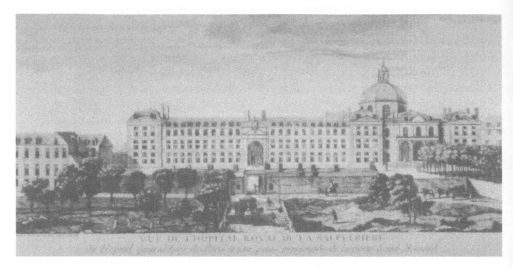

View of the Hôpital royal de la Salpêtrière, by J. Rigaud.

practiced by popular healers and charlatans, and the obsolete, quasi-scholastic medicine taught at the faculties. These were the twin enemies against which the new medicine must struggle – on the one hand, the untrained healers who preyed on an ignorant, superstitious, and credulous populace; on the other, the corporate authority of the old, benighted faculties.[46]

In these prolegomenas to the medical science of man, certain words carry special methodological weight. One is "observation," which functioned at several different levels of meaning. Pragmatically, "observation" meant close physical attention to actual patients as opposed to the armchair theorizing that the medical revolutionaries thought was characteristic of official medicine.[47] Critics from Vicq d'Azyr forward had heaped abuse on the kind of medicine that came from textbooks rather than from physical contact with the sick. Exhortations to observe actual patients went hand in hand, moreover, with the campaign for hospital reform. The most comprehensive of all the hospital reorganization plans, that devised by Jacques Tenon and published in 1788 as *Mémoires sur les hôpitaux de Paris,* emphasized, among other things, that doctor-patient contact was essential both for therapeutics and for medical education.[48] Cabanis's *Observations sur les hôpitaux* (1790) made a similar argument, although, unlike Tenon, Cabanis saw small-scale institutions or even home care as the best practical means for achieving the

46 *Ibid.,* i; Pinel, *Traité médico-philosophique,* xliii, lvi.
47 On this theme, see Triaire, *Récamier et ses contemporains,* 142–43.
48 Greenbaum, " 'Measure of Civilization,' " 44–45.

goals of clear observation and sound clinical practice. Like the Montpellier doctors, Cabanis based his whole therapeutic approach on the view that patients and maladies were endlessly variable, dependent on minute differences in age, sex, temperament, constitution, climate, occupation, and the like. The only possible means by which doctors could hope to gain sufficient information about such variables was by intimate clinical contact, for which a proper therapeutic environment was the first necessity. Only in a small, closely regulated "hospice" could the kinds of clinical documentation be amassed that would allow this kind of observation and encourage the correct therapeutic response.[49]

Observation meant something much more sweeping, however, than clinical practice. Indeed in epistemological terms it constituted one of the foundation stones for the very concept of a medical science of man since it had come to be virtually synonymous with the idea of science itself. In this sense "observation" signified embrace of the whole Baconian-Newtonian-Lockean project to know the world from experience and sense-data rather than from pure ratiocination, received authorities, or revelation. Thus to argue that medicine must become "observational" was to reject both the procedures of antiquated official medicine and the Christian teaching that medicine should restrict itself to the body and leave the soul to theology. True medicine, the medical revolutionaries insisted, could not approach its object with any such preconceived division of phenomena; it must be attuned to the infinitely variable and subtle signs and events presented by the living patient. Observational medicine entailed constant, careful, and rigorous registering and recording of phenomena, and in this sense "observation" was the beginning of scientific practice itself.[50] The completion or fulfillment of that practice was achieved – and this was the second methodological keyword of the science of man – by a series of procedures that the revolutionaries, after Condillac's usage, called "analysis."

From a certain vantage point the high prestige of Condillac among the medical revolutionaries is something of a puzzle. Condillac's topics were those of abstract philosophy, whose study he routinely recommended as a path to piety. Sharing Barthez's horror of controversy, he eschewed all the activities and enterprises of the politically engaged philosophes.[51] Despite the care he took with his own reputation, however, by the end of the century his very name was enough to cause consternation in devout circles. This trick that history played on Condillac resulted in good part from the work of the medical revolutionaries, who in company with the Ideologues

49 Cabanis, "Observations sur les hôpitaux," in *Oeuvres*, 1:1–32; see also "Rapport sur l'organisation des écoles de médecine," in *Oeuvres*, 2:405–24.
50 Moravia, "Philosophie et médecine," 1114–21.
51 Isabel Knight, *The Geometric Spirit: The Abbé de Condillac and the French Enlightenment* (New Haven: Yale University Press, 1968), 2; Arthur Wilson, *Diderot* (New York: Oxford University Press, 1972), 67.

embraced Condillac's philosophy and transformed it into a powerful weapon in their critical arsenal.

Condillac was crucial to the doctors, both as the foremost French interpreter of Lockean "analysis" and as the author of what Isabel Knight calls "the most rigorous demonstration of the sensationalist psychology of his century."[52] Although Keith Baker is right to insist that Condillac was not the sole source of the philosophes' philosophical themes, nonetheless among the medical reformers Condillac occupied high rank indeed, not much below that of Bacon, Newton, or Locke.[53] Condillac's exposition of analytic method was widely regarded as the clearest and most comprehensive available. Alibert wrote, for example, that "the glory of the science of Locke and Condillac is that it has remade all the other [sciences] and has become . . . the universal key to the human mind."[54]

Two passages – one published in 1798 and the other in 1800 – may be juxtaposed to suggest how the methodological procedures constituting "analysis" were understood by the medical revolutionaries. Pinel adapted this definition of "analysis" directly from Condillac:

To analyze is nothing other than to observe in successive order the qualities of an object in order to establish in our minds the simultaneous order in which they exist. . . . What is this order? Nature shows us herself; it is the order in which things are presented. There are some [objects] that are particularly striking and cry out for our attention; these are dominant. All others seem to be arranged around them and to be explained by them.[55]

Another definition appeared in a work much admired by Cabanis, the *Principes de physiologie* (1800–3) of the Montpellier physician C.-L. Dumas:

[A]nalysis . . . is a rigorous method which, interrogating nature by exact observation and experience, restricts itself to gathering facts, noting their analogies and dissimilarities, making deductions from these first simple results and then – by means of calculation – drawing more general conclusions which are themselves so many demonstrated facts to which the first [naturally] led.[56]

These renderings of "analysis" emphasize what the medical revolutionaries generally regarded as the salient features of analytic method: dependence on rigorous observation; reduction of large phenomena to constituent parts; comparison and contrast; and the establishment of "general consequences" whose order was discernible through direct interrogation of nature itself.

52 Knight, *Geometric Spirit*, 12.   53 Baker, *Condorcet*, 117.
54 Alibert, "Discours sur les rapports," lxxv; Brodier, *Alibert*, 242–44.
55 Pinel, *Nosographie*, xi.
56 C.-L. Dumas, *Principes de physiologie, ou Introduction à la science expérimentale, philosophique et médicale de l'homme vivant*, 4 vols. (Paris: Crapelet, 1800–03), 1:158–59.

One important element of "analysis" does not appear in these passages, however, and that is some sense of the crucial importance of language itself.[57] Among medical reformers the problem of language was both philosophical, involving larger epistemological and methodological problems about the correspondence between words and objective reality, and pragmatic, entailing reexamination of the working terminology of everyday medical practice. Thus medical figures engaged the problem of language on various levels, taking direction both from Condillac and from their own medical forebears such as Boissier de Sauvages, who had pressed for reform of medical nomenclature well before Condillac defined science itself as "a well-made language."[58] Medical reflections on the necessity for linguistic clarity addressed diverse problems. Vicq d'Azyr decried the condition of anatomical language and called for general linguistic reform in the field. Pinel ridiculed the "frivolous games of the imagination" indulged in by doctors who described disease in an ever more absurd medical terminology, replete with hyphenated names like "bilious-putrid fevers."[59] Cabanis, always the most philosophically sophisticated of the medical revolutionaries, developed what Sergio Moravia has called a "pragmatic conception of language" that saw words as "altogether arbitrary" and language itself as an "artificial means" for representing the phenomena of sensation: "We may say that words capture sensations; they sum them up and fix them."[60]

For the medical revolutionaries as for scientists in many fields, the chief practical work of "analysis," insofar as it implied the quest for linguistic clarity, lay in classification. The nosological enterprise inspired widespread interest and encouraged some physicians to undertake detailed revisions of the language employed in special disease areas. Pinel's nosology, with its five general "classes" of disease and multitudinous "genera," is perhaps the best known of these projects, but other schemes also attracted the attention of contemporaries. Alibert's famous *arbre des dermatoses* classified all dermatological maladies as stemming from a trunk, branching into diverse limbs, having the minute differences of leaves, and so on.[61]

But classificatory efforts were by no means the only result of the embrace of "analysis" in medicine. Rather, analytic method was brought to bear on

---

57 Of the large literature on the eighteenth century's preoccupation with the origins, ontological status, and quest for reform of language, see Michel Foucault, *The Order of Things: An Archaeology of the Human Sciences* (New York: Vintage Books, 1973), which makes the "rupture" in the relation between "words and things" the critical movement in the epistemic revolution of the late eighteenth century; see also Baker, *Condorcet*, 110–14, 124–27; Moravia, "Philosophie et médecine," 1137–51.
58 Brodier, *Alibert*, 80–85; Moravia, "Philosophie et médecine," 1143.
59 Pinel, *Nosographie,* ix–x.
60 "Les mots saisissent, pour ainsi dire, les sensations: ils les résument et les fixent." Quoted in Moravia, "Philosophie et médecine," 1149.
61 Pinel, *Nosographie;* Brodier, *Alibert,* 146–86.

a range of problems, often by followers of Pinel, who seems to have been its most vigorous advocate among medical teachers of the period. René-Théophile Laennec, who became famous for the invention of "mediate auscultation," attributed this breakthrough to his effort to achieve maximum clarity in observing and analyzing the "signs" of pulmonary afflictions.[62] Xavier Bichat regarded his tissue theory as a product of "analysis" since he settled on tissues as the smallest constituent part of the anatomical complex.[63] Thus Condillacian "analysis," with its emphasis on the isolation of central constituent parts and on the necessity for close attention to and precise labeling of the "signs" that guide observation, was given credit for a variety of innovations, classificatory and otherwise.

Condillac enjoyed high prestige among the medical revolutionaries not only because he provided an exemplary statement of how analysis should proceed but also because his works offered a lucid (and natively French) exposition of sensationalist psychology.[64] The Paris theorists were by no means in complete accord with Condillac's peculiar version of sensationalist philosophy, but they nonetheless regarded sensationalism as their point of departure. "There can be no truths," Cabanis wrote, "except those corresponding to the general manner of sensing [established by] human nature."[65]

Much has been written about the development and use of sensationalist principles by the Paris clinical school and the Ideologues, so it is necessary here only to indicate the specific ways in which sensationalism was incorporated into anthropological medicine.[66] In his immensely influential *Rapports du physique et du moral de l'homme*, Cabanis argued that Locke, Condillac, Bonnet, Helvétius, and "the physiologists" had demonstrated beyond question that sensation was the source of all ideas, although he acknowledged that the problem of how sensation was transformed into thought remained unsolved.[67] Too little, Cabanis held, was known about the structure and functions of the brain to explain the sensation-into-thought process. Yet the fact that all thought resulted from some kind of action by the brain on sensory impressions was undeniable. To express the character of this action, Cabanis drew what was to become a famous

---

62 On Laennec and the stethoscope, see Triaire, *Récamier et ses contemporains*, 128–29; on vitalistic elements in Laennec's work, see Jacalyn Duffin, "Vitalism and Organicism in the Philosophy of R.-T.-H. Laennec," *BHM* 62 (1988): 525–45.

63 Xavier Bichat, *Anatomie générale appliquée à la physiologie et à la médecine*, 3 vols. (Paris: Brosson, Gabon et Cie, 1801), xciii.

64 Knight, *Geometric Spirit*, 12.   65 Cabanis, "Rapports," 143.

66 On the sensationalist epistemology of the Paris clinical school and the Ideologues, see Gusdorf, *La conscience révolutionnaire*, 454–61; Moravia, "Philosophie et médecine," 1105–28; Staum, *Cabanis*, 41–48.

67 Cabanis, "Rapports," 165; see also "Rapport sur l'organisation des écoles de médecine," where Cabanis wrote that medicine was in the process of illuminating "that invisible connection that unites the functions of the organs with the noblest operations of the intellect and will" (2:408).

analogy between the way the brain works on thought and the way the viscera work on nutrients:

> We see . . . impressions arriving at the brain, by the intermediary of the nerves; at this point they are isolated and without coherence. The viscera enters into action; it acts on them and soon it renders them back metamorphosed into ideas that are expressed in the language of physiognomy and gesture, or the signs of speech and writing. We conclude . . . that the brain in some way digests impressions, that it produces organically the secretion of thought.[68]

It was therefore unnecessary to distinguish between sensation as such and what philosophy had long regarded as the distinct "faculties" of reason, imagination, judgment, and the like. "The difficulty no longer exists," Cabanis wrote, "once one recognizes that in its diverse operations the brain *acts on* impressions that are transmitted to it."[69] Because sensations produced thought, Cabanis concluded, medicine alone could explicate matters of consciousness, for it was the only science that investigated the general operations of sensibility and the diverse influences governing them. Medicine could thus lay claim to the whole of human experience and was rendered fundamentally anthropological in nature. Constituted in this fashion, furthermore, medicine had no need to borrow positivity from better-established sciences; medicine was itself the source of all positivity since it alone could render judgment on the validity and quality of intellectual operations. From this perspective, medicine alone could constitute a science of man.

FROM PHYSIOLOGY TO MORAL SCIENCE: PROGRAMS FOR ANTHROPOLOGICAL MEDICINE

Analytic method taught that the first crucial step in any investigation was to reduce a subject to its constituent parts. Thus when Cabanis set out to define the science of man for his most important audience, the Institute's Class of Moral and Political Sciences, he did so by elaborating its components: "Physiology, the analysis of ideas, and *morale* are but three branches of one and the same science, which can be rightly called the science of man."[70] Study of physiology was anterior to all other investigations in the science of man, Cabanis argued, because the body was well known, whereas the mental faculties remained a greatly mystery and the moral faculties had been obscured by the "systems" of metaphysicians and theologians.[71] Starting from this premise, Cabanis elaborated a program for the science of man that foresaw its explaining the physical, intellectual, and moral components of human nature and thus supplying medical guidance in all of human life.

68 Cabanis, "Rapports," 196. 69 *Ibid.* 70 *Ibid.*, 126. 71 *Ibid.*, 125–26.

To grasp Cabanis's rationale for basing the science of man on the study of physiology, it is necessary to examine the term more closely for it had diverse meanings in the era of the medical revolution. John Lesch has argued recently that in the eighteenth century physiology was "institutionally and intellectually" indistinguishable from medicine.[72] Yet, if it is true that all of physiology was in some sense medical, it was by no means true that all medicine was physiological. Some of the greatest clinicians thought the only proper realm of investigation for doctors was therapeutics – pragmatic response to the presence of sickness. In this view close study of the body, anatomical or physiological, was of little value. The functional explanations devised by physiology were thought especially futile since they were largely conjectural and lacked practical medical applications.[73] This view of the relation between physiology and medicine had been forcefully condemned by Bordeu as early as 1747. And because it was the vitalists who most strongly argued for the importance of physiology to medicine, the word itself tended to imply – in medical if not broader scientific circles – some grounding in or sympathetic relation to vitalism.

This does not mean that for the medical revolutionaries the mechanist-vitalist dichotomy, which had sharply divided earlier physiologists, continued to hold in the same form. Mediation between the mechanist and vitalist positions had been one of the principal consequences of the labors of the physiologist Albrecht von Haller, who explained many phenomena by the vital "properties" of sensibility and irritability yet, unlike Montpellier theorists, held that these properties resided in specific anatomical structures of nerve and muscle.[74] Haller's career unfolded principally in Swiss and German centers of biomedical science (Bern, Tübingen, Göttingen), but he lived in Paris on several occasions, had many associates in the Parisian scientific community, and was an important contributor to the *Encyclopédie*. The medical revolutionaries of the 1790s were well acquainted with Hallerian doctrines, which functioned as an important point of reference for them in conceptualizing the physiological basis of the science of man. Although they were much more sympathetic to the observational method and general orientation of Montpellier medicine than they were to Haller's experimentalism, Haller's conception of physiology entailed concern with similar problematics: the character

72 John Lesch, *Science and Medicine in France: The Emergence of Experimental Physiology, 1790–1855* (Cambridge, Mass.: Harvard University Press, 1984), 13.
73 Bordeu condemned this approach to medicine in "Recherches anatomiques sur la position des glandes et sur leur action," in *Oeuvres complètes de Bordeu*, ed. A.-B. Richerand, 2 vols. (Paris: Caille et Ravier, 1818), 1:45–208.
74 François Duchesneau, *La physiologie des Lumières: Empirisme, modèles et théories* (The Hague: Martinus Nijhoff, 1982), esp. 141–70.

of organization, the nature of the vital properties, functional interdependencies, and the like.[75]

For Cabanis the central physiological problem of the science of man concerned the nature of "organization," a term he used (as the Montpellier doctors had) to mean, at the most fundamental level, simply that a body was alive. "Unorganized bodies" were brute, "dead" matter. They consisted of basic chemical elements and their "aggregates," which, as Lavoisier had recently demonstrated, were governed by the "laws of affinity." "Organized bodies," by contrast, were living beings whose composition and fundamental "laws" were unknown.[76] Although "life" itself was variously defined and the precise line between the organic and the inorganic remained a matter of dispute, the central importance of sensibility to any understanding of life was beyond argument. "Sensibility was," Cabanis argued, "a general fact of living nature" and "the ultimate term one arrives at in the study of vital phenomena."[77]

Cabanis defined sensibility only obliquely, in reference to what he saw as the most important eighteenth-century formulations of the nature of the vital properties: Haller's doctrine of the independent properties of sensibility and irritability and, ranged against Haller's conception, the views of the Stahlian "semi-animists," the Edinburgh "solidists," and the Montpellier vitalists. Cabanis believed that the doctrines of the anti-Hallerians were separated only by nuances and that they were all essentially variants on Stahl's teaching that vital actions were uniformly guided by a single animating principle. Although Haller's theories would later be seen as a breakthrough to a properly anatomically based physiology, from the vantage point of 1796 Cabanis dismissed this debate as strictly semantic. He asserted that the Stahlian and Hallerian explanations were fundamentally the same, although Stahl's language was preferable since simpler and more in keeping with the "unity of the physical principle."[78] Thus for Cabanis the capacity to feel – however and from wherever it derived – was the crux of life. He replaced Descartes's "cogito" with a very different aphorism: "from the moment that we feel, we exist."[79]

If sensibility was the acknowledged source of all life activity, its precise workings were nonetheless little understood. Although the nervous structures were clearly "the special seat of sensibility," they could not be re-

75 For a comparison of the teachings of Haller and Montpellier, see William R. Albury, "Experiment and Explanation in the Physiology of Bichat and Magendie," *Studies in History of Biology*, ed. William Coleman and Camille Limoges (Baltimore: Johns Hopkins University Press, 1977), 1:47–131.

76 See Karl M. Figlio, "The Metaphor of Organization: An Historiographical Perspective on the Bio-medical Sciences of the Early Nineteenth Century," *History of Science* 14 (1976): 17–53.

77 Cabanis, "Rapports," 198, n. 1; Staum, *Cabanis*, 177.

78 Cabanis, "Rapports," 166–68.   79 *Ibid.*, 168.

garded as the exclusive source of feeling. In any case the problem of how "impressions" were conveyed in the body and how, generally, the anatomical-functional relation that constituted sensibility was established belonged in works of "pure physiology."[80] An issue that was of central importance in establishing the claims of the science of man, however, was distinguishing between kinds of impressions and defining their respective sources. It was essential in this regard to advance beyond the observations of the "analytic philosophers," who limited their attention to "sensations" coming from outside the body while ignoring all those that originated on the inside. External sensations that were registered via the sense organs as such were crucial to life; they established our relations with the exterior world of people, things, and the general environment. But the "internal impressions" that originated in the viscera – brain, stomach, sexual organs – were equally influential in the life of the organism and as fully deserving of analysis as the "sensations" examined by analytic philosophy. Thus from the larger perspective of the science of man, the most important question to be posed about sensibility was whether, as the philosophers would have it, our mental activity was governed solely by sensation properly speaking, or whether, as physiology suggested, external and internal impressions combined in some way to form our "ideas and determinations":

The new question that presents itself is to know whether it is true, as Condillac and others have established, that ideas and moral determinations are wholly formed and depend uniquely on what they call *sensations* and whether, consequently, . . . our ideas come to us from our *senses* and from exterior objects; or whether internal impressions contribute equally to the production of moral determinations and ideas, following certain laws, whose constancy is revealed to us by study of the healthy and the sick; and whether, the latter case being true, observations directed by this new point of view will not allow us readily to recognize here too the laws of nature, and to state them with exactitude and clarity.[81]

In this formulation, the mind was no longer Locke's clean slate to be inscribed with information from the outside world. Nor was the human organism remotely similar to Condillac's statue wakened to consciousness successively by the operation of touch, taste, sight, hearing, and smell. The mind in this view was not tranquilly, uniformly prepared to receive sense-data but instead was captive to the body and its diverse states, which in turn were governed by a constant interplay between interior and exterior environments.

To support this formulation about the influence of internal impressions on the mental and passional life, Cabanis presented diverse evidence that is striking to the modern reader for its anticipation of major preoccupations of nineteenth-century psychophysiology. He argued that illness, particularly

80 *Ibid.*, 171–72.   81 *Ibid.*, 174.

of the intestinal region, produced disordered thought, bizarre appetites, and often a strange elevation and energy of the spirit. Maladies of other organs, especially the sexual organs, produced true *folie,* which Cabanis defined as "disorder, or lack of harmony in ordinary impressions." Puberty was hastened by an imagination fevered by "the noxious habits of city life." Dreams were produced not by jumbled or poorly recalled external sensations but by digestive and circulatory activity. Ingested substances resulted in peculiar states of well-being or malaise (*mal-être*). The inescapable conclusion was that although these conditions had nothing to do with the sense organs as such, they nonetheless caused "important modifications in the nature of penchants and ideas, and clearly acted with immediacy on the faculties of thought and feeling."[82]

Thus the physical-moral link was even more intimate and powerful than had been suggested by classic sensationalist theory. If it had long been recognized that knowledge was dependent on the proper functioning of our eyes, ears, and other sense organs, physiology was now ready to demonstrate that all mental activity was dependent on the condition – young or old, healthy or sick, weak or strong – of our bodies. Hence the indispensability of medicine and physiology to the science of man:

It is exclusively the domain of these two sciences to indicate, on the one hand, the ordinary modifications that take place in the organs as a result of the life functions themselves and, on the other, the accidental changes produced by morbid affections, especially those that are accompanied by phenomena specifically related to the operations of the brain.[83]

According to Cabanis's tripartite scheme, once the science of man was properly grounded in physiology it would be equipped to fulfill its two other tasks: the "analysis of ideas" and the study of moral problems. Cabanis framed these divisions of the science of man in reference to the "influences" exerted on "ideas and moral affections" by the factors long privileged in vitalist medicine: age, sex, temperament, disease, regimen, climate, and the like. On many points his analysis was like a compendium or handbook of vitalist principles – the dominance of the different vital regions in the successive "stages of life," the heightened and childlike sensibility of women, the continuing utility of the four-temperaments scheme, and so on.[84]

In other respects, however, Cabanis moved beyond classic vitalist doctrines of psychophysiology. He attempted, for example, to differentiate clearly between "vital operations" that were governed chiefly by "instinct" and those that were "reasoned." He thus sought to articulate a distinction in behavior – even moral behavior – between activities that lay outside the

82 *Ibid.,* 174–77. 83 *Ibid.,* 179.
84 *Ibid.,* 248, 252, 258, and generally, Memoirs 4–12 of the "Rapports."

controlling range of reason and those that were directed by will and judgment even when strongly influenced by factors militating against rational control.[85] In so doing, he broke not only with the vitalist science of man but also with analytic philosophy, both of which had continued to uphold the Christian view that human decisions were ultimately under rational direction and that even feelings could be managed with due moral striving. Although the Montpellier doctors had drawn attention to the role of instinct, they never fully departed from this fundamental Christian and rationalist perspective. Cabanis was willing, on the other hand, to give new weight to the role of instinct in human behavior and thus to withdraw crucial human activities from the domain of reasoned action. This was a step that even he took with trepidation, however. While insisting on the importance of instinct in human behavior, Cabanis argued at the same time that the human "moral system" was composed of both innate inclinations and reasoned choices.[86] He observed that the role of instinctual behavior was much greater in animals than in human beings yet held that the role of instinct in human feeling and action could not be eliminated. Instinct was not, as some theorists claimed, a word "void of sense, representing a vague or false idea." Rather it was a word "used in all languages" to express universal observations of "the working [*résultat*] of impressions received by the interior organs."[87] Cabanis argued further that in the best of circumstances neither the rational nor the instinctual element of the moral system would overwhelm the other: "When all these apparatuses [*organes*] enjoy a moderate and more or less proportionate activity, no particular order of impressions will dominate."[88] Thus human "organization" itself set clear limits on the reign of reason. One of the signal benefits of medicine was that it, alone of the sciences, could illuminate these intricate relations of the moral system and establish the limits within which human expectations and ambitions should unfold.

Cabanis's program for a science of man was the most systematic offered within medical circles but it was not the only one. Another prospectus for anthropological medicine was written by Alibert, permanent secretary of the Société médicale d'émulation from 1796 to 1802. Published in the second volume (1798) of the society's *Mémoires* under the title "Discours sur les rapports de la médecine avec les sciences physiques et morales," this work lacked the depth and detail of Cabanis's program but offered fine rhetorical flourishes that were much admired in his circle. The *Décade philosophique* reviewer described Alibert's treatise as "remarkable for its philosophical and imaginative breadth, for its methodical organization and animated composition, for the merits of its science and . . . its style."[89] To Alibert the days when medicine subordinated itself to other sciences were past: "A bet-

85 *Ibid.*, 182–88.   86 *Ibid.*, 188.   87 *Ibid.*   88 *Ibid.*
89 *Décade*, no. 29 (20 messidor, an VII/1799), 79.

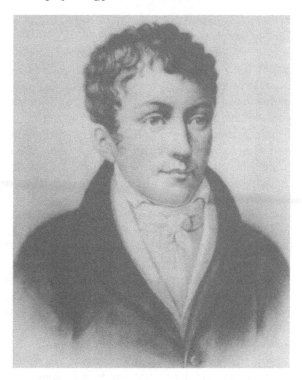

Portrait of P. J. G. Cabanis, by Ambroise Tardieu.

ter fate is reserved to medicine in our day; it is not longer the accessory sciences that have conquered medicine but medicine that has conquered the accessory sciences, . . . rul[ing] their efforts and direct[ing] at will the useful application of their discoveries." Medicine was "infinite in scope," "a science to which no moral question was foreign," "an art designed to watch over all of . . . human destiny."[90] Again the source of medicine's claims was the intimate relation between the physical and the moral. Alibert regarded the link between mental, physical, and moral phenomena as wholly established, even though, like Cabanis, he conceded that the precise "organic means" governing the "intellectual forces" were not yet understood. Yet for Alibert whatever gaps there were in medical knowledge, doctors were the only inquirers who had even begun to comprehend the complicated phenomena of fundamental organization and of sickness and health. They alone could account for the "astonishing variety of mental capacities" that had perplexed metaphysicians since the days of Galen.[91]

Alibert asserted that the services medicine could render to learning and to society were limitless. As the science of sensibility, it would be the

90 Alibert, "Discours," lxxxi, cx, xc.   91 *Ibid.*, lxxix–lxxx.

beacon for metaphysics as "recreated" by Bacon, Locke, and Condillac. It would lead in analyzing and treating the mental illnesses that were inimical to human progress – the "furors, manias, melancholic languors, and thousand other partial or total eclipses of the mind that sadden the heart and cast shame on human reason."[92] Medicine would ground all future work on "sympathy" and "sociability," which were, "for animated bodies, what attraction and affinity were for inanimate matter."[93] It alone could write "the unbounded history of the human heart," curbing and controlling the passions that destroyed all felicity.[94] Lastly, an "alliance between medicine and politics" would be forged in the labors of public hygienists and doctors whose special task was to advise and assist "the judicial art."[95]

References to similar ambitions for the medical science of man are scattered throughout the writings of Philippe Pinel, Xavier Bichat, Jacques-Louis Moreau de la Sarthe, Jean-Noël Hallé, Jean Burdin, and other doctors who were associated with the Société médicale d'émulation and bent on extending the cultural authority of medicine. Among their writings there are differences of both emphasis and doctrinal detail. Moreau, for example, particularly stressed the need for the development of hygiene. Pinel was primarily interested in developing a theoretical framework for treating mental disorders. Bichat was seeking to restructure the whole of medical theory and teaching. Nonetheless, all these figures shared the fundamental view that the human organism was a totality – physical, mental, moral – whose interrelated operations could be grasped only by a medicine that was genuinely anthropological in character.[96]

In this holistic orientation, the doctors of the revolutionary era were functioning within the vitalist perspective that had long been favored in Montpellier. Yet there were crucial differences between the Montpellier science of man and the programs for anthropological medicine advanced in the revolutionary years. The Montpellier doctors had asserted their special capacity to divine the human heart and to comprehend human na-

92 *Ibid.*, lxviii.   93 *Ibid.*, lxxxiii.   94 *Ibid.*, xc–xci.
95 *Ibid.*, xcv; see also Alibert, "De l'influence des causes politiques sur les maladies et la constitution physique de l'homme," *Magasin encyclopédique, ou Journal des sciences, des lettres et des arts* 5 (1795): 298–305.
96 See Pinel, *Traité médico-philosophique*, xxxv, lvi; Xavier Bichat, *Physiological Researches Upon Life and Death* (Philadelphia: Smith and Maxwell, 1809), article 6, "General Differences of the Two Lives Morally Considered" (43–64), in which Bichat demonstrates the applicability of his principles to problems of sociability, intelligence, and the passions; J.-L. Moreau de la Sarthe, "Art de guérir: Traité médico-philosophique sur l'aliénation mentale par Ph. Pinel," *Décade* (20 prairial, an IX/1801): 458–59, n. 1; see also his extract of Jean Burdin, *Cours d'études médicales* in *Décade*, no. 18 (30 ventôse, an XI/1803): 514–21; no. 19 (10 germinal, an XI/1803): 8–73, *idem*, "Encore des réflexions et des observations relatives à l'influence du moral sur le physique," *Décade*, nos. 11–12 (20 and 30 nivôse, an IX/1801): 69–75, 134–41; on Hallé, see Staum, *Cabanis*, appendix E, 381–82.

ture, but their assertions about the powers and benefits of medicine were far less sweeping than those articulated by Cabanis and Alibert. And although this difference may be attributed in part to the inherent conservatism of the Montpellier learned community, it must be explained chiefly in reference to the structural transformation of French medicine effected by the Revolution itself.

In the late Ancien Regime, medicine derived its authority from three principal sources – the social prestige of the medical corporations, the support and legitimation given medical figures and institutions by the crown, and the vague though no doubt crucial authority of medical science. With the coming of the Revolution, the first two of these sources of authority were irrevocably destroyed: the medical corporations were disestablished, and the crown proved incapable even of saving itself. Yet these apparent losses in fact proved to be signal gains for medicine. The chaos of the early Revolution quickly gave way to a general restructuring of authority in which medicine was able to make an independent claim to social efficacy based on its analytic and therapeutic powers. The Revolution's general restructuring of authority, especially the attack on clerical prerogatives and prestige, meant that there was a vast domain of social and cultural experience into which new claimants for authority could step. Medicine was by no means alone in setting forth such claims, as the heightened importance of the law, the military, and the larger scientific establishment indicates. Yet medicine was a crucial element in this struggle, and its key rhetorical and intellectual vehicle was the science of man, with its assertion of medicine's unique capacity to comprehend and direct human efforts. We turn our attention now to one of the most important means by which medicine proposed to arbitrate the extended process of social reorganization necessitated by the Revolution: the classification and analysis of physiologically based human types. In the study of types, the revolutionary doctors again adapted and transformed to new ends an intellectual tendency that was present in vitalist medicine but not yet plumbed for social utility. Again it was the Revolution that encouraged a new intensity and resoluteness in the formulations of the science of man. Where in Montpellier doctrine the construction of types primarily served a diagnostic-therapeutic purpose, and only secondarily constituted a reflection on social organization, in the discourse of the revolutionary doctors the establishment of human types functioned as a new modality of sociomedical authority. In classifying and naming types, doctors asserted a new prerogative to assess social capacities and to assign social tasks. And although their right to perform such a function did not go unchallenged, the very fact that it was asserted changed the social framework of medicine in ways earnestly intended by the advocates of the science of man.

THE DOCTRINE OF HUMAN TYPES

As one of its most important benefits, the medical science of man promised to explain why and how human beings differed. Embedded in the concept of vital force was the idea that spontaneity, variability, and autonomy from the rigid laws of unorganized matter were the very definition of "life." The capacity of the physician to recognize and gauge variability – in both the patient's fundamental constitution and the myriad external factors that made up the patient's milieu – also lay at the heart of vitalist therapeutics. If treatments were not attuned to the particulars of the patient's experience, they were doomed to failure. The rhetoric of both Hippocratism and "observation" demanded close attention to the specific details of particular patients and illnesses.[97]

Yet for the medical revolutionaries this clinical rationale for privileging particulars over generalities was by no means the only source of their concern for the problem of human diversity. Rather, they deliberately brought their medical perspective to bear on larger philosophical debates of the eighteenth century and staked out positions in the fevered political conflicts of the era. Their chosen philosophical antagonists included Helvétius, who in Alibert's construction had "explained everything by the varying character of occupations, by the choice of methods, or by the pure play of circumstances."[98] The doctors criticized Helvétius for many reasons but primarily because his doctrine rested on an inadequate understanding of the "human physical economy."[99] Similarly, Montesquieu was disputed for attributing excessive power to the force of climate and neglecting the effects of "organization." And Rousseau, although cherished by Cabanis as "a great observer of nature," was regarded as deeply flawed in his thinking and given to "antiphilosophical" paradoxes.[100]

Important as this philosophical tradition was to anthropological medicine, however, it was overshadowed by the political context. Working in an environment marked, as G. A. Kelly has written, by "upheaval and *sauve qui peut*," these doctors were all intensely aware of the momentous political and social ramifications of any pronouncement made on the subject of human equality or inequality. Thus Alibert fulminated against the barbarism and rapacity of the early Revolution's "levelers." Bichat rejected the doctrine of human equality as chimerical. Cabanis firmly insisted that hierarchy was the necessary social expression of inequalities inherent in human organization.[101]

97 See Chapter 1.   98 Alibert, "Discours," lxxx.   99 *Ibid.*
100 Cabanis, "Rapports," 253.
101 G. A. Kelly, *Victims, Authority, and Terror: The Parallel Deaths of d'Orléans, Custine, Bailly, and Malesherbes* (Chapel Hill: University of North Carolina Press, 1982), 23; Brodier, *Alibert*, 302–3; on Cabanis, see Picavet, *Les Idéologues*, 218. See also Frank Manuel, "From Equality to Organicism," *Journal of the History of Ideas* 17 (1956): 54–69.

The intensity of such opinions suggests that the medical conception of diversity functioned in part as a theoretical formalization of the profound emotion roused in these theorists by their own experience of the radical Revolution. To them and their associates, the Terror had brought harassment, imprisonment, and death. Memories of the chaos and violence of the Robespierre era remained vivid, as may be seen in accounts such as those published in the *Décade philosophique* describing in detail the hounding, torture, and deaths of Condorcet, Bailly, and other philosophe victims of the radical Revolution.[102] The medical revolutionaries themselves described the events of 1793–94 in language that evoked either untamed nature or humanity in a precivilized state. Robespierre himself was a "mad beast," "a ferocious tyrant." The era was one of "storms and tempests." The crowds around the guillotine were seized with bloodlust and "drunk with furious passion."[103] Thus much medical writing of the period from Thermidor to the establishment of the Empire was marked by a deeply felt need to explain, and where possible curb, the vicious, uncivilized behavior witnessed during the early Revolution. For both Cabanis and Bichat, this disposition eventuated in hierarchies of human types whose differing degrees and kinds of vital force prepared them for distinct roles in society. These hierarchies were presented in works written at about the same time – Cabanis's memoir on sensibility, which was presented to the Institute in 1796 and revised for publication in the *Rapports* in 1802, and Bichat's treatise *Recherches sur la vie et la mort,* which was published shortly before his death in 1802.[104]

Bichat's schematization of human types is best approached by examining his celebrated theory of the two "lives" of animate beings. In Bichat's physiology all living bodies fell into the two large classificatory groups of the

102 The importance of Condorcet to the Ideologues has been documented in Baker, *Condorcet,* 372–74. Bailly, though not an Ideologue, had participated in the prerevolutionary hospital reform movement and was doubtless well known to the medical revolutionaries both for this work and in his capacity as mayor of Paris. See "Eloge de Bailly," *Décade,* no. 4 (nivôse-ventôse, an III/1794–95), 321–30, and *ibid.,* "Détails sur la mort de Condorcet," 62–64.

103 "Eloge de Bailly," 329; Pinel, "Lettre à son frère Pierre, 16 novembre 1792," in René Semelaigne, *Philippe Pinel et son oeuvre au point de vue de la médecine mentale* (Paris: Imprimeries réunies, 1888), 163; P. J. G. Cabanis, "Note sur l'opinion de MM. Oelsner et Soemmering, et du citoyen Sue, touchant le supplice de la guillotine," *MSME* 1 (an VI/1797): 278–93, at 291.

104 The question of the extent to which Cabanis's work, prior in time, influenced that of Bichat is extremely interesting but cannot be dealt with here. Picavet gives priority to Cabanis on many points of doctrine, but his remarks should not be taken as definitive. See Picavet, *Les Idéologues,* 435–37. Given Bichat's pivotal position at the nexus of biomedical and social thought of this era, it is to be hoped that some historian well versed in both of these areas will undertake a thorough study of Bichat's political thinking and connections. The existing secondary literature, while tortuously complex and argumentative on Bichat's physiology, is virtually mute on the political context and implications of his work. One exception is John Pickstone's highly interesting but largely speculative "Bureaucracy, Liberalism, and the Body in Post-Revolutionary France: Bichat's Physiology and the Paris School of Medicine," *History of Science* 19 (1981): 115–42.

vegetable and the animal. The former had but one "mode of existence," which he termed the "organic." The latter had both the "organic," which they shared with vegetables, and the "animal," which was exclusively theirs. To define these two "modes of existence," Bichat elaborated a series of interconnecting dichotomies. The first was the distinction between internal and external; the vegetable manifested internal life but the animal enjoyed as well

> an external life which establishes numerous relations between it and surrounding objects; . . . Its existence . . . [is] entwined with that of every other being. . . . It avoids or approaches these according to its fears or wants, and thus appears to appropriate everything in nature to its exclusive use.[105]

The animal and the organic lives were responsible for distinct functions, the animal for those linking the body's "exterior" to the brain and in turn linking the brain to the locomotor organs and the voice. The organic life consisted of those functions responsible for "assimilation" (nutrition, respiration, circulation) and "dis-assimilation" (excretion, secretion, exhalation).[106] Morphology showed the same division. The organs that maintained organic life were asymmetrical: heart, intestines, muscle fibers. Those responsible for animal life, including the sense organs, nerves, and sides of the brain, were symmetrical. This morphological pattern Bichat took as a privileged sign of the division between the two "lives." "Symmetry is the essential character of the organs of the animal life of man," whereas "the peculiar attribute of the organs of internal life is the irregularity of their external forms."[107] From this basic framework the dichotomies between the two lives multiplied; they are schematized in Table 4.

A separate study would be required to trace Bichat's reasoning in support of all these oppositions, but we must examine at least briefly those underlying Bichat's doctrine of types. It is important to ask first, however, what kinds of questions such an exposition was intended to answer. At one level this work of Bichat's is a contribution to what Cabanis called "pure physiology." Much of the work is devoted to Bichat's version of vital properties theory, which rejected both Barthez's unitary vital principle and Haller's sensibility-irritability doctrine in favor of a five-properties scheme Bichat developed in an attempt to capture the empirical specificity of vital phenomena. The unifying thematic of the work was nonetheless the problem that lay at the heart of vitalist physiology – the distinction between the living and the nonliving – and much of its power resided in Bichat's innovative approach to the question of how the living become the nonliving,

105 Bichat, *Physiological Researches*, 2.
106 *Ibid.*, 4–5; see also Bichat, *Anatomie générale*, xxxv–xxxvi, xl–xli, ci–ciii.
107 Bichat, *Physiological Researches*, 10.

Table 4. *Characteristics of Bichat's "Two Lives"*

Organic	Animal
Internal	External
Asymmetrical	Symmetrical
Unpaired	Paired
Variable morphology	Fixed form, size, and position
Discord possible	Harmony essential
Uninfluenced by habit	Determined by habit
Center of passions	Center of intelligence/understanding
Direct action of passions	Indirect action of passions
Influenced by temperament	Unaffected by temperament
Involuntary	Voluntary
Sensibility inferior	Sensibility highly developed
Contractility involuntary	Contractility voluntary
Product of instinct	Development begins at birth
Uninfluenced by occupation	Influenced by occupation

Source: Based on Xavier Bichat, *Recherches sur la vie et la mort* (1800), 1–117.

how life is transformed into death.[108] It has been suggested that this style of conceptualizing vitality was a reflection of Bichat's "dark counter-revolutionary temper," which predisposed him to see life not as a spontaneous, unified, and powerful force – in the manner of Barthez – but as a condition precariously maintained in the face of ceaseless onslaughts by destructive forces.[109] Hence Bichat's famous definition: "Life is the totality of those functions which resist death."

Whatever the validity of this political reading of Bichat's idea of the struggle for life – a matter difficult to judge given the dearth of knowledge about his political orientation – it is clear that such a conception automatically privileged the problem of the environment in which life was sustained, and encouraged Bichat to explore problems of "milieu" that for others lay outside the domain of physiology. To Bichat, every activity or capacity of an organism was part of its total life-preserving capability and, on the other hand, everything in the environment of an organism was potentially life-threatening. Both subjects – the organism's own activities and the effects exerted on it by its milieu – were "physiological" in character. When Bichat reported that cases of heart disease had multiplied during the Revolution,

108 *Ibid.*, 65–94.
109 Pedro Laín Entralgo, "Sensualism and Vitalism in Bichat's *Anatomie Générale*," *JHMAS* 5 (1948): 47–64. Foucault's peroration on Bichat in *Birth of the Clinic* (pp. 170–72) is oddly similar, though he makes no explicit reference to the theme of counterrevolution; see Michel Foucault, *The Birth of the Clinic: An Archaeology of Medical Perception*, trans. A. M. Sheridan-Smith (New York: Vintage Books, 1973).

he was not merely engaging in a rhetorical flourish or indulging a "counter-revolutionary temper." He was attending seriously to a *physiological* cause of illness.[110]

All this explains in part why, for Bichat, physiology was still and must remain a part of medicine. Physiology engaged a subset of problems that medicine – with its attention to all the circumstances of the organism, the patient – embraced whole. There was no room in such a conception for a wholly autonomous science of physiology that would hive off from medicine – as mainstream physiology was soon to do – and that would enshrine as its chief investigative method the experimental creation of phenomena in the artificial environment of the laboratory. That Bichat was not hostile to experiment as such (something Claude Bernard asserted and historians long believed) has been fully demonstrated by recent scholarship.[111] His receptivity to and readiness to stage experiments does not change the fact, however, that for Bichat the laboratory could never shed light on the essential problem of physiological medicine, that of how an organism manages to live given the myriad, complex, and unpredictable forces that seek to kill it.

This being the case with Bichat's general physiology, we can readily understand why the *Recherches sur la vie et la mort*, which was his most ambitious theoretical work, functioned on another level altogether from that of "pure physiology." Viewed in another light, Bichat's work constituted a direct and timely response to the injunction of the Société medicale d'émulation to tie medicine intimately to the concerns of *morale*, without which, as the society's prospectus stated, "one has of man but an incomplete, crude, and material knowledge."[112] The Société médicale d'émulation was the institutional setting most important to Bichat as a medical scholar, and its prospectus upheld the view that "a medical theory will be the wiser and better established the more fully it is identified with the general science of relations [*rapports*], of which practical medicine is nothing but a corollary or application."[113]

This conviction is evident throughout *Recherches sur la vie et la mort*, which at frequent intervals draws explicit conclusions for the science of *morale* from physiological principles. In a section entitled "General Differences

110 Bichat, *Physiological Researches*, 46.   111 Albury, "Experiment and Explanation."
112 It has been suggested that Bichat himself wrote these words, found in the "Discours Préliminaire" to the *Mémoires de la Société médicale d'émulation*. See, for example, Russell C. Maulitz, *Morbid Appearances: The Anatomy of Pathology in the Early Nineteenth Century* (Cambridge: Cambridge University Press, 1987), 27. Although for the most part the "Discours préliminaire" is consonant with sentiments found elsewhere in Bichat's writings, it seems unlikely that he actually wrote it given the warm tribute paid there to Barthez (vii). Bichat's remarks on Barthez elsewhere were consistently unfavorable. See, for example, *Physiological Researches*, 65, and *Anatomie générale*, 184. It is much more likely the piece was written by Alibert, who was a close friend of Barthez. For an assessment of Barthez's work by Alibert, see the latter's *Nosologie naturelle, ou les maladies du corps humain distribuées par familles* (Paris: Caille et Ravier, 1817), lxvii–lxix.
113 "Discours préliminaire," ix.

of the Two Lives Morally Considered," for example, Bichat explicates his view that the intellect and the passions are wholly distinct, the former seated in the brain and dependent on its health for vigorous activity, the latter seated in and intimately related to the most minute operations of the viscera. Bichat was at pains in this exposition to give the brain (and with it judgment and will) a high degree of autonomy (a concern that he shared with the conservative Barthez). Bichat insisted, for instance, that strictly intellectual activity was unaffected by differences of temperament. All the same, he did not create a physiological ideal of the mind-dominated cerebral type. In company with his medical associates, and like them hearkening back to the classical ideals of balance and moderation, he held that the healthiest and happiest human being was the one in whom the intellectual and the passional, the "animal" and the "organic," were in equilibrium. In his view this happy balance was not, however, generally found in reality. In most human beings either the animal/intellectual or the organic/passional predominated, as dictated by fundamental physiological organization. Disequilibrium was common, while balance was rare and easily upset. Bichat linked his own conclusions in this respect to those advanced by the Dutch anatomist Peter Camper, whose "luminous considerations upon the respective intelligence of animals" showed that animals varied greatly in the "excellence" of their respective functions.[114] The same was true for human beings:

What we observe in the long chain of animated beings, we may remark in the human species taken separately. In the one, the passions which govern them are the principle of the greater number of their motions; the influence of animal life [is] every moment surpassed by the organic. . . . In the other, this [animal] life is superior to the former; hence all the phenomena relative to the sensations, perceptions and intelligence appear to be aggrandized at the expense of the passions which are condemned to silence by the organization of the individual.[115]

In this passage Bichat sets forth what may be called a "principle of limited energy," a vitalist-inspired doctrine that contributed more than any other to establishing a physiological conception of human types. Note in the preceding passage that if the intellectual faculties of an individual are highly developed, the passions are necessarily "condemned to silence." The reverse was true as well: if the passions dominated, the intellect could accomplish little. In a telling image, Bichat acknowledged that although the brain was not directly linked to the viscera, and thus not directly subject to the influence of the passions, the passions could still by various means "snatch from the empire of the will motions which are naturally voluntary."[116]

114 Bichat, *Physiological Researches*, 62. On Camper, see Claude Blanckaert, "Les vicissitudes de l'angle facial," *Revue de Synthèse*, 4th ser., nos. 3–4 (1987): 417–53, at 420–27.
115 Bichat, *Physiological Researches*, 62–63. 116 *Ibid.*, 55.

The fact that Bichat overtly lent assent to a Cartesian division between mind and body has led some historians to assert that he does not belong in company with Cabanis and other "medical Ideologues."[117] To my mind, such an interpretation of Bichat's physiology is mistaken. It takes Bichat's affirmation of mind–body dualism at face value and ignores other evidence (such as his praise for Camper) that indicates the extent to which Bichat did believe intellectual function to be dependent on material structures. More important, it obscures the fact that Bichat and the other vitalist-inspired revolutionary doctors often schematized the physical-moral relation not according to a strict mind–brain correlation but according to a general correspondence between talents, capacities, and faculties and the differential distribution of vital energy. Thus in Bichat's framework, some individuals were dominated by the "animal life" and accordingly given to intellectual activity; some were dominated by the "organic life" and consequently given over to the activities of the passions.[118]

The principle of limited energy was articulated not only by Bichat but, at one point or another in their writings, by all the medical theorists examined in this chapter, and it had crucial implications for the medical science of man. It meant first that, contrary to the theory of limitless perfectibility taught by some eighteenth-century philosophes, human beings could improve their capacities only to a point fixed by their fundamental organization. For some individuals this meant no intellectual improvement at all, because the dominance of the "organic life" was already set and could not be altered. For others, in whom the "animal life" held sway, there was some room for development. That the senses, the brain, and the locomotor apparatus could be improved by "habit," "education," or "practice" was a fact well established by vitalist medicine.[119] But past a certain natural threshold of growth and development, animal functions – sensory, intellectual, locomotor – could be enhanced only at the expense of other physiological activities. Either they improved by drawing force away from essential organic processes such as circulation, nutrition, or excretion, or they improved at the cost of one another. Beyond a point, then, a person could refine his intellect only by ruining his health. An artist could develop eye or ear only by sacrificing mental acuity. An athlete could train to perfection only by dulling sensation. A "fundamental law of the vital powers" decreed, wrote Bichat, that where was "a determinate sum of forces or powers" so that when "[the powers] are increased in one part they are diminished in all the rest of the living economy."[120] The single exception to the principle of limited energy was the "genius," a category Bichat mentioned but did not discuss in any detail.[121]

117 Staum, *Cabanis*, 256–59.   118 Bichat, *Physiological Researches*, 63.
119 See Chapter 1.   120 Bichat, *Physiological Researches*, 109, 113.
121 *Ibid.*, 113–14.

The principle of limited energy and the doctrine of types that followed from it gave the science of *morale* a concrete, useful tool for civic and social improvement. Henceforward any attempts to better the "citizenry" – a concept that still had deep resonance for medical revolutionaries under the Directory despite their disillusionment with the radical Revolution – were the more likely to succeed the more clearly they recognized the true potential of individuals.[122] Of all these doctors Bichat was the most pessimistic about improving the human lot. In his conception, the faculties of the "animal life" could be improved by practice; indeed the intellectual and sensory faculties had to be developed through education and training or else they would remain latent. But nothing could be done to change the character of people who were vicious or lascivious or cowardly because they were dominated by mean passions. To his mind nothing could eradicate or even lessen the influence of the passions in those individuals whose organization supplied no counterbalance. Bichat argued:

The character is . . . the physiognomy of the passions; as the temperament may be said to be of the internal functions: now, both these remaining constantly the same, and having a direction that habit and exercise never discompose, it is manifest that temperament and character must be also withdrawn from the influence of education. . . . To endeavour by [education] to alter the passions . . . or to enlarge or contract their sphere, would be as useless as the attempt of a physician to elevate or abase . . . the ordinary contractile power of the heart in a state of health.[123]

Cabanis's doctrine of types was less grim but it too rested on the view that only limited improvement was possible, and then only under circumstances in which "all the diverse influences" governing temperament and character could be manipulated to "act in concert." Even so, he observed, when the "original imprint is firm and deep, it is only rarely effaced."[124]

Whereas Bichat's doctrine of types was framed by his two-lives theory – one of his chief theoretical innovations – Cabanis's was cast in more traditional terms, drawing upon the doctrine of the non-naturals and Montpellier teachings. Of the eleven memoirs that Cabanis collected and published as the *Rapports,* five (on age, sex, climate, temperament, and regimen) addressed matters that physicians had long isolated not only as critical factors in health and sickness but as major determinants of human personality and behavior. In Cabanis's teaching some of these factors set fixed boundaries to human perfectibility and prescribed narrow social roles; others set flexible, but still limited, ranges of possibilities.

122 Even very early in the Revolution, when Cabanis was associated with Mirabeau, he favored a project for educational reform that sorted elements of the population according to their supposed capacities and the character of their sensitive response. See Staum, *Cabanis,* 130.

123 Bichat, *Physiological Researches,* 125.   124 Cabanis, "Rapports," 631.

Cabanis seems to have regarded the differences established by sex as more rigid than any of the others. Female "organization" was significantly and unalterably different from male "organization," and the consequences of these differences were enormous. As in his physiology generally, Cabanis's consideration of sex-based distinctions was rooted in sensibility theory. Like Pierre Roussel (see Chapter 1), he argued that women differed from men most significantly not in the gross anatomy of the generative organs but in the nature of their sensibility. Like that of children, women's sensibility was easily roused, intense, and unstable. The overall constitution of women fit their tasks as assigned by nature. Cabanis denounced the pretensions of *femmes-savantes* and rejected the view – purveyed by "philosophers" who "have regarded . . . [women's] weakness as the product of the life society imposes on them" – that women were the intellectual equals of men. "These philosophers," Cabanis rejoined, "have relied on certain rare phenomena which only prove that in this respect, as in many others, nature may sometimes accidentally cross her own limits."[125] In company with other legislators and theorists who had observed the political mobilization of women in the early phase of the Revolution, Cabanis had a real horror of women who attempted to move outside their "natural sphere."[126] He buttressed physiological authority with the example of classical heroines when, in his *Lettre à Thurot*, he celebrated the peculiarly female virtues of Andromache:

How touching is this celestial woman who establishes a kind of cult in honor of her husband; [who] in the weakness of a suffering heart demands support and conceives none other than the heart of the great Hector; [who] shows the sweet submissiveness of a devoted soul which exists, feels, and desires only for the unique object of its affections.[127]

If sex difference was absolute in its determination of social role, distinctions caused by temperament, climate, and age were highly significant too. The four temperaments of classical theory – the phlegmatic, melancholic, atrabilious, and bilious – constituted a scheme for which Cabanis had considerable respect. He was well aware of the modifications introduced by "solidists" and stressed that even the ancients regarded the four temperaments as ideal types not to be looked for, unmixed, among living people, but to be regarded as a guide in therapeutics. This guide was all the more useful since the therapeutics of the science of man that Cabanis now pro-

125 This translation appears in *On the Relations Between the Physical and Moral Aspects of Man,* ed. George Mora, trans. M. D. Saidi, 2 vols. (Baltimore: Johns Hopkins University Press, 1981), 243.
126 On women in the Revolution, see Jane Abray, "Feminism in the French Revolution," *American Historical Review* 80 (1975): 43–62; Suzanne Desan, " 'Constitutional Amazons': Jacobin Women's Clubs in the French Revolution," in *Re-creating Authority*, 11–35.
127 Quoted in Picavet, *Les Idéologues,* 270.

posed encompassed not just the sick individual but the troubled social order. Temperament, like sex, set the bounds within which moral and intellectual improvement could be expected.[128]

Cabanis's treatment of the "modifications" caused by age was, as suggested earlier, classic vitalism. He adopted the scheme of the four "stages of life" – childhood, youth, maturity, and old age – each of which was marked by a characteristic condition of humors and solids, by a certain degree of sensibility, by peculiar diseases, and by special "penchants and ideas." In youth the solids grow supple and strong, the blood and humors increase in vitality, the nervous system exhibits its "highest tone," the spirit is dominated by imagination, illusion, and romance. In youth, vital energy was concentrated in the chest and the generative region. It was a well-established, though admittedly mysterious, fact that the diseases of youth (such as consumption) were linked to intense "venereal desire." Cabanis rejected the explanation of "the chemists" that animal heat was generated by combustion in the lungs, a view that might seem to explain the link between *poitrine* and groin. Rather this nexus of desire and disease was "one of the numerous examples presented by the animal economy in which one sees the interweaving [*entrelacement*] of phenomena."[129] The only true interpretation of such phenomena was suggested by the Hippocratic image of life as a circle, without beginning or end. "In the organization all parts are tied one to another; . . . the functions all presuppose one another and are all essential to the order of the whole."[130]

In old age, by contrast, the humors become acrimonious and settle in afflicted areas, the elements separate (hence the creation of stones), the skin hardens, circulation slows, the vital movements are interrupted, mental operations lag, the spirit becomes timid, "fearful," and egoistic.[131] With the old, the task of the physician was to help them achieve nobility in death and to "render it sweet." Death was not to be fended off but to be accepted, gently, as the closing of the "circle of life." Such was "the influence medicine must establish one day in perfecting and achieving the greatest well-being for the human race."[132] The benefits of medicine thus conceived were not technical but moral.

Finally, Cabanis urged vigilant attention to the formative influence of climate. Voyagers and naturalists had proved that "each latitude has its character, each climate its color." The animals characteristic of various regions were the "living image of the locale" and the human beings so different that they might best be thought of as distinct species.[133] Climates formed integrated environments just as the milieu of the body was an interconnected whole: "The nature of the waters is connected to that of the earth; the air is linked to the soil, the direction of rivers and mountains, the combination of

128 Cabanis, "Rapports," 316–58.   129 *Ibid.*, 255.   130 *Ibid.*   131 *Ibid.*, 263–66.
132 *Ibid.*, 270–71.   133 *Ibid.*, 461.

gases and other exhalations. The vegetable productions reflect the qualities of the earth and waters."[134] All these features left an indelible imprint on both animals and human beings.

The physical analogy between man and the objects that surround him and on which he depends for the satisfaction of his needs is so striking that one can by a simple inspection almost always determine the nature and zone of the climate to which each individual belongs.[135]

Hippocrates continued to be the most reliable source on all such matters; "moderns" either denied the role of climate altogether or immoderately exaggerated it. In any event the medical perspective alone could genuinely illuminate such problems for, in this case as in all others pertaining to fundamental organization, the key lay in sensibility: "Human sensibility is, in comparison to that of all other known animal species, the most supple and mobile, so that any [agent] that acts on other living creatures generally acts in much stronger fashion on [man]."[136] This being the case, human beings were more or less irrevocably molded by the complex and interlinked agents – internal and external – that acted on sensibility. Once "constant impressions" modified "organic dispositions," such "modifications [were] fixed in the races." The influence of locale was thus inescapable: "all the industry of man cannot change it."[137]

It would be misleading to try to derive from these typologizing procedures and schemes any final word on whether anthropological medicine was "fixist" or "meliorist" in its orientation, whether it did or did not have a coherent and stable theory of "race," whether it preached "perfectibility" or denied it. Ample evidence can be found in the medical discourse of the period for either side of such dichotomies. In some instances the doctors stressed the irrevocability of "organization," in others the possibilities for altering it. In some passages internal "agents" were given primacy, in others "external." Some individual writers were predominantly "pessimistic," others more "optimistic." And of course the individual theorists themselves went through evolutions of thought dependent on political and personal circumstances of the moment. What counts in all this, then, is not so much the nuances of doctrine or individual opinion as the bedrock of the whole endeavor, which lay in an inherent disposition to typologize deriving from the general theoretical and therapeutic system of vitalist medicine, and in certain hypotheses and assumptions about human organization, of which the doctrine of limited energy is the most significant.

Nevertheless it must be said that the vitalism of the medical revolutionaries did exercise a genuinely conservative influence because of the inherent constraints it imposed on any vision of the human organism and its potentialities. As I argued in Chapter 1, it was impossible within such a system

134 *Ibid.*   135 *Ibid.*, 460–61.   136 *Ibid.*, 473.   137 *Ibid.*, 468.

to embrace any boundless teleological progressivism since limits to progress, perfectibility, and improvement were established by the fundamental character of living economies. In this sense vitalism is a clearly "premodern" system; it postulates as its ultimate values not movement forward, upward, outward, or beyond, but tranquil, uninterrupted, systemic harmony. That men who were "revolutionaries" – as these men were – should have clung to and more fully developed such a system is indicative, I think, of the tensions, paradoxes, and ambiguities characteristic of the larger Revolution. In company with the Ideologues, the medical revolutionaries wanted to change the world in profound ways, not least in replacing the influence of traditional elites with medical authority throughout diverse domains of social experience. Their institutional renovations and enterprises – which transformed the hospitals, medical education, the medical bureaucracy – also make manifest their revolutionary ambitions. But at the core of their vision of the new society and of the relations of those social elements – classes, sexes, generations, families – whose meaning and situation the Revolution threw into question, there was a profound reluctance to leave the past behind. This reluctance was to characterize much of French medicine from the Revolution forward, so that in the era that has been seen to usher in medical modernism what may be perceived instead is a reassertion by anthropological medicine – in language and terms that are sometimes deceptively "new" – of distinctly premodern conceptions both of the human body and of the social body in whose restructuring medicine now sought to play so important a role.

COMMENTARY ON GALL: THE POLITICS OF LIMITED PERFECTIBILITY

The general conception of human nature that underlay the medical science of man becomes clearer if we compare these teachings on human types to those of another system that sparked great interest in medical circles in precisely the years considered here, the phrenology of Franz-Josef Gall. The story of Gall's flight from Vienna, his arrival in Paris, and the excitement caused by his lectures has been told many times.[138] Although less is known of the close texture of Gall's life in Paris – his intellectual friends and enemies, the institutions that received or rebuffed him – the information available indicates, not surprisingly, that among Gall's most attentive listeners were the architects of anthropological medicine. Their commitment to the

138 Erwin Ackerknecht and Henri V. Vallois, *Franz G. Gall: Inventor of Phrenology and His Collection*, trans. Claire St. Leon (Madison: University of Wisconsin Medical School, 1956); Georges Lantéri-Laura, *Histoire de la phrénologie: L'homme et son cerveau selon F. J. Gall* (Paris: Presses universitaires de France, 1970); Owsei Temkin, "Gall and the Phrenological Movement," *BHM* 21 (1947): 275–321; Robert M. Young, *Mind, Brain, and Adaptation in the Nineteenth Century* (Oxford: Clarendon Press, 1970).

"analysis of ideas," revolutionary politics, and Ideology predisposed them to interest in a system whose aim, in Gall's words, was to "determine the relation between intellectual faculties and the organism."[139] The Ideologues' circle gave Gall an early hearing, publishing an account of his doctrines in the *Décade philosophique* as early as 1804. Shortly after his arrival in Paris in 1807, Gall began teaching at the Athénée, one of the ad hoc institutions of higher learning that sprang up early in the Revolution to replace the defunct faculties and academies. The niche Gall carved out for himself may not have been altogether comfortable – his system soon came under strong attack from powerful quarters – but it was spacious enough to allow him to work, publish, and gain a wide reputation. The insights offered by Gall's "organology" were not for the most part congenial to Parisian biomedical circles, but the questions he posed were certainly the right ones in the institutional context established by the medical revolution and the theoretical setting constituted by the science of man.

Gall has frequently been regarded as an opponent of Condillac, sensationalism, and Ideology; Robert Young has argued, for instance, that Gall "rejected the tenets of sensationalism and sought to replace . . . the 'epistemological psychology' of Locke, Condillac, Destutt and Cabanis with a biological one."[140] Although this judgment is accurate in many respects, it obscures important affinities between Gall and the French medical revolutionaries. Gall was their ally in key ways, especially in his commitment to a thoroughly naturalistic approach to the mind–body problem. Like the Paris doctors, Gall banished metaphysical entities, inveighed against "systems," and privileged observation. He was committed, moreover, to methods derived from comparative anatomy and natural history that, if not actually used by the medical revolutionaries, were nevertheless much admired by them. Although most of Gall's references and citations are to authorities in the German world of biomedicine, he also paid frequent and lavish tribute to heroic figures in the French tradition such as Vicq d'Azyr.[141] Finally, Gall was as eloquent as any writer of the period on the obligation of medicine to tie its concerns to those of the larger social world and to become a truly universal *art de guérir*. He invoked the revered example of the Greeks when he bemoaned the modern fragmentation of physiology, medicine, legislation, education, and *morale*. Such a tendency was bad for medicine; it meant that few doctors recognized "the full extent of their sphere of activity and . . . the full dignity of their status."[142] It was equally bad for society, which sorely needed the services of "doctor-observers" whose knowledge of "human nature [was] certain and

---

139 Franz-Josef Gall and G. Spurzheim, *Anatomie et physiologie du système nerveux en général et du cerveau en particulier*, 4 vols. (Paris: F. Schoell, 1810–19), I:iii.
140 Young, *Mind, Brain and Adaptation*, 15.
141 Gall and Spurzheim, *Anatomie et physiologie*, I:lii.   142 *Ibid.*, lix.

profound."[143] Only the doctor – no other – could command that intimate knowledge of physical and moral needs demanded by the healing art:

To whom does human nature reveal herself with less constraint? Who knows better the needs of men? . . . Who has more occasion than the doctor to see men in the state of absolute abandon? Who is more fully obliged to study both the physical and the moral? Who, further, is better prepared by accessory knowledge and the study of nature? Finally, who takes note so often as the doctor of the influence of nutriments, drinks, temperament, climate . . . ? The doctor alone, night and day, is witness to the most secret events and most intimate relations of families.[144]

Above all, the affinity between Gall and the revolutionary doctors lay in their mutual commitment to discerning the somatic basis of mental function. Like Cabanis, who described thought as a "secretion of the brain," and Bichat, who perceived a correlation between brain size and mental acuity, Gall was in search of the material key to the operations of mind. In this respect his break with the classical epistemology of Locke and Condillac was no more radical than that already effected by the medical science of man. Indeed Cabanis had stood Condillac's statue on its head by giving as much analytic weight to the effect of "internal impressions" that were determined by "fundamental organization" as he did to "exterior sensations."[145] In this sense the Paris doctors' science of man and Gall's organology participated in a general biomedical transmutation of the procedures and conclusions of eighteenth-century analytic philosophy. Locke had bracketed the body in the famous opening paragraph to the *Essay Concerning Human Understanding:*

I shall not at present meddle with the physical consideration of the mind; or trouble myself to examine wherein its essence consists; or by what motions of our spirits or alterations of our bodies we come to have any *sensation* by our organs, or any *ideas* in our understandings; and whether those ideas do in their formation, any or all of them, depend on matter or not.[146]

Condillac had reflected on the operations of mind with the help of a hypothetical statue rather than a living body. No biomedical theoretician – from Paris or Vienna – was disposed to do anything similar in the years around 1800.

All this being said, however, it remains true that there were important differences – methodological and substantial – between the psychophysiology of Paris medicine and of Gall. In respect to method, even Gall's most stringent critics – Cuvier, or later Pierre Flourens – hailed Gall's anatomical skill. Flourens, whose own accomplished experiments on the cerebellum

143 *Ibid.*, lvi.   144 *Ibid.*, lvi–lvii.
145 See the preceding section, "From Physiology to Moral Science."
146 John Locke, *An Essay Concerning Human Understanding*, ed. Maurice Cranston (New York: Collier Books, 1965), 25.

launched a highly successful career in the 1820s, wrote in his *Examen de la phrénologie* (1842) that Gall was a great anatomist who had recovered from a debased tradition the proper procedures for dissecting and studying brains.[147] And the famous 1808 report by a committee of the Institute – chaired by the surgeon Jacques Tenon, and including as members Antoine Portal, Cuvier, Pinel, and R.-B. Sabatier – praised Gall's "steady and sure manner" in dissection while dismissing his "physiological doctrine" as unscientific.[148]

In his anatomical skill Gall differed from all the doctors examined here with the single (and certainly important) exception of Bichat. The union between medicine and surgery had just been effected on a nationwide basis, and surgical skill was admired largely in the abstract by medical theorists like Cabanis, Alibert, and Pinel. Consequently, their approach to the problems of psychophysiology was not anatomical but medical and physiological, meaning that they observed sick people and then reflected on their observations. Extracting, slicing, and palpating brains – in Gall's way – was not something they did. Pinel certainly looked at brains on occasion to see if brain damage necessarily accompanied mental disease. (He concluded that it did not. To Pinel the physical component of mental disorder was just as likely to reside in the play of organic sympathies, "regional" distress, or generalized trouble with the whole organization as it was to lie in localized brain lesion.)[149] Thus Gall's disposition to look closely at the brain to find the explanation for mental function set him apart from the Paris reformers. In Paris comparable investigations on the brain were undertaken only by comparative anatomists, and then almost exclusively on animal brains and without any intention to elaborate comprehensive psychophysiological principles – for animals or humans – on the basis of the results.[150] It might be argued that Gall's enormous and to some extent scandalous reputation in France derived precisely from his blending of two research traditions that, to this point at least, had remained rigorously separated there – medical theorizing on physicomoral *rapports* and intensive anatomical investigation of the human brain.[151]

147 Pierre Flourens, *Examen de la phrénologie* (Paris: Paulin, 1842), 28, 102.
148 "Report on a memoir of Drs Gall and Spurzheim, relative to the anatomy of the brain. By M. M. Tenon, Portal, Sabatier, Pinel, and Cuvier, presented to, and adopted by the Class of Mathematical and Physical Sciences of the National Institute," *Edinburgh Medical and Surgical Journal* 5 (1809): 36–66, at 36–37, 51.
149 Pinel, *Traité médico-philosophique*, 3, 16, 111–33.
150 Cuvier was willing, however, to make commonplace observations on the apparent physical basis of "negro inferiority" in his reflections on the "Hottentot Venus." See Georges Cuvier, "Extraits d'observations faites sur le cadavre d'une femme connue à Paris et à Londres sous le nom de Vénus Hottentote," *Mémoires du Muséum d'histoire naturelle* 3 (1817): 259–74.
151 On the state of brain research in France from Descartes to Gall, see Jules Soury, *Le système nerveux central, Structures et fonctions: Histoire critique des théories et des doctrines*, 2 vols. (Paris: Georges Carré et C. Naud, 1899), 1:371–516.

Now it might be objected that Gall's vaunted anatomical skill created no real difference between him and the Paris doctors since his psychophysiology in fact bore little relation to his anatomical work. It is certainly true that he did not find, or even attempt to find, precise "organs" within the brain corresponding to the twenty-seven "faculties" of his psychological theory. But this objection is anachronistic. Flourens was to make this charge – that Gall's physiology had no genuine anatomical basis – in 1842, but only after three decades of experimentation on the brain and nervous system had intervened. In 1807–8, the years of Gall's arrival in Paris and his rebuff by the Institute committee, his work in brain anatomy was as sophisticated as any being done, and it was the methodological foundation for his organology. He was convinced that the precise location and nature of the components of the brain where the faculties were situated would become known. This readiness to look for precise physical points of origin for multiple, discrete psychological faculties set him apart from Parisian theorists, who were much more concerned with systemic relations between the physical and the moral than they were with seeking the precise organological sites of distinct faculties.

The faults that the Paris doctors found in Gall's procedures were spelled out by Moreau de la Sarthe in a series of articles on Gall written for the *Décade philosophique* in an XII (1804). In Moreau's view, the insights and findings of "physiological metaphysics" controverted Gall's brain-centered system for explaining the physical-moral relation. Physiology taught that the passions and the intellectual functions, far from being governed by the brain alone, were influenced by the "whole organization." Gall was in error in

making everything that is linked to instinct, appetites, and moral affections depend on the brain. These last depend almost always on organization in general, or on organic particularities that constitute the diverse modes of constitution.[152]

Proof for the significance of "overall constitution" lay in the role of temperaments, whether interpreted with the humoralists as the result of the character and action of the fluids or with the solidists as the consequence of the nature of the fibers.[153] Nor could Gall's one-to-one organ-faculty psychology explain the diverse effects of substances like opium, coffee, or *vin de champagne,* which produced temporary results not in keeping with Gall's static typology. The role of illness was also neglected in his system. Valuable evidence – such as Pinel's observation that maniacs enjoyed heightened imagination, or the case of Rousseau, which showed that hypo-

---

152 Moreau, "Exposition et critique du système du Dr. Gall, sur la cause et l'expression des principales différences de l'esprit et des passions, lues à l'Athénée de Paris," *Décade*, nos. 12–14 (an XII), 129–37; 194–202; 257–65.

153 *Ibid.*, 261.

chondria could produce "eloquence and sublimity" – found no place in Gall's theory.[154]

Moreau's most profound objection to Gall's ideas lay, however, neither in differences of method nor in the handling of concepts like "faculty" or "organization." Rather, Moreau's opposition to Gall was rooted in a moral repugnance scarcely less intense than that which prompted Cuvier's Institute committee to dismiss Gall's system out of hand. What would be, Moreau asked, the moral consequences of a system like Gall's?

Although we are very far from contesting the influence of the physical on the moral, although we are even forced to admit that there exist temperaments and modes of organic constitution better suited to great development of the intellectual faculties, or to the habit of generous actions, still we cannot dissimulate that if each modification of the heart and spirit [*esprit*] were regarded as a distinct faculty, dependent on a particular organ, there would no longer exist any morality in the actions of men. The unfaithful and adulterous woman, the swindler, the thief, even the murderer – finding themselves such by virtue only of the dominance of their organs of physical love, of ruse, of larceny, and sanguinary penchants – would justify themselves by accusing nature [itself].[155]

The horror of barbarism, immorality, and disorder in the role of women that had characterized medical rhetoric since Thermidor is manifest here again. Moreau strongly denied that such considerations entered into his assessment of Gall. If Gall's system were true, he insisted, then Fontenelle's counsel should be followed: admit the truth but reserve it for the wise. "But it is *not* true!" he exclaimed, and his palpable relief belies the claim that he judged Gall purely on scientific grounds.

Moreau's evaluation of Gall is congruent with the general ideological temper of the medical science of man. Science could guide, it could improve. It could not change fundamental human nature, nor should it try. A society in which the activities of murderers and adulteresses were explained away by the influence of "nature" would be a society with no moral bearings. The science of man gave guidance to morality; it did not supplant it.[156] In this commentary on Gall the tensions and ambiguities in anthropological medicine are again evident. The brain was the organ of thought, but its influence was not determinative. Anatomical and surgical techniques were great boons, but their importance must not be exaggerated. Temperamental, constitutional, and material influences on mind and character were profound, but men and women must be held accountable for their actions. Medical science must replace religion, but the old morality must remain unshaken.

154 *Ibid.*, 259–60.   155 *Ibid.*, 257–58.
156 A similar set of objections was raised by French doctors and social theorists in the 1880s to the theories of Cesare Lombroso; see the Epilogue.

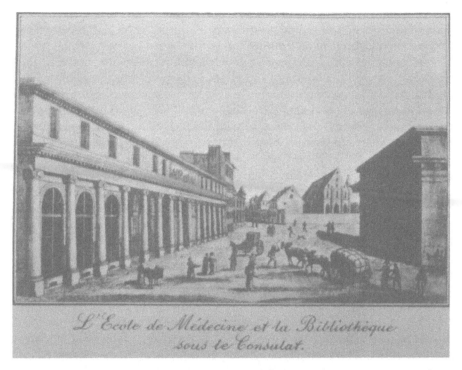

View of the Paris Ecole de Médecine and Bibliothèque under the Consulate.

THE SCIENCE OF MAN IN THE ERA OF BONAPARTE

By the time that Moreau wrote his critique of Gall for the *Décade philoso-phique* (an XII/1804), the position of the Ideologues and the medical revo-lutionaries within the Parisian political, cultural, and intellectual milieu had changed markedly from the days of the Directory. After the fall of Robes-pierre, the adherents of Ideology had come to occupy a range of important positions in the capital: Daunou and Garat sat on the Committee for Public Education; Cabanis was a member of the Council of Five Hundred; Siéyès and Roederer appeared and reappeared in coalitions intended to stabilize Di-rectory politics.[157] In the wake of Thermidor, many Ideologues became in-creasingly conservative in personal temper and in political ideals, often clinging precariously even to the moderate constitutionalism that had typ-ified the politics of Destutt and Cabanis at the outbreak of the Revolution. Then from 1797 on, when the name of Napoleon Bonaparte came more fre-quently to be heard, and as the collapse of the Directory became imminent,

157 Picavet, *Les Idéologues*, 118–19, 401; Staum, *Cabanis*, 151; L. P. Williams, "Science, Ed-ucation, and the French Revolution," *Isis* 44 (1953): 311–30.

the Ideologues were required to make a judgment and take a position on the coming of Bonaparte's military-bureaucratic dictatorship. Some rushed to embrace him, fatigued and embittered as they were by past struggles, or pleased with the opportunities for power and advancement offered in the new meritocracy. Others waited and hoped, rejecting Bonaparte only when his imperial ambitions became wholly evident. Napoleon's attitude to them is well known. His epithet "the Ideologues" held all the contempt of the militarist for the thinker and stamped the lot of them as futile metaphysicians.[158] Although Napoleon recognized and used the knowledge, talents, and skills of those among the Ideologues who did not flagrantly defy him, the institutional base of Ideology was broken. The Second Class of the Institute was abolished in 1803. The curriculum of the *écoles centrales* was rewritten to restore religion and eventually the schools were replaced by the Napoleonic *lycées*. In 1807 the *Décade philosophique* was forced to merge with the pro-imperial *Mercure de France*.[159]

The position of the medical revolutionaries in these developments was mixed. Some key figures had already left the scene (Bichat died in 1802, Cabanis in 1807), while others (Moreau, Alibert, Pinel) retained their positions in the institutions created anew or refurbished by the Revolution. But they all uniformly ceased addressing the larger concerns of the medical science of man and restricted their labors to specialized problems, especially in therapeutics. The altered tone of the publications of the Société médicale d'émulation in these years is unmistakable. The names of contributors were now followed by lengthy lists of imperial posts and titles; the subject matter of the journal excluded any "metaphysical" topics. In short the grand goals of anthropological medicine – deciphering the relations of the physical and moral, rendering clear and distinct the "analysis of ideas," providing exclusive guidance to *morale* – were shelved. All of this was in keeping with Bonaparte's hostility to doctors and to medicine generally, and with his special disdain for medicine tinged with Ideology.[160]

Still, far from bringing the medical revolution to an end, Bonapartism eventually assured to official medicine the most important concrete legal and bureaucratic gains of the whole period. It was under Bonaparte that

158 Léonard cites this charge Napoleon made against doctors: "Voilà comment vous êtes tous avec vos principes d'école, médecins, chirurgiens, pharmaciens! Plutôt que d'en sacrifier un seul, vous feriez périr toute une armée et toute la société" (*Les médecins de l'Ouest*, 255). Léonard also notes, however, Napoleon's interest in medicine and the friendly gestures he made toward individual doctors (254–56). Evidence of his regard for surgeons appears in Jules Coquerelle, *Xavier Bichat (1771–1802)* (Paris: Maloine, 1902).

159 Gusdorf, *La conscience révolutionnaire*, 315–30; Kitchin, *Un journal "philosophique,"* 22–25; Williams, "Science, Education"; *idem*, "Science, Education, and Napoleon I," *Isis* 47 (1956): 369–82, esp. 380.

160 These changes in the *Mémoires de la Société médicale d'émulation* are especially noticeable in vol. 7 (1811). Bonaparte was equally hostile to Gall and his "materialism"; see Soury, *Système nerveux central*, 1:503.

doctors gained a legal monopoly over the practice of medicine. The law of 19 Ventôse, an XI (1803) established new requirements for the training and certification of doctors that gave the medical faculties more power than they had ever had under the Old Regime. Legal structures now excluded from medical practice itinerant empirics, midwives, popular healers, and, perhaps most important to advocates of the science of man, clerical practitioners, whose mix of inept therapeutics and superstitions they particularly deplored.[161]

In 1802 the Bonapartist regime established the Conseil de salubrité de Paris et du Département de la Seine, a council of advisors to the Empire that elaborated the new medical framework that came to be known as "public health."[162] Among the council's early members were a number of doctors and surgeons who were linked to anthropological medicine by personal, pedagogical, and professional ties. Michel-Augustin Thouret, for example, had worked with Cabanis in the hospital reform movement. As dean of the Paris Ecole de santé (later Faculté de médecine) from 1794 to 1810, he was linked to Pinel, Cabanis, and Moreau de la Sarthe, all of whom held posts at the medical school during his tenure. Marc-Antoine Petit had been a close associate of Bichat, with whom he served on the staff of the Hôtel-Dieu. C. C. H. Marc was an active member of the Société médicale d'émulation (as were Thouret and other early members of the Conseil de salubrité). These biographical data would not be of much interest if the work of the Conseil de salubrité had not embodied the program of anthropological medicine in important respects. But this is precisely what it did, both in the practical measures it instituted to control the health "environment" to which anthropological medicine attached so much importance, and in its establishment of the "public" character and mission of medicine.[163]

Yet the gains that were made by medicine in legal and bureaucratic authority under Bonaparte were accompanied by the augmentation of state control over the medical establishment itself. The imperial government moved to achieve centralized control of Paris hospitals, for example, with the founding of the Conseil général d'administration des hôpitaux et hospices de Paris. This move was in some respects a boon to anthropological medicine: it prepared the way for establishment in the hospitals of the intern-extern program, which made available a pool of student labor for the accomplishment of myriad tasks required for proper "observation" (keeping notes of bedside visits, collecting data on climate and other influences). But it also helped to shift the emphasis in medical education away from theoretical subjects toward practical training in surgical techniques, the care of

---

161 Léonard provides an extensive analysis of the *ventôse* law in *Les médecins de l'Ouest*, 261–84; see also Ramsey, *Professional and Popular Medicine*, esp. 78–87.
162 Weiner, "Public Health under Napoleon."   163 *Ibid.*

wounds, and dissections, a deemphasis of the theoretical that was characteristic of the whole Bonapartist approach to medicine and its functions.[164]

In other ways, too, the regime asserted control over medical education. In 1808 the *écoles de santé* were transformed into faculties of medicine of the new Imperial University and their administration was brought under the control of the "Master" and the Conseil de l'Université. Thanks to the fact that the medical schools had already enjoyed some ten years of successful existence, they were left a higher degree of autonomy than the faculties of law and theology. But some powers were lost immediately to the bureaucracy and, more important, a structure and framework of state control – whose impact could increase at any moment – was now in place. From 1806 onward, moreover, the regime moved to create a number of regional medical schools (*écoles secondaires de médecine*) whose purpose was to train second-tier *officiers de santé* rather than full-fledged physicians.[165] This program served not only to attenuate the professional exclusiveness of physicians but to divert resources away from the three great faculties, whose overweening position in the teaching of medicine constituted a potential ideological threat.

These changes of the Bonapartist era significantly enhanced state control over medical education and practice while greatly augmenting the medical bureaucracy. The overall results were mixed. The authority of doctors was increased by the legal safeguarding of their prerogatives and the creation of new bureaucratic structures, especially those for public health. At the same time, however, the intellectual and ideological independence of medicine was undercut. This loss of autonomy occurred, moreover, at a moment when Bonaparte was simultaneously moving to affirm the privileges and standing of the new "Gallican" church, an institution that he believed had greater promise than medicine for service as an instrument of the state. In so doing he created the conditions for a continuing struggle over the nature, role, and dimensions of medicine that would continue for decades. The features this struggle assumed under the Restoration, and its impact on the medical science of man, are examined in the next chapter.

164 Coury, "The Teaching of Medicine in France," 165; J. M. D. Olmsted, *François Magendie: Pioneer in Experimental Physiology and Scientific Medicine in XIX Century France* (New York: Schuman's, 1944), 15.
165 Louis Liard, *L'enseignement supérieur en France (1789–1893)*, 2 vols. (Paris: Armand Colin, 1888; 1894), 2:93–147; Coury, "Teaching of Medicine," 151.

3

Medical politics under the Restoration: The fragmentation of the science of man

Medical historians portray the early nineteenth century as the "triumphal age" of French medicine. The years 1794–1848, isolated as the era of "hospital medicine," have been treated as the period when France made its greatest contribution to the development of modern medicine. The hospital itself is seen as a French creation, and valuable methods and techniques – clinical training, intensive study of cadavers, invention and use of the stethoscope, keeping of medical statistics – are credited to leaders of the "Paris school." In this age that saw what Foucault called "the birth of the clinic," many historians (though not Foucault himself) have seen medicine struggling to pull itself free from metaphysics, speculation, and philosophy. In a typically confident account of medicine's emergence from the prepositive state, Paul Triaire wrote in 1899 that after the Revolution a "new stratum of doctors" – "men of reason and action" – replaced "the pure speculators, the philosophers, the men of letters, the naturalists, the creators of dogmas and systems, the authors of new nomenclatures" who had dominated eighteenth-century medicine and long obstructed its progress.[1] The brilliance of early nineteenth-century French medicine is thus explained by the new vigor imparted by institutional renovation and the new disposition of French doctors to embrace scientific methods and to hone technical skills. Surgical precision, modern chemical analysis, close statistical observation – these were the hallmarks of Paris clinical medicine and the foundation of its stunning achievements.[2]

1 Paul Triaire, *Récamier et ses contemporains, 1774–1852: Études d'histoire de la médecine aux XVIIIe et XIXe siècles* (Paris: J. B. Baillière et fils, 1899), 142–43.
2 Erwin Ackerknecht, *Medicine at the Paris Hospital, 1794–1848* (Baltimore: Johns Hopkins University Press, 1967); David M. Vess, *Medical Revolution in France, 1789–96* (Gainesville: University of Florida Press, 1976); Dora B. Weiner, "Introductory Essay," in *The Clinical Training of Doctors: An Essay of 1793*, by Philippe Pinel (Baltimore: Johns Hopkins University Press, 1980), 3–22. The innovativeness of Paris clinicians is challenged by Othmar Keel, "The Politics of Health and the Institutionalisation of Clinical Practices in Europe in the Second Half of the Eighteenth Century," in *William Hunter and the Eighteenth-Century Medical World*, ed. W. F. Bynum and Roy Porter (Cambridge: Cambridge University Press, 1985), 207–56.

This portrait draws into the foreground those features of early nineteenth-century French medicine that seem most praiseworthy to admirers of modern medical organization and procedures. Yet it blurs, or eliminates altogether, other important elements of French medicine of the period. Accenting the role of medical individualists and innovators such as Laennec, it obscures the extent to which medical institutions – faculties, hospitals, medical press, learned societies – were brought under rigorous state control in this era, first by Napoleonic and then by Restoration bureaucrats. As we saw in Chapter 2, the elaboration of what Jan Goldstein has called a "statist model" of medical organization was pursued diligently by the Consulate and the Empire.[3] Thanks to the work of Napoleonic officialdom, a framework of state control over training, certification, hospital organization, and public health was now in place. The coming of the Restoration did not entail any dismantling of the apparatuses established by the Consulate and Empire to supervise public health and to control medical teaching and practice. The only significant innovation in respect to public health was the establishment within the Ministry of the Interior of the Conseil supérieur de santé, which was dominated by conservatives and functioned for a time as the chief stronghold of contagionist medicine.[4] In the bureaucracy charged with controlling medical education, some names and faces changed from the days of the Empire, although even in personnel there were crucial overlaps (Louis Fontanes continued as director of the university until 1822, for example, but without the Napoleonic title of *grand maître*).[5]

Certain elements of the medical establishment were unhappy with the degree of state control introduced by Bonaparte and looked to the Restoration regime to turn back the clock. The Montpellier professors, for example, requested of the king that they be "separated from the University and allowed to resume the independent existence that they had never ceased to enjoy . . . and to recover the prerogatives that had been granted them by popes and kings as a fitting recompense for their long and painful labors."[6] Similarly, discontented surgeons sought the reestablishment of the independent Collège and Académie de chirurgie. In response to such demands and in keeping with a more general sense that the new regime should put its own stamp on university teaching, a plan devised in February 1815 aimed to decentralize the system, creating seventeen largely autonomous provincial universi-

3 See Chapter 2.
4 Ann Fowler La Berge, *Mission and Method: The Early Nineteenth-Century Public Health Movement* (Cambridge: Cambridge University Press, 1992), chap. 3.
5 Alan B. Spitzer, *The French Generation of 1820* (Princeton: Princeton University Press, 1987), 189–90; the title of *grand maître* was revived in 1822; see Louis Liard, *L'enseignement supérieur en France (1789–1893)*, 2 vols. (Paris: Armand Colin, 1888, 1894), 1:150–51.
6 Quoted in Liard, *L'enseignement supérieur*, 1:139–40.

ties. But the Hundred Days intervened and the Second Restoration spelled the end to all such measures.[7] Despite the regime's initial hesitation in confirming the work of the Empire, few major changes in the university structure ever in fact took place. For a time the university was put under the control of a royal commission, the Commission (later Conseil royal) de l'instruction publique, which was headed by the Doctrinaire philosopher Pierre-Paul Royer-Collard up to 1819 and then by Georges Cuvier. By 1822, however, the title and position of *grand maître* had been revived, the university's Napoleonic constitution reaffirmed, and the university itself established as "a branch of royal power." In 1824 an independent ministry was created for education and religious affairs and the university's *grand maître* thus elevated to ministerial rank.[8] This multilayered bureaucracy served the Restoration as a powerful agent for the surveillance of higher education, including the teaching of medicine.

The significance of all these developments, beginning under the Consulate and continuing into the Restoration, was that medicine was, to a degree it had not been before, intensely politicized. This is not to say that either medical theory or medical establishments were apolitical in the days before Napoleon; certainly the *parti pris* of medical Ideology was manifest. Rather it means that the institutional arrangements now governing medical life made all medical decisions and discourse political acts, if for no other reason than that all medical people were empowered to practice by the state. The corporate or guild status of medicine was a memory, and professional autonomy (to the extent that that was ever achieved by French doctors) lay in the distant future.[9] For the medical elite – the faculty professors, the doctors who practiced and taught at the large hospitals – the situation was rendered extreme by the fact that they owed their appointments to the state and were paid with state money. Misstep could mean dismissal, a fact brought forcefully home to the Faculty of Medicine in 1822, when a purge of liberal professors was carried out. In that year the government, spurred to more systematic repressive measures by the assassination of the duc de Berry in 1820, and by a series of student disturbances, closed the doors of the Faculty of Medicine, suspended all classes for nearly a year, and dismissed one-third of the chairholders for opposition (suspected

7 *Ibid.*, 138–40. Plans to reorganize medical education, principally by again dividing surgical and medical training, are discussed in George Weisz, "Constructing the Medical Elite in France: The Creation of the Royal Academy of Medicine, 1814–20" *Medical History* 30 (1986): 419–43.

8 *Ibid.*

9 Matthew Ramsey, "The Politics of Professional Monopoly in Nineteenth-Century Medicine: The French Model and Its Rivals," in *Professions and the French State, 1700–1900*, ed. Gerald Geison (Philadelphia: University of Pennsylvania Press, 1983), 225–305; George Weisz, "The Politics of Medical Professionalization in France, 1815–48," *Journal of Social History* 12 (1978): 3–30.

or genuine) to the regime.[10] This action came in the wake of a tumultuous student demonstration, disrupting one of the elaborate ceremonies that were a prominent feature of faculty life under the Restoration. The demonstration supplied a handy pretext for action against the liberal professoriate that had already been contemplated by the newly appointed master of the university, the ultramontane Denis-Luc Frayssinous. With this move the government retired eleven professors – Pinel, Chaussier, Dubois, Jussieu, Desgenettes, Deyeux, Pelletan *père*, Lallement, Leroux, Moreau de la Sarthe, Vauquelin – a number of whom had played prominent roles in the medical revolution. The era of Cabanis seemed to be definitively closed.

When the faculty reopened in 1823, several crucial changes had been made in its operation. The government abolished the *concours* for appointments to the professoriate and thus did away with that element of Napoleon's meritocracy. Henceforward appointments were to be made solely on the basis of ministerial decisions, a move that in the view of some observers effectively excluded critics of the regime from the faculty until the close of the Restoration.[11] The carrot offered along with this stick was the establishment of the *agrégé* system, which did function on the basis of the *concours*. By this means some republicans succeeded in gaining access to the faculty citadel; in later years the ranks of the *agrégés* were often filled with young turks whose politics set them at odds with administrators and professors.[12] Despite such measures, however, reorganization of the faculty ensured that the institution would now be dominated by the regime's sympathizers.

Another crucial step in the Bourbon effort to give statist direction to the medical community was the founding in 1820 of the Académie royale de médecine, which was headed by figures friendly to the Restoration cause such as Antoine Portal (1742–1832), who in 1815 had been appointed as First Physician to Louis XVIII.[13] In 1820 Portal was well into his seventies and he had for many years occupied chairs at both the Collège de France and at the Muséum d'histoire naturelle, where he taught human anatomy. Aside from his overtly royalist politics, he was an appealing figure to the government because his teaching was traditionalist and innocuous. Portal made no claims whatsoever for extending medical and anatomical discussion into the

10 An account of the purge appears in Charles Odic, "Les événéments du 18 novembre 1822" (Thèse en médecine, Université de Paris, 1921). See also P. Menetrier, "Le centenaire de la suppression de la Faculté de Médecine de Paris," *Bulletin de la Société française de l'histoire de médecine* 16 (1922): 441–45.
11 Paul Broca, *Eloge de M. P.-N. Gerdy lu à la Société de Chirurgie le 2 juillet 1856* (extract *Moniteur des Hôpitaux*) (Paris, 1856), 25–27.
12 On the rebellious spirit of French medical students and lower faculty, see Francis Schiller, *Paul Broca: Founder of French Anthropology, Explorer of the Brain* (Berkeley: University of California Press, 1979), 16–58.
13 Weisz, "Constructing the Medical Elite," 435–42.

larger zones of metaphysics or morals.[14] The Académie de médecine exerted great influence within the medical community. George Weisz has written of the academy that it "came to serve as the major advisory body to the government on all health-related matters; it evaluated medical publications, awarded prizes, collected and examined epidemiological information, administered smallpox vaccinations, and supervised secret remedies and mineral waters."[15] The academy would later be criticized for the long-winded and pointless debates it sponsored, but in the Restoration years its prestige within the medical community was great.[16]

These institutional strictures on medical life were greatly reinforced by the general tenor of intellectual and cultural life under the Restoration. Napoleon had made censorship a fact of life and in this respect the Restoration reaffirmed his work, although it added prominent Bonapartists to its list of political enemies.[17] The coming of the Restoration renewed intellectual authority for conservative voices that had long been mute or spoken only from exile. The return to the cultural scene of figures such as Louis de Bonald meant that the terms of all intellectual debate were ineluctably changed from the revolutionary era, when Ideology was the byword, and from the Bonapartist period, when only practical or utilitarian subjects even found a forum.[18] The conservative intellectuals and theologians who came to the fore during the Restoration – at first in opposition to its putative moderation, then after 1820 in support of militant reaction – were determined to close the Napoleonic hiatus and rejoin combat with their ideological adversaries over moral and philosophical issues. Bonald's case is illustrative: after years in exile, hiding, and silence, and then a partial accommodation to Bonapartism, he worked ceaselessly to undermine the intellectual and political standing of those he held responsible for the years of revolution and chaos.[19]

Nor were the religiously inspired conservatives of Bonald's variety alone in their attack on the intellectual heritage of the eighteenth century and the revolutionary years. Already under Napoleon, philosophical critics, many of them erstwhile Ideologues, had launched an assault on sensationalism, Ideology, and medical efforts to reduce the moral to the physical. To these

---

14 Later anthropologists regarded Portal's long tenure in his teaching posts as inimical to the progress of anthropology in France; see Ernest-Théodore Hamy, "La collection anthropologique du Muséum national d'histoire naturelle," *L'anthropologie* 18 (1907): 257–76, esp. 262–65.

15 Weisz, "Constructing the Medical Elite," 440.

16 For one such critique, see *Archives générales de médecine*, 4th ser., 11 (1846): 115.

17 The predicament of Bonapartist intellectuals is lamented in Jean-Baptiste Bory de Saint-Vincent, *Justification de la conduite et des opinions politiques de M. Bory de Saint-Vincent*, 2d ed. (Brussels: Chez les Marchands de Nouveautés, 1816).

18 On the constraints placed on scientific inquiry by the Bonapartist regime, see L. P. Williams, "Science, Education, and Napoleon I," *Isis* 47 (1956): 369–82.

19 Henri Moulinié, *De Bonald: La vie, la carrière politique, la doctrine* (1916; rpt. New York: Arno Press, 1979).

sources were imputed all the philosophical and moral horrors conveyed by the word "materialism," which in this period functioned less as a philosophical concept than as a term of abuse hurled at medical theorists by their detractors.[20] Former Ideologues were in several cases the bitterest critics of materialism and the revolutionary past. Cabanis's old friend François-Pierre Maine de Biran came to embrace a thoroughly Catholicized doctrine of human nature that posited the existence of three autonomous "lives" – the material, the intellectual, and the moral. Pierre Laromuiguière, once a close associate of the Ideologues, rejected sensationalism on the grounds that it took account only of the "passive" reception of sensations and denied the force of human "activity."[21] This emphasis on the active character of mental function had been prefigured in the work of the Montpellier physiologist Charles-Louis Dumas who, though in many respects a great admirer of Cabanis, nonetheless tried to find some middle course between Cabanisian materialism and conservative interpretations of the legacy of Bordeu and Barthez.[22] Like many other critics of Ideology, Dumas insisted that sensations were transformed into thought only once the mind had done its multiform work:

> The mind reacts on [sensations] and works on them in diverse ways. It links, disposes, ties, and combines some of them; others it distinguishes, separates, divides, and reduces. All of them it submits to its own operations. Multiplying and augmenting them, it adds the fruit of its own considered reflections [*connaissances réfléchies*]. These last operations depend on a faculty that must not be confused with that of feeling. . . . Such is the work of reflection, which combines with sensation to create all the knowledge [*science*] of which the human understanding is capable.[23]

Physiological formulations that, like this one, drew on classical Lockeanism had some appeal to those who were in retreat from Ideology. But ultimately the most influential antimaterialist doctrine was the work of the philosopher Victor Cousin who, as Jules Simon later wrote, was regarded by many as having utterly demolished "the Ideologues and the sensationalists."[24] From 1817 to 1820, Cousin taught at the Ecole normale supérieure as *suppléant* for Royer-Collard. From his lectern Cousin attacked the sensationalist principle that all knowledge is sense-derived and hence dependent on the sensory apparatuses of the body. According to his interpretation of "psychology," a word and concept he privileged since it de-

20 L. S. Jacyna, "Medical Science and Moral Science: The Cultural Relations of Physiology in Restoration France," *History of Science* 25 (1987): 111–46, esp. 113–14.
21 Quoted in George Boas, *French Philosophies of the Romantic Period* (New York: Russell and Russell, 1964), 37. See also F. C. T. Moore, *The Psychology of Maine de Biran* (Oxford: Clarendon, 1970).
22 Charles-Louis Dumas, *Principes de physiologie, ou introduction à la science expérimentale, philosophique et médicale de l'homme vivante,* 4 vols. (Paris: Crapelet, 1800–3).
23 *Ibid.,* 1:9.
24 Jules Simon, *Victor Cousin,* 2d ed. (Paris: Hachette, 1887), 76.

marcated a special branch of inquiry for the mind alone, sensationalism was based on false, abstract reasoning that denied the universal human experience of an innate, interior sense of unity and continuity constituting the "self" (*moi*). Without the structural, organizing principles given in consciousness, Cousin held, sense experience was meaningless. Intellectual function had its origin, then, not in the workings of the material, sensory apparatuses but in unitary consciousness as given natively to human beings in creation. Accordingly, psychology must be rigorously divided into two domains: the study of sensory operations in the body, which was properly the concern of medicine and physiology, and the study of consciousness, which must be reserved for philosophy. Method too was to be tailored to suit these mutually exclusive endeavors. "Observation" was appropriate to investigations of sensation and the material apparatuses of the body, but only a kind of rational intuition, the "spontaneous . . . pure apperception of reason," could shed any real light on the workings of mind.[25]

Of course, Cousin was himself too liberal for Restoration Ultras. His "eclectic" position, which took psychology away from materialist physicians and returned it to metaphysics, was unacceptable to clerical supporters of the regime. To the genuine theocrats, philosophy had no greater authority than medicine on matters of intellect. As the instrument of human rationality, judgment, and moral choice, intellect belonged to the domain of theology. In 1821 Cousin was eased out of his teaching position and then in 1824 he was arrested when crossing the border back from Germany, where he had gone to visit his friend and mentor G. W. F. Hegel. His six-month imprisonment caused an "explosion" of indignation against the government.[26] Throughout most of the 1820s Cousin himself was officially silenced, but his attack on sensationalism, Ideology, and "materialism" was carried on by associates and disciples who were all the more devoted to Cousin, given the bitterness of his "martyrdom."[27]

In such a climate the moral, political, and ideological conflicts within and surrounding medicine were once again violently engaged. All the problems raised but left unresolved by anthropological medicine – the nature of mind, sensibility, and passion; the role of the physician in society; the possibilities for medicosocial perfectibility – returned with force. In this environment the term science of man came to serve as an enabling rubric for diverse, always highly charged medical programs and polemics that spanned the political and ideological spectrum from Right (turncoat Ideologues, Montpellier conservatives) to Center (eclectics, hygienists, advo-

25 Lucien Lévy-Bruhl, *History of Modern Philosophy in France* (1899; rpt. Chicago: Open Court Publishing, 1924), 330–51, at 339.
26 Simon, *Victor Cousin*, 22; see also Alan Spitzer, *Old Hatreds and Young Hopes: The French Carbonari against the Bourbon Restoration* (Cambridge, Mass.: Harvard University Press, 1971), 206–9, 268.
27 Simon, *Victor Cousin*, 22.

cates of mental medicine) to Left (Broussais's "physiological medicine"). Yet although the term science of man ceased to have any single or precise signification, its fragmentation and dispersal entailed not a loss but a heightening of rhetorical power. We customarily think that intellectual traditions gain authority as they move in a linear development toward the conquest of coherence. This view may be by and large correct, but I argue in this chapter that anthropological medicine developed within a fragmented discursive field and that this very process was the condition for its widespread influence. Disagreements about the overt content of the science of man – often centering on the notorious problem of the body-mind relation – tended to obscure the extent to which there were deep layers of consensus on the existence of an intimate physical-moral relation, on the social character of medicine, and on medicine's capacity to sift, sort, and classify the physicomoral types produced by diverse modes of physiological and social organization. To a large extent, medical disputation during the Restoration was locked inside the framework of old battles, and the heat generated by attempts to gain new victories on old ground obscured the extent to which physicians across the ideological spectrum shared the common intention and goal of medicalizing French society. To this end, the assertion that medicine constituted a general science of man was diversely useful.

RENOUNCING IDEOLOGY

Aside from Cabanis himself, no individual of the revolutionary era more fully typified the medical Ideologue than J.-L. Alibert (1768–1837). As a youth in Aveyron he was a friend to Laromuiguière and the Abbé Sicard. On his arrival in Paris in 1794 he studied at the Ecole normale and at the Muséum d'histoire naturelle with Volney, Monge, Garat, and other prominent figures of the Ideologue circle.[28] His contacts at the Autueil salon, especially with Cabanis, Pinel, and Roussel, inspired him to take up medical studies. As a student at the Ecole de santé in its critical formative years of the mid–1790s, Alibert was a founding member of the Société médicale d'émulation and made important contributions to its Mémoires.[29]

In medical philosophy and method, Alibert typified the blend of Montpellier doctrine and Condillacian philosophy characteristic of anthropological medicine. He embraced the expectant posture of Montpellier medicine

---

28 On these figures, see Georges Gusdorf, *Les sciences humaines et la pensée occidentale*, vol. 8, *La conscience révolutionnaire: Les idéologues* (Paris: Payot, 1978); Volney has received extended attention in Jean Gaulmier, *L'Idéologue Volney, 1757–1820: Contribution à l'orientalisme en France* (1951; rpt. Paris: Slatkine, 1980).

29 L. Brodier, *J.-L. Alibert, médecin de l'Hôpital Saint-Louis (1768–1837)* (Paris: A. Maloine, 1923), 291–362.

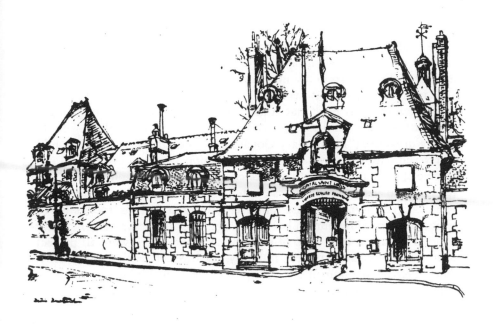

Sketch of the Hôpital Saint-Louis, with inscription "Liberté, Egalité, Fraternité" above the entrance.

and worked to develop natural therapeutics such as hydrology.[30] Alibert was also deeply impressed by the merits of "analysis," whose procedures he learned chiefly from his cherished friend Pinel. Alibert was in sympathy with the goals of the early Revolution, but he was appalled by what he judged the fanatical violence of the Terror.[31] The exact course and pace of Alibert's turning away from Ideology and liberal politics are not known, but the change was already complete by 1815, when, on the return of Louis XVIII to the throne, Alibert was appointed as medical consultant to the king. In 1821 he was favored by an appointment to the Paris Faculty of Medicine as professor of botany, an appointment that was interrupted by the 1822 purge. When the faculty reopened in 1823 with its new conservative appointees, Alibert's place was secure, though in a new slot: from 1823 to his death in 1837 he was professor of therapeutics and *materia medica*. In these years he continued to hold a prestigious hospital position, as *médecin-en-chef* at the Hôpital Saint-Louis, to which he had been appointed during the Napoleonic years.[32] In the early years of the Restoration Alibert seems to have been known chiefly for his work on diseases of the skin and for his clinical teaching. For a long time he wrote nothing on the medical science of man, but in 1825 he published the two-volume *Physiologie des passions, ou*

30 *Ibid.*, 227–28.   31 *Ibid.*, 302.   32 *Ibid.*, 306–16.

nouvelle doctrine des sentimens moraux, a work that went through many editions in several languages and established Alibert as a prominent spokesman for the kind of medicosocial moralizing that found favor with the regime.[33]

Alibert opened the *Physiologie des passions* with an immediate reproach to the "materialists": "To know man, one must seek him in his soul and not in the material organs that make up his bodily envelope."[34] Yet it was apparent from the first page that Alibert had no intention of abandoning to materialist science the language and constructs of "physiology." In his opening discourse ("Preliminary Considerations on the Sensitive System"), Alibert laid bare the flaws in classical sensationalism and proposed a new doctrine of mental function that reconciled the findings of physiology with "fundamental verities."[35] The catchphrases and ritual exhortations of the medical science of man – praise for observation and analysis; recognition of the necessity to know human beings by age, sex, and temperament; determination to unveil the "laws of the animal economy" – were all present, but in a new context supplied, tellingly, by Bossuet. Following Bossuet, Alibert averred that human physiology must be joined with "la morale" to form "true philosophy."[36]

Yet for true philosophy to prevail, the false philosophy of materialism had first to be destroyed, and to that end Alibert revived and reasserted the theologically sanctioned doctrine of innatism. Against Locke and Condillac he argued that although some of our "ideas" were acquired through the sensory apparatuses, those that were the most elevated and the most characteristically human constituted the "inspired" knowledge of the soul. Thus the soul was the "true source of our most intense joys" and of the most basic truths, whereas the senses were the stuff of our lower nature and indeed formed that part of human makeup that was shared with the animals.[37] Indeed human sensory capacities were much inferior to those of the beasts, whose wondrous sense accomplishments had long been admired by natural historians.[38]

33 J.-L. Alibert, *Physiologie des passions, ou nouvelle doctrine des sentimens moraux,* 2 vols. (Paris: Béchet jeune, 1825). All references here are to the 1827 edition.
34 *Ibid.,* 1:i.   35 *Ibid.,* lxxxiii.
36 *Ibid.,* xv. On Bossuet as defender of absolutism, see Keith Michael Baker, *Inventing the French Revolution: Essays on French Political Culture in the Eighteenth Century* (Cambridge: Cambridge University Press), 113–14, 225–26.
37 Alibert, *Physiologie des passions,* 1:xv–xx.
38 *Ibid.,* xvii–xx. Scattered throughout the book are illustrations of the sense superiority of animals, which became a hallowed element of conservative physiology. In the 1860s anthropologists of the Broca school would make much of this principle in the context of a debate over "man's place in nature" set off by T. H. Huxley's book of that title. By then the argument that the great distance between humans and animals was evident from the inferiority of human sensory response was something of a truism, especially as it had come to be coupled with the principle of limited energy discussed in Chapter 2: the high development of sensory apparatuses in animals precluded their further intellectual development while human intellectual power necessarily implied diminished sensory acuity. See my discussion in the Epilogue.

This was the stuff of old-fashioned moralism: man's higher and lower nature, senses against mind and soul, and so on.[39] But Alibert was eager to show that innatism meant not only the existence of a soul, and a preordained awareness of moral truths, but also that it embodied the only correct understanding of sense-derived knowledge itself. Here he drew on arguments advanced by the Scottish faculty psychologists to hold that prior to sense information – and essential to its processing – were the innate mental "faculties" of curiosity, attention, and perception.[40] Curiosity was the "first attribute" of the *système sensible* and the "first active faculty of the understanding"; it functioned involuntarily, without any effort of will. All human beings were naturally curious, though the object of their curiosity varied with their level of moral development; "civilized men" were restlessly drawn to the arts, "savages" to the merely useful.[41] Closely related but subsequent in actual operation to curiosity was "attention," which was the result of deliberate, voluntary mental activity. Focusing and directing sensory equipment, attention gave resolution to multitudinous impulses and thus made learning possible. Without the proper fixing of attention, individuals suffered either from sporadic or pathologically intense relations to the phenomena of the exterior world, a fact Alibert believed to be demonstrated by observation of the "manias" of the mentally ill, maladies he attributed to defects in this essential mental faculty. Finally, and most critically, perception itself was no pure act of "appropriation" of the exterior world but rather, as Charles Bonnet had defined it, "the reaction of the soul on objects" grasped by the senses. The precise nature of this "reaction," however, Alibert did not explore.[42]

While the "exterior life of the sensitive system" was guided by curiosity, attention, and perception, the "interior life" was directed by the innate faculties of reflection, "reverie," memory, imagination, conscience, will, and "habit."[43] In explicating these mental "attributes," Alibert sometimes followed Cousin ("one of the most illustrious professors of our age"), as when he defined reflection as a "reverse operation" that follows once "attention settles." Sometimes he drew from medical colleagues such as Frédéric Bérard (professor of hygiene at Montpellier), who had "carried the science of man to new heights" by destroying the view of "Locke's sectarians" that memory was nothing but recovered sensation.[44] These partisans of true physiology had destroyed the absurd "mechanist" contention that memory

39 On the moralist tradition, see Louise K. Horowitz, *Love and Language: A Study of the Classical French Moralist Writers* (Columbus: Ohio State University Press, 1977).
40 On the Scottish school, see James McCosh, *The Scottish Philosophy: Biographical, Expository, Critical, from Hutcheson to Hamilton* (1875; rpt. New York: AMS Press, 1980); Louis Schneider, ed. *The Scottish Moralists on Human Nature and Society* (Chicago: University of Chicago Press, 1967).
41 Alibert, *Physiologie des passions*, 1:xxiv–xxv.
42 *Ibid.*, xxviii–xxxii, xxxv–xxxviii.   43 *Ibid.*, liii.   44 *Ibid.*, lxvii–lxx.

works by leaving "*physical traces* of objects . . . in the pulpy substance of the brain."[45] Alibert's scorn for these mere "anatomists" was intense: "What can the anatomist's scalpel teach us? What can our doctrine have in common with [one that urges] dissection of an organ whose unique destiny is to intensify the fires of the soul?"[46] Alibert's examination of the remaining faculties of the "interior life" was cursory: imagination got some seven pages; conscience, ten; will, nine; habit, six (and this in a two-volume work whose total bulk was over a thousand pages). Surveying these innate faculties, whose existence and functioning Alibert trumpeted as overturning the whole of sensationalist and materialist psychology, provided him with an occasion for little more than praise of conservative authors (the baron de Massias, the comte de Sabran) and for *aperçus* about the absence or overabundance of key intellectual faculties in children, animals, savages, *aliénés*, and women.[47] From these summary observations, Alibert then moved to the principal subject matter of the book, the investigation of the passions, a line of inquiry that would yield the "facts bearing most directly on our happiness."[48]

In writing on the passions, Alibert was working within a venerable tradition of French moralists. His seventeenth-century predecessors included the Montpellier graduate Marin Cureau de la Chambre, whose famous *Les charactères des passions* was published in 1640 and whose work *L'art de connaître les hommes* (1659) supplied a title to the Ideologue Moreau de la Sarthe when the latter translated Johann-Caspar Lavater's physiognomical treatise into French in 1820.[49] Descartes's *Les passions de l'âme* (1649) served as Alibert's anti-model: "When one reads the Treatise on the Passions of Descartes, [a writer] who seeks to submit the finest and subtlest operations of our understanding to his calculations, one cannot help deploring the feebleness of the human mind."[50] Eighteenth-century treatments of the passions appeared in Vauvenargue's famous *Introduction à la connaissance de l'esprit humain* (1746), and works by two Montpellier physicians – de Beauchene's *De l'influence des affections* (1781) and Laroque's *De l'influence des passions sur l'économie animale* (1798).[51] At the turn of the century the momentous writ-

45 *Ibid.*, lxxiv, italics in the original.   46 *Ibid.*, lxxiv.
47 *Ibid.*, xxiv–cx. Baron Massias (an "honorable thinker," in Alibert's characterization) was the author of a treatise entitled *Rapport de la nature à l'homme, et de l'homme à la nature, ou Essai sur l'instinct, l'intelligence et la vie* (Paris: F. Didot, 1821).
48 Alibert, *Physiologie des passions*, 1:cvi.
49 Marin Cureau de la Chambre, *Les charactères des passions* (Paris: P. Rocolet and P. Blaise, 1640); *idem*, *L'art de connoistre les hommes* (Paris: P. Rocolet, 1659); Johann-Caspar Lavater, *L'art de connaître les hommes*, ed. and trans. Jacques-Louis Moreau de la Sarthe (Paris: L. Prudhomme, 1806–9). See also Robert Doranlo, *La médecine au XVIIe siècle: Marin Curin de la Chambre, médecin et philosophe, 1594–1669* (Paris: Jouve, 1939).
50 René Descartes, *Les passions de l'âme* (Paris: H. Legros, 1649); Alibert, *Physiologie des passions*, 1:1, 5.
51 Luc de Clapiers Vauvenargues, *Introduction à la connoissance de l'esprit humain* (Paris: A. C. Briasson, 1746); Edmé-Pierre Chauvot de Beauchène, *De l'influence des affections de l'âme dans les maladies nerveuses des femmes, avec le traitement qui convient à ces maladies* (Montpellier:

ings on the passions of Cabanis, Bichat, and Pinel inspired interest in the subject among medical students; four medical theses on the passions appeared between 1802 and 1805 alone. Then from 1805 to the appearance of Alibert's work, medical treatises on the passions proliferated.[52] Thus Alibert was scarcely controversial in claiming for medicine a privileged role in study of the passions; medical authors had long been prominent in the field. Indeed Alibert argued that it was precisely Descartes's lack of "physiological knowledge" that explained the "defective and incomplete" nature of his work.[53]

Still, Alibert thought it important to insist on the preeminence of physicians in investigation of the "moral sentiments" (a term he used interchangeably with passions): "Is it not to doctors that this study must especially belong? One has only a glimpse so far of how much a deepened knowledge of our physical infirmities can clear the way to a true theory of the passions" and ultimately to an understanding of "the most precious and noble attributes of man's being."[54] This claim to medical primacy in the study of the passions supported both Alibert's general view that physicians must assume greater responsibility in surveying behavior and morals, and the theoretical particulars of his reworking of the science of man. Only the medical science of man could offer a complete understanding of the passions since the passions were intimately connected to the activities and functions of the body. Physical ailment or defect was a primary cause of disordered passion, and its remedy lay only with medicine. Just as medicine would illuminate the passions, furthermore, study of the passions would enlighten medicine: "To know man profoundly and well, it does not suffice to view him in the full exercise of his reason; one must follow him in all the ailments of his spirit [*esprit*]."[55]

Although Alibert's physiology was intended to be synonymous with the science of man, it nonetheless marked a radical departure from that conceived by the Ideologues and especially by Cabanis. In Alibert's conservative conception, there was no physiology of intellect as such nor any prospect or possibility of one since intellect was independent of the "corporal envelope." The passions, on the other hand, were grounded in and often determined by the body. Multiple, powerful, and subtle interrelations linked body and passion, and Alibert's chief task was to explain these interrelations. He did so primarily with the aid of the concept of instinct, a

Méquignon, 1781); Raimond Laroque, *De l'influence des passions sur l'économie animale, considérée dans les quatre ages de la vie* (Montpellier: Fontenay-Picot, 1798). For other titles, see Kathleen Grange, "Pinel and Eighteenth Century Psychiatry," *BHM* 35 (1961): 442–53.
52 These *thèses* were written by M. F. R. Buisson (1802); G.-M. Royer (1803); Jean-Etienne-Dominique Esquirol (1804); and Léon Simon (1805); see Brodier, *Alibert*, 267. Some *thèses* on the passions written during the 1830s are listed in *Journal hebdomadaire des progrès des sciences et des institutions médicales* 4 (1834): 246–50. See also Albert O. Hirschman, *The Passions and the Interests: Political Arguments for Capitalism before Its Triumph* (Princeton: Princeton University Press, 1977).
53 Alibert, *Physiologie des passions*, 1:1.   54 *Ibid.*, 1.   55 *Ibid.*, xxx.

term for which he offered not a definition but a classification. In his doctrine, four primordial instincts – "conservation," "imitation," "relation," and "reproduction" – functioned as the source of all the passions, good and bad, noble and ignoble. Thus the instinct of "conservation" was the font of egoism, avarice, vanity, courage, fear, prudence, and intemperance; "imitation" of emulation, envy, and ambition; "relation" of *bienvaillance*, consideration, pity, ingratitude, resentment, hate, and love of one's native land; and "reproduction" of the four varieties of love – conjugal, maternal, paternal, and filial.[56]

Each of these passions was discussed in expository prose and then the more colorful among them were illustrated by moral tales. These tales were of humble folk ("le pauvre Pierre" at the Hôpital Saint-Louis; Anselm, "le fou ambitieux," at Bicêtre) who showed innate goodness or who were ruined by unwonted ambitions. Others were of heroic national figures ("La Perouse à la Baie d'Hudson") who were moved by a passion for glory, or of philosophers ("Entretien d'Epicure avec Pythagore") who reflected in dialogue on the natural moral virtues. In the tradition of "médecine galante," Alibert offered several stories particularly for his female audience, one of "the serving-girl Marie" (see the illustration "La servante Marie") who though born to a humble condition devoted every free moment to cultivating a talent for sculpture (in this she was aided by a learned and generous doctor). Another feminine tale ("Couramé ou l'Amour de la Terre Natale") concerned a beautiful, quick-witted Guyanese girl who was adopted and educated by a kindly French-born widow (see the illustration "Couramé"). Although trained to play and to speak excellent French, Couramé continued to exhibit "a sort of savagery beyond the elegant manners imparted by civilization." When visitors from her native village appeared, Couramé fled with them. She later recounted to a doctor who came to work among the Indians (a "physician of the soul as well as the body") how she had never ceased yearning to return to her homeland.[57]

Such exotic settings for Alibert's moral tales were not accidental but rather were deliberately selected to illuminate, from the experience of peoples close to nature, the character of universal passions:

I believe that the knowledge of noncivilized peoples is singularly useful in proceeding to a profound examination or, so to speak, an anatomy of the most intimate of our passions. . . . It is by such study that we can form a proper idea of our native penchants as well as of the primitive nature of our sensitive system.[58]

56 These are partial lists of the particular passions linked to the four instincts. For others, see
   ibid., "conservation": 1:13–84, 149–218; "imitation": 1:279–308, 331–52; "relation": 2:1–
   100, 189–246, 301–20, 377–98; "reproduction": 2:445–522.
57 *Ibid.*, "pauvre Pierre": 1:94–148; "Entretien": 1:221–78; "servante Marie": 1:311–30; "le
   fou ambitieux": 1:355–84; "La Perouse": 2:321–76; "Couramé": 2:399–44.
58 *Ibid.*, 2:403

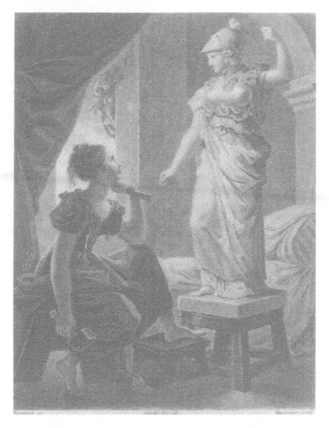

"La servante Marie." Illustration from J.-L. Alibert's *La physiologie des passions* (1825).

Alibert concluded that physicians would consult with profit the excellent work on the peoples of the *pays chauds* by such learned men as Chateaubriand, von Humboldt, and Bernardin de Saint-Pierre.[59]

Alibert's scheme of the four "instincts" appears to be of his own creation, though the term had been in use for some time. In eighteenth-century texts, "instinct" was not readily differentiated from the related terms "need" and indeed "passion" itself, which often had been employed to denote human inclinations that were thought to be universal (such as maternal love) as opposed to "faculties," "capacities," or "powers" (intellect, talents) that were regarded as highly variable.[60] There are echoes in Alibert of Montpellier doctrine, in which instinctual activities, such as the baby's urge to suckle or

59 *Ibid.*, 401.
60 Alibert does not cite Lamarck, whose theory of instinct was developed in *Philosophie zoologique*, 2 vols. (Paris: Dentu, 1809).

an animal's natural tendency to seek foods appropriate to it, were seen as manifestations of the vital principle and as proofs of the "preestablished harmony" between the life principle and organization.[61] There are strains too of Cabanis – who tended to equate instinct with the "interior sensations" that formed the basis for his challenge to Condillacian sensationalism – and of Bichat, whose conception of the "organic life" of the body (innate, interior, involuntary) subsumed processes that others captured with the term instinct. Though Bichat did not use the term himself, his conception of nonwilled, life-preserving activity was nonetheless an important element of the context for all physiological discussions of instinct.[62]

Despite his hostility to Cabanis's materialist sensationalism, Alibert's very affirmation that the human "animal economy" was propelled by instinctual drives validated the perspective of anthropological medicine over and against an orthodox tradition that denied instinct any role in human behavior and that held the opposition intellect–instinct to be essentially equivalent to the antinomy between the human and the animal.[63] Alibert's borrowing from Bichat was direct: his concept of the instinct of "relation" was an extrapolation from Bichat's theory of the organism's unceasing need to regulate and to adapt its relations with the exterior environment.[64] In Bichat's theory, however, relational functions were not instinctual but acquired: the infant had to learn to eat, walk, smile, and perform all the other activities by which it established relations with its milieu.[65] On this crucial point Alibert departed from Bichat. Sentimentalizing the concept of "relation," he rendered it as an instinctual inclination to enter into concourse with others. It thus became essentially synonymous with what the Scottish school had called "sociability." This maneuver allowed Alibert to claim instinctual status for the good passions – kindness, esteem, respect – and

61 Paul-Joseph Barthez, *Nouveaux éléments de la science de l'homme*, 2 vols., 2d ed. (Paris: Goujon, 1806), 1:101–5.
62 Cabanis defined instinct in these terms: "Some of these determinations [of vital movements] cannot be referred to any sort of reasoning . . . they are formed the most often without the will of the individual having any other role than in best directing their execution. It is the ensemble of such determinations that has been given the name instinct." See P. J. G. Cabanis, *Rapports du physique et du moral de l'homme* in *Oeuvres philosophiques de Cabanis*, ed. Claude Lehec and Jean Cazeneuve (Paris: Presses universitaires de France, 1965), 1:165. Cabanis held that all instinctual activities are caused by internal excitation and that together instinct and reason formed "the moral system of man" (see *ibid.*, 188). On Bichat's conception of the "organic life," see Chapter 2.
63 Condillac upheld this view in his *Traité des animaux* as did Buffon in the *Histoire naturelle et générale;* see Michèle Duchet, *Anthropologie et histoire au siècle des Lumières: Buffon, Voltaire, Rousseau, Helvétius, Diderot* (Paris: François Maspéro, 1971).
64 Xavier Bichat, *Physiological Researches upon Life and Death* (Philadelphia: Smith and Maxwell, 1809) : "Every organism establishes numerous relations between it[self] and surrounding objects; its existence is entwined with that of every other being, it avoids or approaches these according to its fears or wants, and thus appears to appropriate everything in nature to its exclusive use (2).
65 *Ibid.*, 103–4.

thereby to assimilate the physiological concept of instinct to sentimental ideas of the innate benevolence of human nature. Where the materialist Bichat had perceived the relational life of the organism as a constant and bitter struggle with a harsh, godless environment, Alibert construed it as a playing out of man's natural, God-given inclinations to the good.[66]

Yet there was an obverse to Alibert's cheerful construal of instinct and passion. Conceiving the instincts in medical context, he held that they could be deranged or perverted by physical disease or infirmity. Thus the maladies of old age turned natural self-love into egoism. Sensory deficit produced "continual egoism" in deaf-mutes and the blind. "A temporary alienation of the brain" caused "fatuity" (a species of vanity). A "state of delirium" explained the absence of maternal love manifested in infanticide.[67] Precisely how disease and physiological states could derail instinct Alibert did not clarify, which was perhaps fitting in a work one reviewer saw as uneasily suspended "between poetry and science."[68]

Despite Alibert's claim that medicine had a special task in guiding the passions, his work was short on therapeutics and amounted to little more than medical reinforcement for the idea that virtue lies in leading the good life. Still, his performance of this task was sufficiently skilled to recommend the book to churchmen and to like-thinking doctors. Clerics including the archbishop of Paris praised the work highly, and Alibert's conservative colleague Etienne Pariset paid it tribute as the labor of "a pure intelligence, who, freeing us from the gross bonds of matter, draws us near to divinity itself with the aid of virtue."[69]

Although Alibert's book reproduced a seemingly antiquated discourse on the passions, its advocacy of a purely medical approach to physiology in fact fit well with certain regnant principles of Paris clinical medicine. When Alibert contended that to know what was healthy in the passional life one must understand what was sick, he affirmed the Paris clinicians' view that to understand "normal physiology" investigators must observe the phenomena of disease, infirmity, and defect directly in patients, both living and dead.[70] Observation of the sick had long been regarded as the most important element of the physician's labor, and exhortations to undertake accurate observation as well as praise of results thus obtained were staples of all medical doctrines. In the Paris school this sense of the clinical ideal had been extended to include widespread use of postmortem dissection in med-

66 On this feature of Bichat's physiology, see Pedro Laín Entralgo, "Sensualism and Vitalism in Bichat's *Anatomie générale*," *JHMAS* 5 (1948): 47–64.
67 Alibert, *Physiologie des passions*, 1:19, 26, 55, 2:507.
68 Reviewer in *Le Globe* (July 2, 1825); cited in Brodier, *Alibert*, 283, n. 2.
69 *Ibid.*, 269, n. 1; on Pariset's favor with the Restoration government, see George Sussman, "Etienne Pariset: A Medical Career in Government under the Restoration," *JHMAS* 26 (1971): 52–74.
70 Georges Canguilhem, *On the Normal and the Pathological*, trans. Carolyn Fawcett, intro. Michel Foucault (Boston: D. Reidel, 1978).

ical investigation. Thus reinforced by the techniques of pathological anatomy, clinical observation (of both living and dead) was expected to yield results not only about strict morphology – the aim of the old anatomy – but also about the dynamics of disease and ultimately the full range of physiological function.[71]

Although Alibert was by no means a tribune of pathological anatomy, he was one with the *ouvreurs de cadavres* in arguing that only the study of pathology as it naturally occurred in living beings could lead to any true knowledge of the animal economy. This was a welcome perspective within the medical community because it buttressed medicine against encroachments on its domain by the emergent discipline of experimental physiology. In France the new experimental physiology was chiefly associated with François Magendie and his followers, who gave primacy to vivisectionist investigations designed to illuminate minute problems of animal function. Magendie himself was trained at the Faculty of Medicine and worked there for several years as an *aide* and prosector, but after an altercation with a superior in 1813 Magendie resigned his post, never to return to the faculty in any capacity.[72] Beginning with his famous "manifesto" of 1809, Magendie led a concerted attack on Bichat's vitalism, especially the principle that physiological phenomena were fundamentally different in kind from those subject to physicochemical laws. He continued this attack in his synthetic treatise, *Précis élémentaire de physiologie* (1816), and in notes he wrote for editions of some of Bichat's writings.[73] In 1816 Magendie unsuccessfully bid for a place in the Académie des sciences (for an opening created by the death of the hospital reformer, Jacques Tenon). In 1821, however, he triumphed in a competition with the aged physiologist and associate of the Ideologues, François Chaussier. That same year he founded his own journal, the *Journal de physiologie expérimentale et pathologique*, in which he vigorously affirmed the importance of the physical sciences to medicine. He was also appointed to the committee that awarded the Montyon prize, a position that allowed him to become "the arbiter of opinion on practically all memoirs of a physiological nature."[74]

71 Russell C. Maulitz, *Morbid Appearances: The Anatomy of Pathology in the Early Nineteenth Century* (Cambridge: Cambridge University Press, 1987), 9–35.

72 Magendie sought a chair in anatomy and physiology at the Faculté de médecine in 1818 but it went to Pierre Béclard. See J. M. D. Olmsted, *François Magendie: Pioneer in Experimental Physiology and Scientific Medicine in XIX Century France* (New York: Schuman's, 1944), 81; see also 8, 16–17, 48.

73 François Magendie, *Précis élémentaire de physiologie*, 2 vols. (Paris: Méquignon-Marvis, 1816); see also William R. Albury, "Experiment and Explanation in the Physiology of Bichat and Magendie," in *Studies in History of Biology*, vol. 1, ed. William Coleman and Camille Limoges (Baltimore: Johns Hopkins University Press, 1977), 47–131. It is wrong to see Magendie as a clear and simple "antivitalist," a tradition in Magendie scholarship inaugurated by Claude Bernard. Yet the vitalism that remained in Magendie was different in scope and explanatory intent from that examined here as the foundation of conservative physiology and the science of man in the 1820s and 1830s.

74 Olmsted, *François Magendie*, 90. Magendie's journal appeared between 1821 and 1831.

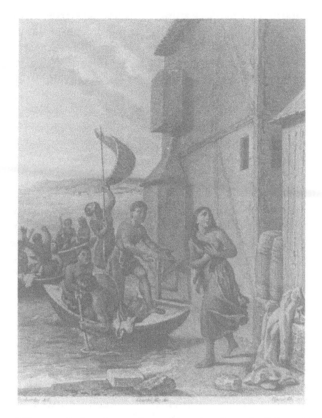

"Couramé abandonne la maison de Mme de Sainte-Croix." Illustration from J.-L. Alibert's *La physiologie des passions* (1825).

The prominence and prestige of experimental physiology caused considerable unease in medical circles, for the questions Magendie asked (and, worse, answered to the satisfaction of prestigious scientists) earlier would have been medical questions: the effects of emetics, poisons, and other substances on the animal economy; the functioning of the liver; the role of the cranial nerves in sensation and movement.[75] Doctors like Alibert responded to Magendie's successes by making special claims for a peculiarly medical physiology whose methods and results differed radically from those of experimental, vivisectionist, laboratory-based physiology. They argued that medical physiology, which relied exclusively on observation of the sick, would always yield different and inherently more valuable results for medical science than the minute and fragmented proce-

75 On physiology's grounding in medicine before the 1820s, see John Lesch, *Science and Medicine in France: The Emergence of Experimental Physiology, 1790–1855* (Cambridge, Mass.: Harvard University Press, 1984), 5–8, 13.

dures of experimentation on hapless animals. What was true in the general medical domain, moreover, was truer yet in the physiology of the passions. It was inconceivable that the techniques of the laboratory, used as they were on enfeebled or dying animals, could say anything about the multiple, subtle, profoundly complex phenomena of the body and the passions.[76]

Thus in the 1820s and 1830s the medical science of man, as developed by a conservative like Alibert, constituted a rallying cry for physicians who saw in the new physiology a threat to the medical preserve. It would continue to fulfill this function within the Paris faculty for several decades after the publication of Alibert's treatise.[77] The central point to bear in mind in all this is that, although Alibert broke with the medical Ideologues on the vexed problem of the body-mind relation, and thereby on a spectrum of issues connected to the physical-moral relation, he continued to promote the medical science of man and to reinforce claims it staked for the independence of medicine in the face of challenges posed by modern, reductionist physiological science. In this respect Alibert made common cause with physicians who stood at the opposite end of the medicopolitical spectrum and whose "materialism" he denounced.

Another one-time Ideologue who has generally been seen as effecting a radical break with medical Ideology was Anthelme-Balthasar Richerand (1779–1840), who, like Alibert, held a prestigious post (as surgeon in chief) at the Hôpital Saint-Louis. Like Alibert, Richerand had been associated with the Ideologues at the salon d'Auteuil and had been closely tied to Cabanis. His 1801 work, *Nouveaux éléments de physiologie,* which Olmsted calls "the best-known text-book of physiology of the day," went through ten editions by 1833.[78] This work was in some respects a classic text of medical Ideology. Richerand followed closely Cabanis's teaching on the nature of sensibility, agreeing that all mental phenomena were dependent on it and that there was a "strict relation between the physical and the mental." Richerand refrained, however, from attempting any comprehensive analysis of the character of mental function, instead referring his readers to Destutt de Tracy's *Eléments d'idéologie.* He also embraced more heartily than Cabanis had ever done the vitalist principle of the irreducibility of life to material determinants.[79]

76 On the superiority of the clinical method over all others, see J.-L. Alibert, *Nosologie naturelle, ou les maladies du corps humain distribuées par familles* (Paris: Caille et Ravier, 1817), v. For a tribute to Alibert's blending of physiological with moral concerns, see "J. L. Alibert," in *Biographie médicale par ordre chronologique d'après Daniel Eloy, etc.,* ed. A. L. J. Bayle and Thillaye, 2 vols. (Paris: Adolphe Delahays, 1855), 2:933–35.

77 See Chapter 4, esp. "Seeking Middle Ground."

78 A.-B. Richerand, *Nouveaux éléments de physiologie* (Paris: Rochard, Caille et Ravier, 1801); Olmsted, *François Magendie,* 16.

79 Martin Staum, *Cabanis: Enlightenment and Medical Philosophy in the French Revolution* (Princeton: Princeton University Press, 1980), 251–52.

Richerand flourished under the Bonapartist regime, achieving appointment in 1807 as professor of external pathology at the Paris faculty. By 1815 he had moved ostentatiously into the Bourbon camp, and he was rewarded for his fidelity to the monarch with the title of baron.[80] Three years later Richerand published a much-praised edition of the works of Bordeu. He presented Bordeu's work as an attack on "mechanism," which in the semantic world of the early Restoration functioned essentially as a synonym for the much-despised "materialism." Richerand was one of the first Paris doctors of the period to begin reconstructing the work of the Montpellier doctors as a conservative bulwark against materialism, Ideology, and other eighteenth-century errors. He praised Bordeu for recognizing more clearly than any other physician of the era the strict division that must be upheld between medicine and the "accessory sciences." He construed Bordeu's Hippocratism as a denunciation of the search for "explanations" in medicine. Medicine, he argued, was a "historical science" based on observation rather than pointless theorizing. "Let us abandon the search for causes in favor of the study of phenomena; in so doing our epoch will merit the name Hippocratic."[81]

Though he lived to 1840, and during the Orleanist period wrote some rancorous pieces against the philosophes, Richerand never bothered to revise his work of 1802 to excise or alter his Cabanisian version of sensibility.[82] This would seem peculiar if we regarded the science of man tradition as necessarily tied to the ideological and political configuration that Cabanis represented circa 1800. In fact, as is clear from the case of Alibert, the turncoat Ideologues did not seek to overturn or demolish the science of man of the revolutionary years but to cleanse it of its philosophically and ideologically objectionable elements and then rework it to their own ends. That there was much in Cabanis that was valuable to medicine and that medicine was properly regarded as one of the principal foundations of *morale* – these were views Richerand upheld as firmly after his shift to the Right as before. In the 1820s and 1830s Richerand threw himself with great energy into the continuing campaign of physicians against "charlatanism." He sided with those who supported the institution of the *officiat de santé* against its many critics because he believed the general population required the ministrations of trained medical men, even the ill-trained *officiers*, if their level of physical and moral well-being was ever to be improved. Thus Richerand – like Alibert and, as we will see, like many physicians who moved into the domains of hygiene and mental medicine – renounced the philosophical extremes of medical Ideology but continued all the same to

80 *Ibid.*
81 A.-B. Richerand, ed., *Oeuvres complètes de Bordeu*, 2 vols. (Paris: Caille et Ravier, 1818), xxiii.
82 Staum, *Cabanis*, 251–52.

insist on the physician's prerogatives and special role in safeguarding the physical and moral health of the people.[83]

MONTPELLIER AS THE BULWARK OF ORTHODOXY

Richerand's revival of Bordeu notwithstanding, the real work of rethinking the legacy of Montpellier and appropriating the science of man for conservative purposes was done in Montpellier itself. The most important figure in this endeavor was the physician Jacques Lordat (1773–1870), a prolific writer who over the five decades from the 1810s to the 1850s nurtured the Montpellier legacy and defended the Montpellier Faculty of Medicine against its Parisian critics and antagonists. Much of his work was devoted to defending the true, "Barthezian" science of man against what he viewed as misinterpretations and distortions of it by Parisian physicians. Lordat's first important work in this vein was the *Exposition de la doctrine médicale de P.-J. Barthez,* which appeared in the same year, 1818, as Richerand's new edition of Bordeu.[84]

In attempting to turn the science of man to conservative ends, Lordat saw himself as upholding the tradition and spirit of Montpellier. There was some justice in his view: as seen in Chapter 1, the Montpellier physicians never drew the revolutionary theoretical conclusions from their work that Diderot saw implied in it. It was a natural step, then, for Lordat to perceive in the charged atmosphere of the early Restoration a favorable opportunity to enhance Montpellier's reputation by identifying its teachings with the defense of religious orthodoxy. Lordat's efforts in this regard make all the more sense if viewed in the context of a continuing institutional struggle between the Paris and Montpellier faculties. Although the Paris faculty was in some respects on the defensive in these early years of the Restoration, it was nonetheless an institution that had been given new vigor by developments from 1789 to 1815. Both statistical indicators and impressionistic accounts demonstrate that the Paris faculty of the early Restoration bore little resemblance to the moribund institution that went by that name under the Ancien Regime.[85] In vaunting the merits of the new organization of medicine in the capital, the Paris professors frequently emphasized the new position Paris occupied vis-à-vis the provincial medical schools, especially Montpellier, whose status had been downgraded by revolutionary-era legislation from that of an autonomous "university" with its own charter to

83 A.-B. Richerand, *De la population dans ses rapports avec la nature des gouvernemens* (Paris: Béchet jeune, 1837); see also Jacques Léonard, *La médecine entre les pouvoirs et les savoirs: Histoire intellectuelle et politique de la médecine française au XIXe siècle* (Paris: Aubier, 1981), 86.

84 Jacques Lordat, *Exposition de la doctrine médicale de P.-J. Barthez, et mémoires sur la vie de ce médecin* (Paris: Gabon, 1818).

85 Jacques Léonard, *Les médecins de l'Ouest au XIXème siècle*, 3 vols. (Lille: Atelier des reproduction des thèses, 1978), chap 8.

that of a "faculty" subordinated like all others to the larger structure of the University of France.[86] Thus in the early Restoration Montpellier was smarting under the impact of these institutional changes and of repeated charges from Paris that Montpellier was witnessing the disappearance of its "ancient splendor."[87] It is scarcely surprising that in such a setting Montpellier theorists would seek to enhance the standing of their establishment by contrasting their own orthodoxy to the materialist errors of the Paris professoriate, and more understandable yet that they did so by reclaiming for themselves authority in discussions of the science of man, which they regarded as one of the finest achievements of their own tradition.[88]

Lordat's 1818 treatise on Barthez's doctrine of the science of man was in many ways a throwback to eighteenth-century debates between mechanists and vitalists, with Haller being generally portrayed as Barthez's principal antagonist. Presenting Haller's physiology as a crudely mechanical doctrine, Lordat attacked Haller's failure to understand Barthez's more thoughtful and nuanced theory of the vital principle. Lordat was equally concerned, however, to demonstrate that Barthez's vital principle was in no way to be identified with the "substantial Soul" of Stahlian physiology or with Van Helmont's famous *Archeus*.[89] Such arguments were rather faded by 1818, and are to be explained only by the fact that after Barthez's *Nouveaux Eléments* appeared in its second edition in 1806, critics had assailed his teaching by comparing its "obscurity" to that of classic vitalist doctrines.[90]

Yet if Lordat's favored targets were the old enemies of eighteenth-century debates, there are nonetheless sufficient references to "moderns" who failed adequately to respect Barthez – Cabanis, and especially Bichat – to indicate that Lordat was as much concerned to save Barthez's reputation from current misinterpretation as he was to reestablish eighteenth-century battle lines. Indeed his decision to treat Haller as Barthez's most formidable opponent seems to have served the principal end of casting Cabanis and Bichat as Haller's epigones. His most important reference to Cabanis, for example, appears in the context of an exhaustive discussion of sensibility, in which Haller is portrayed as the source for all modern "mechanist" views, including those of Cabanis.[91] According to Lordat's reconstruction of the writing

86 Liard, *L'enseignement supérieur*, 2:139.
87 H. Pétiot, "Notice historique sur la vie et les ouvrages de Bérard," in *Esprit des doctrines médicales de Montpellier: Ouvrage inédit de F. Bérard*, by Frédéric Bérard (Paris: J.-B. Baillière, 1830), 47.
88 On the similarity of Barthez's teachings to those of the church fathers, see Lordat, *Exposition*, 263; Montpellier's claim to primacy in the science of man was argued forcefully in Jacques Lordat, *Réponse à des objections faites contre le principe de la dualité du dynamisme humain* (Montpellier: Martel; Paris: J. B. Baillière, 1854).
89 Lordat, *Exposition*, 52–54, 58–59, 110–11, 205–6, 262–63.
90 For Barthez's response to these critics, see *Science de l'homme*, 1:"Notes," 23–25.
91 Lordat, *Exposition*, 145, 149–50, 211.

of *Nouveaux éléments de la science de l'homme,* the cardinal error to which Barthez had responded was Haller's view that sensibility was conveyed only through the nervous system and therefore restricted to parts of the body that were well supplied with nervous structures. Contesting both this Hallerian view as well as the competing hypothesis that sensibility was conveyed by nervous fluid or animal spirits, Lordat then assimilated Cabanis's teaching on sensibility to these older "mechanist" doctrines. With no regard for the nuances of Cabanis's teaching and no acknowledgment of Cabanis's essential agnosticism on the fundamental character of sensibility, Lordat asserted that Cabanis believed sensation was ultimately reducible to movement and life itself "derived solely from organization."[92] Having recast Cabanis as a mechanist in the style of the eighteenth century, Lordat then denounced the absurdity of such a doctrine and reiterated Barthez's dictum that "our minds cannot conceive the slightest connection between the notion of movement and that of sentiment."[93] He reasserted in place of mechanist doctrine the Barthezian view that sensibility was a primordial vital force, diffused throughout the organism and in no way dependent on mechanical structures for its own operation or for the influence it exerted within the animal economy.

Reviving this Barthezian teaching positioned Lordat to refute what he saw as the materialists' distortion of the crucial medicomoral concept of temperament. According to this construction, Cabanis and "modern physiology" generally taught that temperament was dependent purely on organization and therefore that essential elements of character and moral inclination were fatally determined. Barthez's doctrine of sensibility was the bulwark against such a maneuver. If sensibility were a diffuse and original "force," rather than a localized function dependent on specific corporal structures, then temperament too, which was influenced most decisively by the nature of individual sensibility, was something other than a derivative of material apparatuses.[94] This did not mean there was no link between physical constitution and temperament but rather that the nature of the link was not so clearly unidirectional, so obviously causal, as the materialists claimed:

If one resolves to regard the coincidence of a given temperament and a determinate constitution not as the necessary result of a causal relation, but as a rather common fact known through experience, one can profit from the latter mode of investigation without risk of abuse.[95]

Lordat acknowledged without difficulty that Barthez had investigated the importance of "natural causes" such as climate in the formation of "endemic temperaments," defined as "particular modifications of the vital forces

92 *Ibid.,* 145.   93 *Ibid.*   94 *Ibid.,* 233–42.   95 *Ibid.,* 239.

characterizing diverse nations."[96] That such facts were common Lordat did not deny. But Barthez's handling of them was different in spirit and intent from that of the mechanists:

His principal aim in gathering observations about the influence of physical causes is to accustom the mind to expressing in an aphoristic manner the modifications that these causes introduce in the vital power without intermixing the prejudicial view that such modifications are caused by mechanical changes.[97]

To safeguard the science of man from the charge of materialism, Lordat was even prepared to question Barthez's own judgment. In a rare passage directly addressing the question of the materialist basis of thought, Lordat gently chided Barthez for lending credence (in the second edition of *Nouveaux Eléments*) to Samuel Soemmering's contention that intellectual capacity varied according to the ratio (in size) of brain to nerves. He first questioned whether the topic was even properly relevant to the science of man: "it is for the zootomists to pronounce on the accuracy of this judgment."[98] He then argued that if the hypothesis were valid at all, it could be so only for animals. In any event it appeared to Lordat "prodigiously difficult to estimate the degree of intelligence of brutes" or to decide whether they "had any intelligence at all."[99] This whole matter of the material signs of intellectual function had not troubled Barthez himself when he revised *Nouveaux Eléments* for publication in 1806. But by 1818, in the circumstances of Lordat's refashioning of the Montpellier legacy, the problem struck him as being of great moment. Even if it meant diverging from Barthez himself, Lordat was not prepared to see the vitalist science of man – the product of Montpellier's peculiar genius – associated with the irreligious materialism of German and Parisian "anatomists."[100]

To prove the unassailable orthodoxy of Barthezian doctrine, Lordat recounted in detail the reception clerics gave Barthez's *Nouveaux Elémens* when it was published in 1778. He noted that when the work originally appeared, an embittered former student of Barthez had denounced the work to medical and clerical circles in Rome for its "bold, heterodox principles." After an unfavorable reading by three theologians, the work had gone to the congregation of the Index, which, granting the imprimatur, rendered the judgment that the work, "far from favoring materialism . . . [or] presenting the body as capable of thought, instead cast doubt on the view that the body could sustain the vital functions with its own powers."[101] A similar intrigue had been started by a jealous academician in France, but again Barthez had been vindicated by the authorities. Thus the orthodoxy of Barthez's teaching was not open to question: "He teaches the dogma of the duality of man . . . of the existence of two individualities, one purely vital

96 *Ibid.*, 239–40.　97 *Ibid.*, 240–41.　98 *Ibid.*, 198.　99 *Ibid.*　100 *Ibid.*
101 *Ibid.*, 281.

and the other intellectual, a dogma he could have found in Plato, Saint Paul, or Saint Augustine."[102] This was the ultimate defense: Montpellier doctrine differed in no essentials from the teachings of the church fathers or from scripture itself.

In defending the Montpellier legacy, Lordat thus recast the writings of Barthez in a rather un-Barthezian light. We have seen that the Montpellier physicians, though ideologically cautious and invariably respectful of religious teaching and feeling, were secular and "enlightened" in disposition. They never exceeded the ordinary and ritual pieties of much of eighteenth-century discourse. If history has come to remember Montpellier as theocratic in spirit, it is not so much because of the work of the original vitalists but because of the labor of reconstruction and reinterpretation of nineteenth-century commentators, of whom Lordat was the first and most important. In the late 1840s, Lordat would again defend Montpellier, in this instance against Paris professors who were seeking to close the Montpellier faculty altogether.[103] By that point the champions of Parisian prerogatives had made real strides toward establishing the existence of a dichotomy between Paris medicine, styled as progressive, forward-looking, and determinedly scientific, and Montpellier medicine, represented as archaic, backward-looking, and avowedly subordinate to religious doctrine. Lordat's own writings played no small part in this reshaping of Montpellier's public image.

ECLECTICISM IN MONTPELLIER

Just as in Paris a sustained philosophical attack on the eighteenth century and on Ideology was undertaken not only by full-blown Catholic reactionaries but also by conservative liberals like Cousin, in Montpellier a vigorous effort to rescue the science of man from the materialists was undertaken not only by conservatives like Lordat but by self-styled eclectics, including the Montpellier professors Frédéric Bérard, François Ribes, and Fulcrand-César Caizergues.[104] The emergence of a medical version of eclecticism in Montpellier seems to have been roughly contemporaneous with similar developments in Parisian medical circles, where through the 1820s and early 1830s eclecticism gained many adherents among physicians.[105] It is difficult to define precisely what eclecticism meant in either locale since the eclectics eschewed the elaboration of a fully developed "system." Writing for the Paris-based *Journal hebdomadaire de médecine*, J.-B. Bouillaud defined eclecticism as "a system that includes all the knowledge and all the truths

102 *Ibid.*, 263.
103 See Chapter 4, "Mutations of Vitalism."
104 Pétiot, "Notice historique," 53–54.
105 On the eclectic movement, see Ackerknecht, *Medicine at the Paris Hospital*, chap. 8; Léonard, *Médecine entre les pouvoirs et les savoirs*, 123–26.

scattered throughout other systems."[106] The definitions given by the Montpellier professors were similarly vague. In his *Discours sur l'éclectisme médical,* Ribes characterized eclecticism simply as an approach that rejected "both the partisans of spirit and those of matter."[107] His colleague Caizergues argued that eclectics, since undogmatic in spirit, could glean some truth from all earlier doctrines:

Systems are like so many rays of light shining in turn on the different faces of an object, illuminating them and enabling us to perceive their minutest features. Thus in drawing all systems together we may form the most precise and complete idea of these objects that is possible with present knowledge. We must study these systems as eclectic physicians, for each of them is founded on a certain number of true observations made without regard to sectarian loyalties.[108]

That there were multiple connections between the medical eclectics and the larger philosophical movement is clear from the physicians' repeated references to Cousin, Laromuiguière, Degérando, and Royer-Collard, although the detailed history of this link remains to be written.[109] In any event, the Montpellier eclectics took up many of the themes that, as one physician put it, were first broached by "metaphysicians" who charted a course between the extremes of Condillac's sensationalism and Kant's innatism.[110] Denouncing the "destructive materialism" of the eighteenth century, the Montpellier eclectics deplored all attempts to reduce mental functions to material operations, especially the powerfully influential doctrines of Cabanis and Gall. They acclaimed Laromuiguière for insisting that sensation could not be transformed into thought without the work of the innate faculty of attention. They applauded Cousin's handling of the concept of a unified self whose operations differed fundamentally from those of the body's "material apparatus," a view they readily adapted to the hallowed vitalist concept of the "harmony" and "unity" characteristic of the healthy human organism.[111]

Of the Montpellier eclectics the figure who enjoyed the greatest success in bridging the increasingly wide Paris-Montpellier gap was Frédéric Bé-

106 J.-B. Bouillaud, "Examen du Traité de l'irritation et de la folie, ouvrage dans lequel les rapports du physique et du moral sont établis sur la base de la doctrine physiologique; par F. J. V. Broussais," *Journal hebdomadaire de médecine* 1 (1828) : 359–77, at 361n.

107 Quoted in Léonard, *Médecine entre les pouvoirs et les savoirs,* 123.

108 Fulcrand-César Caizergues, *Des systèmes en médecine, et de leur influence sur le traitement des maladies* (Paris: Gabon; Montpellier: Sevalle, 1827), 5.

109 Pétiot, "Notice historique," 65; Amédée Dupau, *Notice historique sur Frédéric Bérard* (Paris: Gabon, 1828), 12.

110 Dupau, *Notice historique,* 12.

111 On Cabanis, see my subsequent discussion. Bérard developed an extensive critique of Gall in "Cranioscopie," *Dictionaire des sciences médicales,* 60 vols. (Paris: Panckoucke, 1812–22), 7:300–09. For Gall's response, see Franz-Josef Gall, *Sur les fonctions du cerveau et sur celles de chacune de ses parties,* 6 vols. (Paris: Chez l'auteur, Boucher, etc., 1822–25), 2:64, 252–54, 361–62, 383–85, 403–5, 425–27, 463–74; 3:32–41. For Bérard's defense of the unitary *moi,* see "Cranioscopie," 7:311–13, and Dupau, *Notice historique,* 5.

rard (1789–1828). After medical studies at Montpellier around 1810 (and a thesis entitled "Plan for a Natural Medicine, or Nature as Physician"), Bérard moved to Paris, where he threw himself into the medical life of the capital. He forged close ties with medical conservatives in the Société de médecine as well as with the *équipe* engaged in editing the great medical encyclopedia of the era, the *Dictionaire des sciences médicales*.[112] In 1824 he caused a considerable stir when he edited and published Cabanis's *Lettre à Fauriel*, a document Cabanis wrote shortly before his death in 1808 in which he reflected on the inadequacy of science to meet the primordial human need for a sense of certainty and meaningfulness.[113] In the early 1820s Bérard collaborated with F. J. L. Rouzet, Antoine Miquel, Jean-Baptiste Bousquet, and Amédée Dupau in putting out the *Revue médicale*, a journal that was consistently antagonistic to mechanism, materialism, and organicism.[114] In these varied forums and in a series of much-praised works, Bérard articulated a version of Montpellier doctrine that was intended to defeat materialism, reassert the value of a holistic science of man, and restore Montpellier's fading reputation.

Bérard's first major work was a summary of Montpellier teaching published in 1819 under the title *Doctrine médicale de l'Ecole de Montpellier*. This work was necessary, he argued, to respond to those who claimed that Montpellier had fallen from its "ancient heights," especially "certain fanatical disciples who believe they are serving the Ecole de Paris."[115] The task was urgent, for at the very moment he wrote (a footnote specified May 1819) there were those who said the school of Montpellier should be abolished and Paris given all authority in medicine.[116]

This work of Bérard's youth seems to have been an uneasy mix of things he learned in Montpellier, where he was a disciple of the physiologist C.-L. Dumas, and views he imbibed from Paris medicine and from the larger intellectual life of the capital.[117] In it Bérard celebrated Montpellier's achievement in establishing a middle way between the dual errors of spiritualism and materialism. He observed that although some Montpellier teachers had veered in the direction of Stahlian spiritualism and others toward Cabanis's and Bichat's "organicism," generally they adhered to sound scientific

112 Bérard contributed the articles "Contemplatif," "Cranioscopie," "Elément," "Extase," and "Force musculaire"; see Pétiot, "Notice historique," 19.
113 P. J. G. Cabanis, "Lettre à M. F. sur les causes premières" in *Oeuvres*, 2:256–98. The circumstances of Bérard's publishing the letter are described by the editors of Cabanis's *Oeuvres* at 2:256, n. 1. See also Staum, *Cabanis*, 299–300.
114 Pétiot, "Notice historique," 62–63; Dupau, *Notice historique*.
115 Frédéric Bérard, *Doctrine médicale de l'Ecole de Montpellier, et comparaison de ses principes à ceux des autres écoles d'Europe* (Montpellier: Jean Martel, 1819), 4.
116 *Ibid.*, 9–10.
117 Dumas too was characterized by Dupau as a *Montpelliérain* who attempted to straddle both worlds, blending Montpellier-style "analysis" with "the organicist ideas of another school"; Dupau, *Notice historique*, 3.

method and to the only genuine "philosophy" in recognizing that the essential nature of the "cause of life" could never be defined.[118] In other respects too Montpellier steered a difficult course between false antinomies. It was neither humoralist nor solidist. It depended neither on "routine" nor on "dogma." Imbued with "a wholly experimental spirit even when it rose to the sublimities of transcendental physiology," Montpellier had "a practical spirit, always directed toward the progress of true medicine, which for it is never an object of vain and sterile contemplation."[119]

Still, no one could deny that progress in medicine had always resulted from progress in philosophy: "the great revolutions in medicine have come from philosophy itself, and . . . all important ameliorations still to be hoped for can be sought nowhere else but at this original source."[120] Elsewhere it might be thought that "art" alone mattered, but in Montpellier it was understood that good medicine could result only from long and arduous consideration of "the science of method."[121] Reversing himself again, however, Bérard then dismissed the view that theory alone could stand as the foundation of medicine: both *médecine-pratique* and *médecine transcendentale* were necessary. If the "bold theories of the one" were not "always weighed by the severe standards of the other," one ended only with "sterile utopias or false applications."[122]

Bérard asserted that Montpellier was perfectly situated for guiding medicine in a "conciliatory and eclectic spirit": it was free from the distractions of the capital and did not suffer the interference of sciences that were more admired and prestigious.[123] Developing an extended analogy between Hippocratic and Montpellier medicine, Bérard argued that the historical circumstances of the two schools were similar in all important respects. Like Cos, Montpellier was not the capital but an important provincial center; it was a meeting ground for diverse commercial and intellectual influences; it enjoyed a balmy, generous climate in which nature could easily do its healing work. Thanks to these favorable conditions, Montpellier replicated Cos's independence of spirit and freedom from dogma.[124]

Like many self-conscious proselytizers for the science of man, Bérard eventually, if rather against his will, turned to Cabanis as the focal point of his meditations. To Bérard, Cabanis was a figure of immense prestige, a revered *maître*, yet at the same time the source of many of the intellectual woes of the age. It was he who, in fulfilling the work of the eighteenth century, had "materialized everything." In 1823 Bérard published a major treatise on the science of man, *Doctrine des rapports du physique et du moral,*

118 *Ibid.*, 80–91; this comment referred specifically to Barthez. Bérard argued that although Barthez was guilty of some confusion and obscurity, he had nonetheless cleansed Montpellier doctrine of both spiritualist and materialist errors and thus succeeded in "generalizing" Montpellier principles. See *ibid.*, 105–8.
119 *Ibid.*, 5, 391–95, 446–49.   120 *Ibid.*, 14.   121 *Ibid.*, 15.   122 *Ibid.*, 439
123 *Ibid.*, 24–32.   124 *Ibid.*, 270–98.

whose title immediately evoked Cabanis. The work opened with a lament for the "metaphysical sciences," on which the eighteenth century had performed a sustained work of destruction. Any subsequent advance in moral science had proved impossible: "Since then everything has been materialized and all principles of moral action have been destroyed. Ideas – and indeed the whole of moral man altogether – have been reduced to sensations."[125] Cabanis and all the others who had contributed to "an incomplete or false ideology" had left the moral sciences in ruin.

Yet despite his antagonism toward Cabanis, Bérard embraced the central claim of the science of man that medicine held the key to understanding human nature and providing guidance on moral questions. Denying that "pure philosophy" could accomplish such a task, he argued that the damage done to moral science by the eighteenth century and the Ideologues could be repaired only by physiology itself:

Only physiology – ever more secure in its progress, measured even in its errors, and complete in its theories – can repair the evil done in its name. It alone can correct itself. No other science has the right or the mission to discover the secrets of *l'homme tout entier*. Only physiology can probe the mystery of sensation, which holds the sure key to human reason that has been vainly sought in abstractions. It can serve metaphysics, if only in declaring itself incompetent on the subject. Devoted especially to the study of organization and life, physiology alone can fix the limits of its domain and give itself laws. Better than any other science, it can – if it refuses to give over to pretensions contrary to observation, its sole guarantee – distinguish that portion of man which belongs to the tomb, and render to metaphysics and religion . . . that portion of man which alone makes him great, noble, and immortal.[126]

Thus Bérard meant to give moral science over to physiology, only for physiology to return to metaphysics and religion what were properly theirs. Yet despite the seemingly prominent role accorded the latter, the preliminary work of classifying, dividing, and demarcating the domains of knowledge lay with physiology because physiology alone could illuminate sensation. In Bérard's view the major challenge of the age was to devise "a theory, more exact and more complete, of the understanding itself and especially of ideas."[127] This task rested with the new generation of physiologists who, "happier or wiser," were ready to build where their forebears had destroyed.[128]

This introduction opened a work whose successive chapters were devoted to sensation, ideas, judgment, reason, and method; memory and imagination; appetites and passions; will and moral freedom; the moral

125 Frédéric Bérard, *Doctrine des rapports du physique et du moral* (Paris: Gabon, 1823), 11. Pétiot notes that Bérard had hurried to complete this work to please the "Minister-Bishop [Frayssinous] who directed the University of France"; see "Notice historique," 64.
126 Bérard, *Doctrine des rapports*, 18–19.   127 *Ibid.*, 16.   128 *Ibid.*, 20–21.

sense; will and muscle movement; habit, imitation, and sympathy; sleep, dreams, delirium, and mental alienation; personality; and, lastly, the soul and psychology. Of these topics Bérard devoted some two-thirds of his text to the problems connected to "sensation and ideas." He began by attacking earlier false doctrines of sensibility, especially those of the medical Ideologues:

Sensation has been viewed as the necessary result of organization (Cabanis), but [we must ask] what is meant by organization. Science must leave behind such vague notions that so easily lead it astray. Organization is nothing but the arrangement of the molecules of matter. What relation can be established between this arrangement, with all its possible combinations, and sensation?[129]

It was impossible to establish a causal relation between organization and the most basic "life properties" (which even Bichat, Bérard noted, regarded as "hyperorganic or added on to matter"), much less the complicated phenomena of sensation.[130] Bérard rejected as utterly groundless Cabanis's teaching that conscious sensation was equivalent to the unconscious impressions generated by vital activity. It was "ridiculous and dangerous" to give the name "sensation" to something that was not felt:

Conscious sensibility and vital sensibility can coexist or replace one another in the same organ; but facts of this order do not prove that the one derives from the other or that one is but an exalted version of the other. . . . All such facts . . . indicate an intimate relation, a powerful influence, or a close linkage between the two properties, but no more. However one regards this relation, this influence, this linkage, and to whatever laws one refers it, such facts will never authorize us to conclude that there is an absolute identity between these two properties.[131]

Scholars and philosophers had attended closely to all phenomena tending to prove the power of the physical over the moral. But they had ignored any facts suggesting the independence of the moral from the physical – and more significant still, the power that the moral exerted over the physical ("those [phenomena] in which moral sensibility augments physical or vital irritability").[132] Given this tendency, it was crucial that moral and physiological science be held separate:

The distinction that we have drawn . . . divides forever the two orders of . . . vital and moral phenomena, vegetative and moral life. Confusion between the two has led ideology and physiology astray through all time. . . . So long as one confounds conscious sensibility and vital sensibility, physiology and metaphysics cannot even exist: one has hypotheses, fictions [*romans*], but not a scientific system. . . . Neither physiology nor metaphysics will exist until each is . . . autonomous and until each has its own laws.[133]

129 *Ibid.*, 55.   130 *Ibid.*, 56.   131 *Ibid.*, 58.   132 *Ibid.*, 59.   133 *Ibid.*, 59–60.

Yet Bérard was not prepared to relinquish physiology's role in creating a moral science: "the relations of the physical and moral will be investigated," he concluded, "but always and only in accordance with the facts given by experience."[134]

As Lordat had done, Bérard sought to undermine the view that sensibility was dependent on the material apparatus of brain and nerves. Unlike Lordat, however, he did not simply recite from Barthez to prove his case. Rather he adduced medical and experimental evidence showing that sensation sometimes survived the sectioning of nerves and paralysis; that some highly sensitive parts of the body had only minimal nervous apparatuses while others that were amply supplied with nerve-endings "show[ed] little sensibility in either health or illness"; and that "a whole class of creatures, zoophytes," had no nervous structures at all, yet had sensibility sufficient for all their needs.[135]

In place of the materialist doctrine that overemphasized the role of the brain and nervous system, Bérard held that sensibility was concentrated in various centers that were located throughout the body and that were, in mechanical terms, wholly independent of one another. This was not to deny the unity of the whole but to make that unity dependent on the general harmony of the organism rather than the directing or guiding action of the brain. The proper relation of the brain to the rest of the body could be understood, Bérard asserted, only if it were conceived in light of the general laws of organization. "All living organs have two sorts of action, one functional and the other dynamic. Sometimes they fulfill the material and organic conditions of life; sometimes they excite the play [*provoquent le jeu*] of vitality, augmenting and supporting the energy of the vital forces."[136] Thus the stomach sometimes presided mechanically over the formation of chyle, but it also, in a general process, "revived, animated, and maintained the tone of all the other organs."[137] If the dual functions of the organs were taken into account, it became clear that "the organs do not all have an equal influence over the others, nor over each individually." Rather there were "nuances, variations, . . . caprices" in these relations, which altered with age, sex, climate, temperament, idiosyncrasy, the state of health or illness."[138] Any doctrine – of the brain or any other organ – that failed to recognize the simultaneous functioning of material operations and vital processes was defective:

It is from this dual series of actions just examined that life results. Materialist physicians, *organicians*, have . . . known only the material of organization and the instruments of life. . . . They have not acted as physiologists properly speaking, whatever the glorious heights to which they have been raised by popular opinion. They have never developed, on the strength of an ensemble of facts, any exact notion

134 *Ibid.*, 60.   135 *Ibid.*, 70–187.   136 *Ibid.*, 157.   137 *Ibid.*   138 *Ibid.*, 158.

of the living forces that govern this inert machine which, without them, would be delivered up to putrefaction and to the murderous action of elements that unceasingly assault it.[139]

It is curious to see Bérard adducing amid these hallowed vitalist tenets an argument from the study of zoophytes, for one of the usual features of the medical science of man in this period was to stress the fact that medical science was necessarily and properly human-centered. But in a typically eclectic spirit Bérard was ready to use whatever arguments and observations were at hand, including comparativist studies, so long as they strengthened his own case. Interestingly, the comparativist to whom Bérard paid the highest tribute was not Cuvier, who has so often been regarded as the iconic figure of conservative life science. Rather, Bérard turned to the man who later was to become Cuvier's chief antagonist from the liberal camp, Etienne Geoffroy Saint-Hilaire.[140] At the moment of Bérard's writing (early 1820s), Geoffroy was still free of the taint he was to acquire in his famous debate with Cuvier, and his "philosophical anatomy" shared some clear affinities with the antireductionist and "metaphysical" tendencies of anthropological medicine.[141]

Drawing on Geoffroy's doctrine of the unitary plan of organic creation, Bérard asked how it could be that the brain and nervous apparatus were essential in higher creatures when they were altogether lacking and unnecessary in the lowest orders. "All animals of the diverse classes are arranged according to the same plan; they do not differ altogether, but only by nuances. The essence of animality is the same in all."[142] Thus, in human beings as in the lower orders, sensibility must be dependent on overall arrangement, not merely on the activities of the nervous system or brain alone. Only those who neglected or were wholly ignorant of comparative anatomy could give so much emphasis to the cerebronervous structures: "Today when we are as preoccupied with other animals as with man himself, when general zoology takes the lead, when one is approaching the general laws of animality, when comparative physiology is establishing the most significant analogies, how can one maintain opinions that are so narrow and that fit so poorly with the ensemble of facts."[143]

This attempt to align Montpellier medicine with modern zoology was a tack that fit well with the larger strategies of eclecticism as a movement.

---

139 *Ibid.*, 158–59.

140 Dorinda Outram throws this traditional representation of Cuvier into question in her *Georges Cuvier: Vocation, Science and Authority in Post-Revolutionary France* (Manchester: Manchester University Press, 1984); cf. Toby Appel, *The Cuvier-Geoffroy Debate: French Biology in the Decades before Darwin* (New York: Oxford University Press, 1987).

141 On Geoffroy's antispecialist inclinations and "synthetic" bent, see Appel, *Cuvier-Geoffroy Debate*, 5–6, 38. For a favorable commentary on Geoffroy's *Philosophie zoologique* by a medical conservative, see Etienne Pariset's review in *Revue encyclopédique* 3 (1819) : 32–40.

142 Bérard, *Doctrine des rapports*, 144–45.   143 *Ibid.*, 81.

Cousin and company never presented themselves as antagonists of science, learning, or rationality, whose prestige they were eager to appropriate. They were openly disdainful of the reactionaries and theocrats (and, as we have seen, persecuted by them). Eclecticism aimed to show science its proper way, to demarcate its zones, to reconcile it with spiritual and metaphysical truths, not to overthrow it. Thus eclecticism was determinedly and avowedly "modern."[144]

This eclectic disposition helps to explain Bérard's stance in a controversy that developed in the later 1820s over the medical effects of the advance of civilization.[145] In this controversy too, Bérard assumed a "modern" and "progressive" position, arguing against critics of industrialism and urbanism that the net social effects of such innovations were beneficial to both individual and public health. Bérard's own contribution to the debate took the form of a treatise published in 1826 in which he denied the Rousseauist view that the progress of civilization damaged health by rendering the body sedentary and weak, and exposing the spirit to the iniquitous influence of inequality of fortune, excessive passion, and exaggerated needs.[146] The keynote of "harmony" was again sounded as Bérard waxed lyrical on the benefits to be gained from an ever more perfect and cooperative division of labor. In this context the traditional Montpellier image of the integrated body economy was refashioned to conjure a smoothly functioning industrial society whose parts cooperated to achieve common ends. Bérard argued that, although human beings were weak when alone, they were strong when the "powers" of men and women, adults and children were united in "joyous harmony." Only "industry" (in the broadest sense) could alter "the agents capable of modifying men" – diet, clothing, lodging, exercise, *aisance*, a feeling of moral dignity, and "security of property and person."[147] Health was dependent on all these conditions, and civilized society alone – by harnessing and channeling human energies – could mold them.

To Bérard the benefits of civilization were obvious: famine and all its accompanying diseases had been ended, slavery was almost everywhere abolished, inequality was either on the wane or restructured for the greater public good ("if [civilization] permits or favors certain natural inequalities, that is to the advantage of industry and public prosperity.")[148] In all cases, "the illumination given by medical philosophy" was the "purest source of the most important truths."

144 Spitzer, *French Generation of 1820*, 81–82.
145 William R. Coleman, *Death Is a Social Disease: Public Health and Political Economy in Early Industrial France* (Madison: University of Wisconsin Press, 1982), 292–302.
146 Frédéric Bérard, *Discours sur les améliorations progressives de la santé publique, par l'influence de la civilisation* (Paris and Montpellier: Gabon, 1826).
147 *Ibid.*, 18.   148 *Ibid.*, 45.

It is never an excess of civilization that harms the human species, physically or morally. Yet it is always in its imperfection – in a state marked more or less with the taint of barbarism – that a solution is, erroneously, sought for human misery.[149]

Thus on all these matters, Bérard emerged as a champion both of the form of social and economic organization favored by conservative liberals and of the essential role that physicians must play in ushering in a new era of moral, physical, and social health.

Throughout the early 1820s Bérard tried repeatedly to win appointment to a chair on the Montpellier faculty but was blocked by what one biographer called his "protected" rivals (probably candidates who were more unambiguously conservative than Bérard).[150] Finally in 1825, Bérard was named to the chair in hygiene and returned to Montpellier to teach. Bérard's program for his hygiene course distinguished between "hygiene-art" and "hygiene-science," and promised to trace the "different hypotheses that had reigned within the science of living man and then been introduced into hygiene proper." The course was divided into three parts: the "effects of external agents on man"; the "effects man exerts on himself through the exercise of his functions"; and "the effects one sex has on the other." This classification provided space for a great range of topics. Bérard opened with the general problem of "life," treated both "individually and collectively," and then turned to all "physical and moral agents that modify human life," including air, climate, habitation, clothing, baths, foods, drinks, and water. In considering how "humans affect themselves," he devised the three classes of, first, Excreta (saliva, bile, feces, transpiration, sweat, mucus); second, Percepta, which included the general nature of sensibility, overall functioning of the individual senses, the faculties of the intellect and understanding, the passions, and sleep; and, third, Gesta and Acta, where he considered exercise, gymnastics, and the physical effects of the professions. His last great division, peculiarly entitled "Genitalia," addressed the reproductive act, conception, pregnancy, childbirth, nursing, and "cessation of the sexual life." In all instances, Bérard examined not only the subject itself but variations caused by age, sex, temperament, constitution, idiosyncrasy, state of health, national difference, and race, as well as the applications of all this knowledge in "public and private" hygiene and specific "prophylactic methods."[151]

Although Bérard always referred to hygiene as but one part of the larger science of man, the part in this case subsumed the whole. Having at last

149 *Ibid.*, 18. The bulk of the work was devoted to the population question since population growth was widely regarded as the best measure of the health or sickness of society; see Léonard, *Médecine entre les pouvoirs et les savoirs*, 159–60.
150 Pétiot, "Notice historique."
151 *Faculté de Médecine de Montpellier. Année scolaire 1825. Semestre d'été. Programme du cours d'hygiène privée et publique. M. F. Bérard, Professeur* (Montpellier: Faculté de Médecine, 1825).

gained his professorial post, Bérard was perhaps reluctant to omit from his instruction anything of real interest to the general science of man. This prospectus would seem to reflect a strong ambition to train a new generation of Montpellier physicians for all the tasks of anthropological medicine, but as Bérard died less than two years after his appointment to the Montpellier faculty, this was an ambition he had no opportunity to fulfill.

The hygiene chair at Montpellier was later held by another physician of eclectic temper, François Ribes, who opened his course with an address entitled *Discours sur l'éclectisme médical.*[152] Like Bérard, Ribes too was more interested in "hygiene-science" than in "hygiene-art." Indeed in his book *Fondemens sur la doctrine médicale de la vie universelle* – an amalgam of vitalism, "associationism," and homeopathy – he held that all physicians were either theorists or practitioners, and clearly lodged himself with the former. Theorists were by nature devoted to the study of "general facts" rather than minute particulars and to the "nonmaterial" rather than the "material." For Ribes the principal attraction of hygiene lay in the opportunity it presented for addressing the fundamental problems of medical philosophy and method.[153]

As the cases of Bérard and Ribes indicate, during the Restoration hygiene became one of the principal preserves of physicians who wanted to realize the public ambitions of anthropological medicine while evading its identification with materialism and Ideology. The hygienic movement was in many ways the perfect medical corollary of philosophical eclecticism for it too presented itself as forward-looking, untroubled by the ideological divisions of the past, and loyal to the values of the emergent bourgeois order. And just as the ideologists of Orleanism portrayed the new regime as embodying the measure, balance, and moderation of the *juste milieu,* the hygienists set themselves the task of transcending quarrels over medical dogma.[154]

Yet there were important differences between the Montpellier hygienists-eclectics and those in Paris. The hygienists in Montpellier sought to transcend dogma by devising a conciliatory approach to medical philosophy. In Paris, on the other hand, the promoters of hygiene vigorously repudiated philosophy as such and directed hygiene toward practical problems presented by concrete social life. Hygiene was different in Montpellier not only because of what Bérard's colleague Dupau saw as the natural division between Paris medicine's dedication to "experiments and observation" and Montpellier's devotion to "methods and general principles."[155] Much more important was the absence in Montpellier of the social and institutional con-

---

152 François Ribes, *Discours sur l'éclectisme médical* (Montpellier: Sevalle, 1829).
153 François Ribes, *Fondemens sur la doctrine médicale de la vie universelle* (Montpellier: Sevalle; Paris: Deville-Cavellin, 1835), 19–20.
154 Coleman, *Death Is a Social Disease,* 22–24.   155 Dupau, "Notice historique," 4.

ditions that in Paris encouraged the pragmatic development of hygienic science. As Coleman has shown, Paris hygiene focused on problems caused by the new industrial order and was thus a medical movement rooted in congested, noisy, dirty urban life. Many of the problems addressed by the Paris hygienists did not even exist in Montpellier, which in the 1820s had some thirty thousand inhabitants and almost no industry. Furthermore, the medical bureaucracy that had been established in Paris under the Consulate and the Empire for the medical surveillance of the population was lacking in Montpellier. Nothing comparable to the Paris Health Council and its city-wide bureaucratic substructures existed there. And as Colin Jones has shown in examining treatment for the mentally ill in Montpellier, even in the hospitals the professional medical establishment had difficulty asserting its authority against the entrenched nursing sisters and other representatives of the old medical order.[156] Thus the Montpellier hygienists remained theorists rather than practitioners of anthropological medicine despite their ritual salutes to *médecine pratique*. It is to Paris, then, that we must turn to see how doctors of the era sought to divest the science of man of its metaphysical pretensions both by undertaking intensive empirical investigations and, no doubt equally important, by articulating a new rhetoric of pragmatism and practice.

THE SCIENCE OF MAN AT WORK: HYGIENE AND MENTAL MEDICINE

Although hygiene had long been central to medical theory and practice, it was institutionalized as a scholarly and pedagogical field only during the Revolution. The first hygiene chair, established in the Paris Ecole de santé in 1794, went to Jean-Noël Hallé, an active and vocal member of the Société médicale d'émulation and a figure whose writings reflected the preoccupation of revolutionary medicine with the public and social dimensions of the healing art.[157] In the 1822 purge, Hallé was replaced by R. H. Bertin, a conservative appointee who held the chair during the crucial years 1822–28 but who wrote little and generally avoided the spotlight.[158] Bertin's inactivity helped to displace the development of hygiene to institutional loci outside the Faculty of Medicine, a move further encouraged by the work of two men in particular, Jean-Baptiste Parent-Duchâtelet and Louis-René Villermé. Parent-Duchâtelet was a long-time member of the Paris Health Council. Along with other members of the council, he was instrumental in founding the *Annales d'hygiène publique et de médecine légale*, which rapidly came to be the authoritative tribune on all matters hygienic. Unlike Parent-

156 Colin Jones, "The Treatment of the Insane in Eighteenth- and Early Nineteenth-Century Montpellier," *Medical History* 24 (1980) : 371–90.
157 See Chapter 2. 158 Coleman, *Death Is a Social Disease*, 18.

Duchâtelet, Villermé had no permanent official position in the medical bureaucracy. After ten years as a military surgeon in Napoleon's army, he worked briefly as a private practitioner and then devoted himself to matters of public health while living on private means. His introduction to the capital's medical establishment was through the Société médicale d'émulation, whose meetings he attended regularly from 1815 to 1824 and which he served as secretary and as editor of its publications.[159]

These two figures, in company with such regular contributors to the *Annales* as C. C. H. Marc, J. P. J. d'Arcet, and François Leuret, elaborated a view of hygiene and public health that to a large extent was inspired by earlier formulations of the medical science of man but that eschewed political and philosophical imbroglios of the sort that had bedeviled medical Ideology. A programmatic statement of the intentions and mission of hygiene appeared in the opening volume of the *Annales d'hygiène publique:*

Medicine has for its object not only to study and heal the sick, it has intimate relations with social organization; sometimes it lends aid to the legislator in the formulation of laws, often it enlightens the magistrate in their application and always it attends, with the administration, to the maintenance of public health.[160]

Together these kinds of pursuits constituted "public hygiene and legal medicine," whose absence from the French medical scene thus far amounted to a "true lacuna in our medical literature."[161] These new fields would investigate a range of problems including conditions in the workplace, hospitals, barracks, prisons, and madhouses; the quality of ingesta (food, water, drugs); and environmental conditions that encouraged disease. Legal medicine was narrower in scope but not less important; its charge was to enlighten the authorities on questions of "moral liberty" in criminal actions, and on judgments required in cases of infanticide, suicide, homicide, and other acts of violence against persons.[162]

Hygienists were committed to the "perfecting of our institutions," reforms that would contribute in turn to "the progress of the human spirit" and to the "noble task of diminishing the number of social infirmities."[163] Thus the state must function as physician to the ills of society, a task that depended on the work of hygienic medicine:

159 *Ibid.,* 5–6; see also Dora Weiner, "Public Health under Napoleon: The Conseil de Salubrité de Paris, 1802–15," *Clio medica* 9 (1974) : 271–84; Ann F. LaBerge, "The Paris Health Council, 1802–1848," *BHM* 49 (1975) : 339–52.

160 "Prospectus," *AHPML* 1 (1829) : v.   161 *Ibid.*

162 *Ibid.,* v, xx, xxxv. That contemporaries saw legal medicine as developing out of the science of man is clear from a *thèse* written by the Montpellier graduate J.-J. Barthez in an XI. He defined legal medicine as "the part of the science of man that is devoted to assisting the upholders of the laws in distributing justice." See J.-J. Barthez, *Essai médico-légal sur l'infanticide* (Montpellier: Tournel, an XI), 7.

163 "Prospectus," v–vi.

Faults and crimes are ills of society that we must work to cure or at least to diminish, and the means of cure will never be so powerful as when they derive their *mode d'action* from discoveries concerning both physical and intellectual man and when physiology and hygiene lend their enlightenment to the science of government.[164]

The hygienists' readiness to collaborate with administrators and magistrates was a constant theme of this prospectus and was reiterated frequently in later issues of their journal. Doctors working under the aegis of hygiene thus sought not an independent role but an intimate working relationship with public authorities, a position that was bitterly criticized by populist physicians such as François Raspail who argued that the people must take responsibility for their own health.[165]

Although the hygienists said little about the larger rationale for their intervention, the theoretical justification for the hygienic enterprise derived entirely from the principles of anthropological medicine. It was only because French physicians had been assuming for decades that there was an intimate relation between physical well-being and *morale* that the hygienists could so easily assert a connection between hygienic improvement and the forward march of civilization. The high degree of attention given to "external agents" was justified not only by recourse to the doctrine of the nonnaturals (a connection William Coleman has demonstrated), but to the general disposition of anthropological medicine to interrogate the environment as an integral part of both diagnostics and therapeutics. The eagerness of hygienists to categorize the population according to diverse physical and social variables (height, occupation, neighborhood) reflected their thorough grounding in the doctrine of types preferred by the medical science of man. Thus it was anthropological medicine that allowed the hygienists to claim as part of their purview any substance, general environmental condition, or activity that contributed to the maintenance of the life of the organism (all ingesta), formed its milieu (air, water, climate, the Hippocratic "places"), or conditioned its own response (exercise, work, habits). Within such a rubric virtually anything could be said to impinge on health or sickness and therefore to fall under the authority of the doctor.[166]

The extent to which the environmentalist prescriptions of the science of man had become generally accepted is indicated by the triumph of "infectious" and "miasmatic" theories over contagionism in the famous Académie de médecine debate of 1827–28. As Erwin Ackerknecht has shown,

---

164 *Ibid.*, vii.
165 See Dora B. Weiner, *Raspail: Scientist and Reformer* (New York: Columbia University Press, 1968).
166 Villermé conceived hygiene as divided into three domains – the moral, physical, and intellectual; its coverage of the circumstances impinging on "[man's] physical and moral atmosphere" was comprehensive. Villermé, "Sur l'hygiène morale, considérée particulièrement dans le royaume des Pays-Bas," *AHPML* 4 (1830) : 25–47, esp. 25, 47. (This article was devoted particularly to demonstrating connections between the incidence of crimes against property and persons and the spread of industrial-commerical civilization.)

the contagionist-anticontagionist debate made a great stir partly because of its economic consequences (the quarantine recommended by contagionists meant erecting barriers to trade) and partly because of its political implications (in the 1822 yellow fever epidemic quarantine meant sending Bourbon troops to the border with revolutionary Spain).[167] Yet the attention historians have given to the bitter divisions caused by this split has obscured the extent to which even the staunchest contagionists, such as Etienne Pariset, embraced the broadly environmental posture of anthropological medicine. After his defeat in the contagionist-anticontagionist struggle, Pariset went on to function as an important member of the hygienist *équipe* that was called upon by the Orleanist regime to attack a range of environmental ills.[168] Thus physicians who were contagionists rather than environmentalists in the specific context of the spread of epidemic disease might well appear as environmentalists in other contexts, for example in linking disease to poverty, vicious habits contracted in unsavory living circumstances, and so forth.

The environmentalism encouraged by the science of man was to take on even more complex dimensions as time went on. Although the hygienists of the 1820s through the 1840s were "environmentalists" in the context of debates over the etiology of disease, hygiene as a general medical movement in France came to have distinctly "antienvironmentalist" implications – the word shifting meaning – in the increasingly important context of the delineation of physiological, pathological, and racial types. As Coleman and others have shown, the hygienists saw "filth" as the source of many of the medicosocial ills suffered by the laboring classes, and thus blamed the environment for a range of pathological phenomena and for variable rates of mortality.[169] Yet in the long run the hygienic movement served as one of the most important medical sources for the view that medicosocial maladies should be attributed not so much to external influences as to the fixing of vice and pathological inclinations in bloodlines. This tendency was already evident in the 1820s in the work of Julien-Joseph Virey, who was an important theoretician of hygiene, although he stood outside the inner circle of the hygiene movement dominated by Parent-Duchâtelet and Villermé. During the Restoration Virey elaborated a doctrine of physiological types that suggested there was relatively little hygienic medicine could do to alter proclivities created by the variable distribution of vital force in the body economy.[170] By the 1840s hygienists were increasingly sympathetic to such views. Drawing in some cases on phrenology and in others on emergent

---

167 Erwin Ackerknecht, "Anti-contagionism between 1821 and 1867," *BHM* 22 (1948): 562–93.
168 Léonard, *Médecine entre les pouvoirs et les savoirs*, 210.
169 Coleman, *Death Is a Social Disease*, 149–80.
170 Julien-Joseph Virey, *Des métamorphoses physiologiques de l'homme dans l'éducation* (extract *Gazette médicale de Paris*) (Paris, 1815).

heredity theory, they increasingly tended to argue that pathological patterns became fixed as inherited "tendencies" or "dispositions," even if they were originally prompted by unfortunate environmental influences. The ultimate product of this "fixist" tendency in hygienic science was the creation of the type of the "degenerate," the individual whose heredity predisposed him to a range of medicomoral ills and whose potential for therapeutic management was severely limited.[171]

But this is to anticipate later developments. Throughout the Restoration and into the Orleanist era, the theoretical assumptions and imperatives of the science of man remained well in the background of hygienic discourse. In the 1820s hygienists showed little interest in elucidating the philosophical, epistemological, or even methodological rationales for their endeavor. In its review section, the *Annales d'hygiène publique* showed itself hostile to works of medical philosophy and ridiculed works the editors regarded as overly speculative.[172] Eschewing theory, the hygienists sought authority instead in numbers. They greeted enthusiastically the appearance in 1837 of a new journal, *Mémoires de la Société médicale d'observation*, founded by P. C. A. Louis, who in the late 1820s had become an insistent advocate of the use of statistics in medical investigation. Louis was "cleverer than anyone in the art of diagnosing maladies," the *Annales* reviewer stated, and "thanks to the severity of his method, [he has] discovered many important truths."[173] Louis's particular findings on disease were not relevant to hygiene, but the method he taught was precisely the one "that gave so much value to the works of . . . Parent-Duchâtelet."[174] The *Annales* proudly published excerpts from the writings of the Belgian statistician Adolphe Quetelet, who was regarded in the medical community as the supreme authority on statistical questions. In 1831, for example, it published an extract from a memoir Quetelet had delivered to the Brussels Academy on "the law of human growth" in which he demonstrated that the "penchant for crime" hit its maximum between the ages of twenty-five and thirty. In that piece Quetelet made favorable reference to the work of François Chaussier, Virey, and Villermé himself, thus indicating the commonality of interest between his own statistical endeavors and French anthropological medicine.[175]

171 Robert A. Nye, *Crime, Madness, and Politics in Modern France: The Medical Concept of National Decline* (Princeton: Princeton University Press, 1984), 119–31; Daniel Pick, *Faces of Degeneration: A European Disorder, c.1848–c.1918* (Cambridge: Cambridge University Press, 1989).

172 See, for example, *AHPML* 9 (1833) : 235, for a review of J.-J. Virey's *Petit manuel d'hygiène prophylactique contre les épidémies*, and *AHPML* 17 (1837) : 455, where the reviewer attacks Casimir Broussais's *Hygiène morale*.

173 *AHPML* 17 (1837) : 464–65.

174 *Ibid.* Parent-Duchâtelet had died the previous year.

175 *AHPML* 6 (1831) : 88–113. On the friendly personal relations between Quetelet and Villermé, see Coleman, *Death Is a Social Disease*, 9, 120, 136.

It is instructive to note that in his famous work of 1835, *De l'homme,* Quetelet adopted an attitude toward medical philosophy and the usefulness of statistics very similar to that espoused by the Paris hygienists. He insisted that his work was limited to "physical man" and did not extend to subjects that were "dependent on moral phenomena."[176] Statistics were essential to medicine for it was only by knowing what was normal that pathological anomalies could be recognized: "in order to recognize whatever is an anomaly, it is . . . necessary to have established the type constituting the normal or healthy condition."[177] The establishment of types was thus an essential endeavor, and to this end only statistics would serve.

Though it will carry us a bit beyond the chronological limits of this chapter, it is important at this point to try to sort out the attitude toward statistics that came to characterize anthropological medicine in the late 1820s and into the 1830s. The medical vitalism from which the science of man derived was inherently hostile to the idea that the phenomena of health and sickness could be pinpointed with precision or reduced to rigid laws. This was one of the chief ways in which vitalism differentiated itself from mechanist medicine. According to vitalist teaching, medical phenomena were characterized by particularity, spontaneity, and variability. Since each case of disease was individual, medicine had to recognize and interpret minute nuances, something that mechanist procedures could never do. This disposition to see medicine as the study of particularistic phenomena continued with medical Ideology. Cabanis repeatedly stressed the necessity of recognizing that vital phenomena did not exhibit the regularities characteristic of the physical actions of brute objects.[178] Such a viewpoint would seem to preclude any recourse to numbers, and it is true that in the writings of the Montpellier doctors and their emulators in Parisian medicine of the revolutionary years, statistical data have no great prominence.

Yet statistics were not altogether lacking in these works, and it would be wrong to see vitalist and anthropological medicine as completely hostile to the use of numbers. Barthez counted and measured when it suited him, and it was the medical Ideologues Cabanis, and especially Pinel, who first insisted most vigorously on the need to keep clear and accurate clinical records.[179] When vitalists insisted on the variability of medical phenomena, then, they did not rule out the use of numbers. Rather they urged that what was to be expected of numbers was fairly limited. Physicians could, indeed

176 Adolphe Quetelet, *A Treatise on Man and the Development of his Faculties* (1842; rpt. New York: Burt Franklin, 1968), v.
177 *Ibid.,* vi.
178 See Chapters 1 and 2.
179 See, e.g., Barthez's references to Peter Camper's facial angle in *Théorie du beau dans la nature et les arts,* 2d ed. (Paris: Vigot, 1895), 70–71. For Cabanis's views on the use of statistics, see Staum, *Cabanis,* 105, 135. See also Philippe Pinel, *Résultats d'observations et construction des tables pour servir à déterminer le degré de probabilité de la guérison des aliénés* (Paris: Baudouin, 1808), esp. 6–10.

must, seek generalizations and patterns; otherwise therapeutics would be wholly haphazard. Yet they must not expect to find complete, or even a high degree of, uniformity in vital phenomena. Above all, they must not anticipate the discovery of invariable "laws." It is only within the context of this attitude toward numbers that the vitalist injunction to seek and delineate "types" (of disease, of treatment, of constitution or temperament) makes any sense. If no regularity was to be expected at all, there could be no medically established types since phenomena would be seen as merely accidental or capricious. Yet it had always to be recognized that organized beings showed markedly less regularity than those made up of unorganized matter.[180]

By around 1830 it was increasingly difficult for physicians to maintain this skeptical and nuanced view of the use of statistics. As experimental and statistical procedures grew in prestige in the other sciences, doctors who were intent on making medicine properly scientific began to insist with new vehemence that medicine must adopt statistical procedures. The Société médicale d'observation made the informed use of statistics its most important criterion for judging diagnostic and therapeutic claims. The society's prospectus noted that its sole purpose was to "train observers" and asserted that the importance of "numerical analysis" in this work was so great that it required no discussion.[181]

The vehemence of the "medical observers" evoked a strong response from other medical quarters. In 1837 an angry debate took place in the Académie de médecine in which traditionalists, some of them frankly vitalist in orientation, denounced the recourse to numbers and insisted on the particularity and irreducibility of medical phenomena. An important spokesman for this point of view was Frédéric Dubois d'Amiens, who spent much of a long career as perpetual secretary of the academy inveighing against medical statistics in particular and the whole attempt to scientize medicine in general.[182]

The response to the statistics campaign among those physicians who worked within the orientation of the science of man cannot be characterized simply. Some physicians working in an anthropological vein were hostile to numerical procedures (Virey, the Montpellier eclectics, Dubois himself);

180 On the difficulties involved in attempting to find statistical guides to mental alienation, see Philippe Pinel, *Traité médico-philosophique sur l'aliénation mentale, ou la manie* (Paris: Richard, Caille, Ravier, 1801), 108–33.
181 *Mémoires de la Société medicale d'observation* 1 (1837) : xi–xii. Cf. the address by Jean Cruveilhier to the Société anatomique in which he declared that that society's work was more valuable to medicine than any other since it emphasized "palpable facts, independent of all theory, representing the mathematical side of a science that is not wholly conjectural." Quoted in *Archives générales de médecine*, 2d. ser., 4 (1834) : 252.
182 "Discussion sur la statistique médicale," *Bulletin de l'Académie royale de médecine*, no. 13 (April 15, 1837) : 684–714; and see, on that debate, F. L. I. Valleix, "Avant-propos," *Mémoires de la Société médicale d'observation* 2 (1844) : xv–xxxv.

others, like the Paris hygienists, were not only enthusiastic advocates of numbers but sought energetically to appropriate statistical authority. All of this raises the interesting question of why in this period statistics became so problematic and their use in medicine a subject of such highly charged debate. One answer is simply to see the problem as a result of the incremental spread of statistics in medicine and the pressure exerted by determined advocates of statistics. It is more enlightening, however, to situate the issue in relation to the discourse of anthropological medicine. From this perspective, numbers in medicine became a peculiarly weighty problem for many physicians precisely because their use was first suggested by the visionaries of anthropological medicine such as Cabanis and Pinel. There thus lurked in the enterprise of making medicine numerical the danger that such procedures would be used not only to characterize corporal phenomena but the phenomena of mental and passional life as well. Once the possibility was admitted that mental phenomena could be reduced to numerical regularities, the room left for the exercise of moral capacities (judgment, free will, self-control) was severely diminished.

This interpretation is borne out by a reading of Quetelet, who in opening *De l'homme* felt compelled to insist against his critics that the discovery of numerical patterns in "phenomena affecting man" lent no support to "materialist" or "fatalist" perspectives on morality. "If certain deplorable facts present themselves with alarming regularity, to whom," he asked, "is blame to be ascribed?"[183] It was because anthropological medicine cut such a wide swath – encompassing not only organic but mental and passional phenomena as well – that numbers were to be feared. For the "medical observers," whose journal restricted its coverage to topics such as pulmonary emphysema, cataracts, cardiac disease, and phthisis, the legitimacy of statistics was clear.[184] Yet for those who wanted medicine to encompass not only physical function and malady but also a broad range of psychosocial matters, the medical embrace of numbers opened yet another domain of conflict over the implications of "materialism."

This whole problem is related, furthermore, to conflicts over physicians' constructions of their public identity, especially to problems raised by incipient specialization. In the Académie de médecine debate François-Joseph Double argued that if doctors chose their therapeutic approach purely by counting the number of times a technique had been successfully applied, the practice of medicine would inevitably decline in stature:

If in so many cases of smallpox, we have obtained infinitely greater success with bleeding than with the analytic method, then [it is said] one must always bleed for

183 Quetelet, *Treatise on Man*, vii.
184 See, for example, the first three volumes of the society's *Mémoires*, published in 1837, 1844, and 1856. Theoretical issues in medicine were treated, if at all, only in the introductory preliminaries to each volume.

smallpox. Such examples could be multiplied, and if so the practice of medicine would no longer be a science, it would no longer be an art, it would scarcely be a *métier*. . . . The physician would then resemble a shoemaker who after measuring the feet of a thousand individuals . . . takes an average and insists on fitting everyone by the measure of this imaginary client.[185]

The true doctor did not limit his art to counting similarities and differences but in each case brought to bear a complex body of knowledge that made possible both the recognition and interpretation of the nuances of disease. This dimension of the contest over statistics reproduced at another level the conflict over whether medicine should be embracive in its purview or restricted to discrete, small-scale, seemingly soluble problems. The use of statistics thus raised once again the same issues of self-definition – both theoretical and, as Double's statement suggests, social – that were prompted by the techniques of pathological anatomy and laboratory experimentation. In this instance too techniques whose prestige would later be unquestioned at this point suggested to many doctors not an enhancement but a humbling of medical science. None of this is to say, however, that those doctors who embraced the tradition of the science of man should be uniformly relegated to some kind of antimodern camp where statistics, autopsy, and innovation as such were abhorred. As Jan Goldstein has observed, the tradition of anthropological medicine always encompassed the two competing tendencies of grandiose generalization and increasing specialization.[186] If the imperatives toward medical specialization came from diverse quarters, not least among them was the need perceived by many physicians within the science of man tradition to get about its manifold tasks by focusing on particular domains of the larger enterprise. So it was with hygiene, which became a highly successful specialty in good part by adopting the increasingly authoritative procedures of statistics.

All the same, the controversy over statistics meant that the hygienists' recourse to and valorization of statistics had to be undertaken with real care. Hygienists expected that statistical regularities were to be found in a broad range of human phenomena – even in matters such as the physical disposition to crime – where the search for patterns might appear to vitiate individual moral responsibility. They insisted that the discovery and interpretation of such regularities were tasks best performed by doctors. They linked their statistical enterprise to the aims and projects of the most determined medical statisticians like Louis. Yet for an *équipe* that sought at one and the same time to extend the domain of medicine as far as possible into sociomoral concerns and to avoid the charges of materialism and fatalism, this purchase of authority from statistics had to be carefully negotiated and

185 "Discussion sur la statistique médicale," 702.
186 Jan Goldstein, *Console and Classify: The French Psychiatric Profession in the Nineteenth Century* (Cambridge: Cambridge University Press, 1987), 55.

ideologically problematic themes to be avoided. Thus in the early years of its existence, the *Annales* took up such matters as mortality rates in prisons, the influence of tobacco on workers, meteorological readings taken at the Royal Observatory, the diet of sailors, the height of Frenchmen, the many techniques of poisoning, and the like.[187] In their handling of such subjects, the hygienists assumed outright the fundamental principles of anthropological medicine – the interrelation of physical and moral phenomena, the necessarily social character of medicine, the value of medical typologizing. But they refrained uniformly from articulating these principles or, in mobilizing statistical indicators, from exploring the implications and meaning of the numerical patterning of physicomoral phenomena.

A similar reticence about the great questions of the science of man is evident in the discourse of mental medicine, the other practical medical endeavor that flourished on the terrain of the science of man from the 1820s. The historical origins of psychiatry have been explored in considerable detail in recent decades, and the link between mental medicine and the medical science of man is clearly established. In the broadest sense, of course, the lineage of all investigations into mental phenomena can be traced to eighteenth-century inquiry into sensation and sensibility, which engendered both those questions about the brain and the nervous system that ushered in modern psychiatric and neurological science and those considerations of the diffuse, systemic, and holistic relations between physical and mental experience that were central to the vitalist tradition. The Montpellier doctors had insisted on the immediate and powerful relations existing between mental phenomena and physical states – whether of humors, solids, or the general body economy – relations that were expressed in "sympathies" operating among the various vital centers and in the generalized effects of temperament and constitution.[188] The medical Ideologues reiterated on diverse occasions the need for a fully elaborated science of mental phenomena both to fulfill the potential of Ideology to become "the science of ideas" and to devise a therapeutics for those maladies that, as Alibert expressed it, "put humanity to shame." Cabanis had argued against the autonomy of reason by pointing to the diverse influences that physical states, especially those caused by disease, exercised over mental function, and had called for intensive inquiry into those phenomena – dreams, instinctual actions, madness – that most clearly manifested these relations.[189]

Of the medical Ideologues who made this plea, it was Pinel who set mental medicine on its course, both with his theoretical work on the classification of nervous disorders and with the therapeutic innovations he summed up as the "moral treatment." In the nineteenth century the story of Pinel's

187 These matters are treated in *AHPML*, vols. 1–10.
188 See Chapter 1, esp. "Vitality and Variability."
189 See Chapter 2, esp. "From Physiology to Moral Science."

responding to the humanitarian impulses of the age by unchaining the mad-
men at Bicêtre constituted French psychiatry's most cherished myth of
origins.[190] Yet as Jan Goldstein has shown, the key figure in the institutional development of French psychiatry was not Pinel but his favored pupil
Jean-Etienne-Dominique Esquirol, who during the Restoration offered
clinical instruction in mental medicine at the Salpêtrière and formed a circle
of young physicians who specialized in the field. The process by which
mental medicine achieved professional and scientific standing was by no
means an untroubled one, but throughout the 1820s and especially in the
Orleanist years the field gradually became entrenched. The Law of June 30,
1838, gave mental medicine the seal of government approval, providing for
the establishment of a nationwide system of asylums under the supervision
of the minister of the interior and providing for the clinical training of new
practitioners.[191]

During the Restoration, however, psychiatry's bureaucratic success story
lay in the future, and it was only because the promoters of mental medicine
successfully maneuvered around ideological pitfalls that the field ultimately
earned its institutional rewards. Clearly in the atmosphere of the Restoration a formulation of mental medicine that openly styled itself heir to the
Cabanisian science of the physical and the moral would have been anath-
ema. Thus the advocates of mental medicine had to chart ways to investigate the problems posed by the science of man without giving ideological
offense and thereby jeopardizing their own opportunities for winning institutional positions and bureaucratic authority. One path taken by a number of young physicians who wanted to pursue the general problem of the
physical basis for mental action was to take refuge in strictly delimited neuroanatomical and neurophysiological studies, the kind of investigation of
the brain and nervous system that for some time naturalists had undertaken
for the "lower orders." By the diverse routes that Dorinda Outram has surveyed, Cuvier had come by 1812 to focus on the nervous system as the key
to animal classification (at least in theory if not always in actual practice).[192]
Then in the two decades after Cuvier's own shift in this direction, more and
more naturalists – many of them Cuvier's protégés – took up problems in
the comparative anatomy of the nervous system. The most celebrated result
was the publication by Pierre-Marie Flourens, who enjoyed Cuvier's approbation and the benefits of his patronage, of the results of his experiments on
cerebellar function. Flourens relied on the still-controversial techniques of
vivisection in these experiments, as did François Magendie in his work on

190 Goldstein, *Console and Classify*, 209–10. Goldstein discusses too the simultaneous usage of
such symbolism by clerics and nuns whose work was part of an intensified religious effort
to offer treatment for the insane.
191 *Ibid.*, 276 (chap. 8 is devoted to analyzing the passage of this law).
192 Dorinda Outram, "Uncertain Legislator: George Cuvier's Laws of Nature in Their Intellectual Context," *JHB* 19 (1984) : 323–68.

the roots of the cranial nerves. As Robert Young has pointed out, this kind of experimental work was narrowly restricted in range and purpose, focusing on closely defined problems of sensorimotor function to the exclusion of less tractable, and ideologically more compromising, problems of personality and behavior such as those Gall had approached.[193]

Flourens, Magendie, and other physiologists undertook this kind of work in the institutional settings that supported the comparativist work of naturalists: Faculté des sciences, Muséum d'histoire naturelle, Collège de France. But at the same time, there were medical investigators who were determined to pursue similar investigations for human beings by searching in autopsy for the physical lesions corresponding to clinically documented mental malady. This group included such figures as Achille Foville, Léon Rostan, Pierre-Augustin Béclard, and Etienne-Jean Georget, all of whom published works in the 1820s treating human neuroanatomy.[194] Of these, Foville and Georget were associated with Esquirol's circle and undertook neuroanatomical investigations in part within the context of psychiatric inquiry and therapeutics. A brief look at Foville's work will indicate the relation of such labors to the larger impulses and requirements of the science of man.

In 1828 Foville, who had pursued clinical study with Esquirol at the Salpêtrière from 1822–24 and then taken up a post at an asylum in Rouen, submitted to the Académie des sciences a work entitled "Recherches sur l'anatomie du cerveau" whose principal purpose was to clarify the organization and purposes of the *cordon*, which in his view was continuous with the spinal cord proper and divided in the region of the brain itself into three "superimposed plans: upper, lower, and middle."[195] This work was reported on by Henri de Blainville, with whom Foville had studied at the Muséum d'histoire naturelle while pursuing his medical studies, and by

193 Robert Young, *Mind, Brain and Adaptation in the Nineteenth Century: Cerebral Localization and Its Biological Context from Gall to Ferrier* (Oxford: Clarendon Press, 1970), 55–94. See also Edwin Clarke and L. S. Jacyna, *Nineteenth-Century Origins of Neuroscientific Concepts* (Berkeley: University of California Press, 1987), 111–12, 212–14, 244–66, 279–86, 291–307; Judith Swazey, "Action propre and action commune: The Localization of Cerebral Function," *JHB* 3 (1970) : 213–34. Although no precise record remains, it seems that Flourens did take up some larger psychological and philosophical problems connected to study of the nervous system in a course he presented to the Athénée in 1821. See Georgette Legée, "M. J. P. Flourens (1794–1867) et Destutt de Tracy (1754–1836)," *Histoire et nature* 2 (1974) : 95–98.

194 Achille-Louis Foville and Félix Pinel-Grandchamp, *Recherches sur le siège spécial des différentes fonctions du système nerveux* (Paris: A. Borée, 1823); Foville, *Traité complet de l'anatomie, de la physiologie et de la pathologie du système nerveux cérébrospinal* (Paris: Fortin, Masson, 1844); Léon Rostan, *Recherches sur le ramollissement du cerveau,* 2d ed. (Paris: Béchet, Gabon and Crévot, 1823); Pierre-Augustin Béclard, *Elémens d'anatomie générale, ou description de tous les genres d'organes qui composent le corps humain* (Paris: Béchet, 1823); Etienne-Jean Georget, *De la physiologie du système nerveux, et spécialement du cerveau,* 2 vols. (Paris: J.-B. Baillière, 1821).

195 The *rapporteurs'* summary is reprinted on pp. 43–51 of Foville's *Traité complet.*

A. M. C. Duméril, who was the sole comparativist on the medical faculty.[196] The report applauded Foville's efforts, observing that it was not "surgical anatomy" that could lead to advances in "the physiology of the brain" but instead "the minute anatomy, superficial and profound, of the human brain in its adult, fully developed, and healthy state." Only such inquiry could establish what the *rapporteurs* called "the rule, the *norm* by which all the rest must be measured."[197] They continued:

> How is one to say whether a symptom . . . corresponds to a certain alteration in the development or tissue of a certain part of the brain if the normal state of this part is not rigorously known, and what is more, if one does not know the limits of variations to which this part is susceptible? Can one establish the movement down the animal series [*la marche de la dégradation animale*] for this important system of the organism if the point of departure is not exactly established? How can we draw conclusions about the usage of these parts from experiments made on animals in which it is not certain that the parts exist? . . . [F]or this, it is essential to undertake researches on the human species. Only in studying that species can we analyze the functions that are given to humans alone, and . . . the alterations and maladies of the brain whose effects can be appreciated by comparison.[198]

The report anticipated that anatomical investigation of this kind would clarify "which parts [of the brain and nervous system] are in particular relation with which faculties of the intelligence or with general sensibility and locomotility." Yet it held out little hope that even this "elevated, physiological anatomy" could resolve other "questions that the human mind cannot approach: the seat of the soul, its mode of action, and its relations with the material substratum."[199]

Thus work like Foville's was seen to rest on a strict bifurcation between approachable and unapproachable problems. It encompassed both gross and fine structure as well as the diverse operations of sensory and locomotor function, but it could not aspire to solve the great problems of the science of man, chief among them the physical-moral relation. In this way human neuroscience of the Restoration retreated into the ideological and philosophical safe haven of Christian dualism, which gave carte blanche to inquiry into all problems of mechanism, apparatus, and somatic process but rejected any possibility of scientific understanding of "man's higher nature." This meant that inquiry into the determination and meaning of mental and behavioral phenomena was restricted from the outset to matters that lay outside theological discourse on the soul and its capacities. The boundaries between theological and medicoscientific discourse on mental phenomena remained to be determined, as mental science and medicine further developed. In practice the limits came to be tested not by the neuroanatomists

196 On Blainville and Duméril, see Appel, *Cuvier-Geoffroy Debate*, esp. 65–67, 115–16, 119–21, 212, 213–15.
197 *Rapporteurs'* summary, in Foville, *Traité complet*, 44.   198 *Ibid.*   199 *Ibid.*

and neurophysiologists – who up to the era of Charcot concentrated on closely defined problems of anatomy and function and eschewed psychology – but in therapeutics, where patients presented themselves whole and where the "higher and lower natures" were not readily differentiated.[200]

As the history of mental medicine – its diagnostic procedures, treatments, and institutions – has been closely examined elsewhere, it remains to be said here only how mental medicine responded or failed to respond to the larger imperatives of the science of man. An older literature, represented by a work such as Henri Bon's *Précis de médecine catholique* (1936) saw in mental medicine a powerful antagonist to Christian teaching on sin, the temptations and tricks of the devil, healing miracles, the prophetic character of dreams, and a host of other subjects.[201] Yet here again, this portrait of a stark antagonism between the medicoscientific and theological domains must be rejected. It is true that there were dramatic contests between the medical and clerical establishments charged with caring for the mentally ill and, more important to this history, between those representatives of medical science and religious orthodoxy who claimed the authority to say what was and what was not mental illness. It is also true that doctors working in mental and legal medicine roused profound antipathy when they insisted on their special capacity to render judgment on the psychological and moral responsibility of the criminally accused. None of this means that there was always a direct clash between orthodox and medicoscientific teaching on the physical-moral relation. It is now amply proven that in many instances the conflicts between doctors and their antagonists in the clerical and legal establishments were mainly disputes over professional, institutional, and broader social prerogatives.[202] Furthermore, there are many cases of the doctors modulating, nuancing, and softening their pronouncements on mental phenomena to avoid giving offense and, as Goldstein has persuasively shown, of religious figures adapting medicoscientific concepts to their own ends rather than challenging them directly.[203]

Nor does this process of reconciliation and rapprochement mean that the medical science of man was dead, as has been argued by historians who think its principal importance lay in its asserting the dominance of the physical over the mental.[204] It means rather that anthropological medicine came

---

200 For some later developments in neuroanatomy and neurophysiology, see Clarke and Jacyna, *Nineteenth-Century Origins*. On Charcot's career, see Ruth Harris, "Introduction," in *Clinical Lectures on Diseases of the Nervous System*, by J.-M. Charcot (London: Tavistock/Routledge, 1991), ix–lxviii.
201 Henri Bon, *Précis de médecine catholique* (Paris: Félix Alcan, 1936).
202 Goldstein, *Console and Classify*, 4–5, 168, 180–82, 216–19, 286–87, 301–07.
203 *Ibid.*, 206–09, 229.
204 Staum, *Cabanis*, where it is argued that the science of man was not taken up by physicians after Cabanis, who retained the traditional division between body and soul (245).

at least partially to fruition by shifting into a different ideological register, one from which the determinedly confrontational language of philosophical materialism had been eliminated. Once this was done, the way was clear – even for those physicians who repeatedly denounced eighteenth-century excesses, Cabanis, materialism, and all medicoscientific attacks on free will – to investigate at length and with diverse tools what they nonetheless took to be the intricacies of the physical-moral relation.

This point of view was best represented by Laurent Cerise who in company with J. G. F. Baillarger and François-Achille Longet founded the first specialized psychiatric journal in France, the *Annales médico-psychologiques*.[205] During his career Cerise published many treatises on the problem of the physical and the moral; he also edited and wrote a series of introductions for works by Pierre Roussel, Cabanis, Bichat, and others in which he took great pains to point out what in the science of man was acceptable and what was not. His edition of Cabanis's *Rapports du physique et du moral* was intended to "define and circumscribe the domain of the science of the relations of the physical and the moral" which, he regretted, "still rested on uncertain foundations."[206] Lamenting "the chaos of theological, cosmological, and anthropological doctrines in which the diverse elements of the science of man move confusedly," he attributed this state of things to the failure of previous investigators to distinguish clearly between the realms of the physical and the moral. Cabanis in particular had ignored any phenomenon demonstrating "an active cause beyond passive sensibility, everything that puts above the organism a motive capable of moving it with power, energy, and liberty."[207] Against this primal Cabanisian error, Cerise argued that only when the unbridgeable dualism of the physical and the moral were recognized could the true science of their *relations* get about its work. And if the things of the soul were rightfully excluded from the sphere of this science, as Cerise insisted they must be, still its purview was vast, including as it did the "physiological bases" for the aptitudes, temperaments, and *moeurs* of peoples and individuals; "the effect of climates and institutions"; the genesis of ideas (*idéogénie*); laws, education, and the fine arts; the nether world of "secret penchants . . . sympathies and antipathies"; and the whole gamut of "mental and nervous affections."[208] This construction of mental medicine even allowed for inquiry into "the structural conditions and special aptitudes of the brain."[209] Once the specter of materialism was banished by a forthright declaration of faith in dualism, mental medicine was safely set on its course. If this course differed from that followed by materialists

---

205 "Introduction," *Annales médico-psychologiques* 1 (1843) : i–xxvi.
206 Laurent Cerise, "Notice sur Cabanis," in *Rapports du physique et du moral de l'homme*, by P. J. G. Cabanis (Paris: Fortin, 1843), xi.
207 *Ibid.*, xli.   208 *Ibid.*, xxix–xxx.   209 *Ibid.*, xxxi.

only in its statement of first principles, then so much the better for all those who sought to bridge the gulf between "pantheists" and "materialists," "animists" and "organicists."[210]

By means of vehicles such as the *Annales médico-psychologiques,* mental medicine conquered its own broad terrain of legitimacy even among those who were determined to leave religious discourse and authority intact. By detaching "the science of the physical and the moral" from what many regarded as its foundations in Cabanisian materialism, physicians such as Cerise and his collaborators encouraged broad acceptance for that blending of medical and moral concerns that was the hallmark of anthropological medicine. That a work such as Bon's *Médecine catholique* could even appear in the France of 1935, with its argument that there was and should be a distinctly Catholic kind of medicine, itself attests to the staying power of conceptions in which medicine and morals were profoundly linked.[211]

THE "PHYSIOLOGICAL MEDICINE" OF F. J. V. BROUSSAIS

Of all the Restoration medical theorists who placed themselves under the rubric of the science of man, the one who was the least willing to mask or moderate his materialism was F. J. V. Broussais, who, in his famous and provocative book *De l'irritation et de la folie* (1828), declared his intention to rescue "the physical and moral science of man" from the obfuscations and obscurities of those who sought "to plunge us once again into the illusions and chimeras of ontology."[212] Broussais was in some respects an unlikely candidate for such a task. His medical career had begun at Saint-Malô in his native Brittany, and he found his first institutional home within military medicine, a sector of the profession that was regarded with some contempt by the high theoreticians.[213] Yet despite these initial impediments to a career as a medical theorist, Broussais had nonetheless turned the medical world on its head with the 1816 publication of *Examen des doctrines médicales* and by the late 1820s had already enjoyed some years of great reputation and notoriety.

Broussais's *Examen* engendered a shift in French medicine that Erwin Ackerknecht once called "a forgotten medical revolution" but that Canguilhem and Foucault have isolated as the decisive moment when the nosological enterprise of the eighteenth century was undermined and the

210 *Ibid.,* xv–xvii.
211 "To attempt to do medicine without considering metaphysics is as impossible as to do chemistry without physics" (Bon, *Précis,* x).
212 François-Joseph-Victor Broussais, *De l'irritation et de la folie, ouvrage dans lequel les rapports du physique et du moral sont établis sur les bases de la médecine physiologique* (Paris: Delaunay, 1828), xv, xxxi.
213 Jean-François Braunstein, *Broussais et le matérialisme: Médecine et philosophie au XIXe siècle* (Paris: Méridiens Klincksieck, 1986), 14–16.

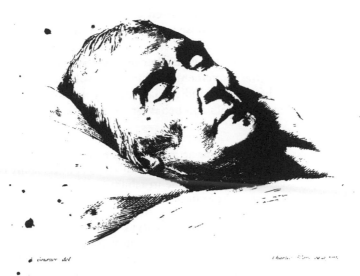

i vourier del   *Charti. ... ...*

Deathbed portrait of F. J. V. Broussais, by A. Gourlier and C. Blanc.

localist conception of disease established.[214] Broussais's chief (though unnamed) target in the *Examen* was Pinel, whose name was intimately associated with nosology thanks to his universally read *Nosographie philosophique* and who was widely perceived as exercising absolute sway over Paris medicine.[215] Broussais denounced the nosological viewpoint, charging that it established a false ontology of disease by transforming mere clusters of symptoms into actual disease entities. In the nosological framework, such disease entities were seen as somehow invading the general organism when in fact, he argued, symptoms should be taken to indicate only a pathological state affecting specific organs in localized sites. Broussais's "localism" was offered in particular as a replacement for the "essentialist" doctrine of fevers, according to which fevers (carefully classified according to duration, degree of heat involved, and so on) were themselves full-blown maladies rather than signs of some underlying affliction.[216] Broussais did not claim sole credit for undermining nosology; indeed he reiterated Cabanis's argument that nosology transformed the myriad, unclassifiable details of sickness into artificial categories whose stability was imposed by the observer.[217] Yet while acknowledging his theoretical debts, Broussais did

214 Erwin Ackerknecht, "Broussais or a Forgotten Medical Revolution," *BHM* 27 (1953) : 320–43; Canguilhem, *On the Normal and the Pathological*, 17–28; Michel Foucault, *The Birth of the Clinic: An Archaeology of Medical Perception*, trans. A. M. Sheridan-Smith (New York: Vintage Books, 1973), 184–92.
215 See, for example, Dupau, *Notice historique*.
216 Braunstein, *Broussais et le matérialisme*, 17, 23–33.   217 *Ibid.*, 27, 32.

develop a unique doctrine that was identified exclusively with his name. His "physiological medicine," as he chose to call it, replaced the nosological perspective with the view that all disease is a result of a general state of "irritation" that could be caused by any number of operative factors including purely physical agents (the movement of fluids and solids, electricity), upsets in the passional life of the individual (misery in love, political passion), and the ill-effects of habits and behavior (overwork, excess in sex or drink).[218]

The word irritation means to doctors the action of irritants or the state of living parts that are irritated. One calls irritants everything that acts on our economy [*tous les modificateurs de notre économie*] in exalting the irritability or sensibility of living tissues and raises these phenomena above their normal levels.[219]

Ostensibly this definition encompasses both hypo- and hyper-excitation, but in practice Broussais attributed little importance to states of deficient irritability. Instead he saw irritation or actual inflammation of a particular organ – in most cases the organs of the gastrointestinal system – in virtually all disease. Hence Broussais developed a reputation for tracing all ills to the stomach, and for his intense commitment to a narrow therapeutic program that counseled copious bleeding for just about everything.[220] Although Broussais was intensely critical of doctrines such as Barthez's that rested on what he saw as an ill-defined vital principle, his own concept of irritation had clear affinities with vitalist teachings: the general force of irritability was found in all living bodies; it was primordial, not the result of mechanical action; it operated through sympathies, moving about in the body from site to site, sometimes in accordance with ancient correspondences that linked ostensibly disparate phenomena – for example, sexual irritation to maladies of the throat; it was closely bound to the intellectual-passional life and hence was a manifestation of the holism of the animal economy.[221]

All these features of Broussais's doctrine of irritation made it suspect to doctors who saw localism as a path away from speculative medical systems in general and from vitalism in particular. Broussais's harshest critic in this respect was Louis, who, committed to a "severe" use of quantitative methods in medicine, accused Broussais of ignoring any fact that threw his "system" into question.[222] Broussais was just as bitterly attacked for his

218 Broussais, *De l'irritation*, 1–4, 61–63, 77–78, 208, 332–40.   219 *Ibid.*, 1.
220 *Ibid.*, see also Ackerknecht, "Forgotten Medical Revolution." The influence of Bordeu is evident in Broussais's emphasis on the stomach as the source or site of most illness; see Théophile de Bordeu, "Recherches sur les maladies chroniques," in *Oeuvres complètes de Bordeu*, 2:797–929, esp. 839.
221 Broussais, *De l'irritation*, xxx–xxxi, 1–4, 59–63, 332–40.
222 P. C. A. Louis, *Examen de l'examen de M. Broussais relativement à la phthisie et à l'affection typhoïde* (Paris: J.-B. Baillière, 1834), 14–15, 19–21.

therapeutics, which to some doctors seemed little better than criminal in emphasizing bleeding to the exclusion of other, gentler remedies.[223]

At one level, then, the notoriety of Broussais is to be explained by his doctrinal iconoclasm and his therapeutic boldness. Broussais was, however, much more than a medical figure and Broussaisism as a doctrine had much more than a medical content. As Jean-François Braunstein has forcefully argued, Broussais was notorious chiefly because during the Restoration he was virtually the sole champion of the materialist philosophical tradition that contemporaries identified with the eighteenth century and with the Ideologues. If even Broussais usually avoided the term "materialist" in favor of the more modern "physiological," this was so much more because he hoped to give materialism the specificity and positive content of medical science than because he hoped to avoid controversy or to dissociate himself from his ideological antecedents.[224] Although *Irritation et folie* was principally styled as an application of his larger doctrine to the study of mental illness, it functioned simultaneously and explicitly as a rehabilitation of sensationalism and Ideology. Broussais embraced as his progenitors Descartes, Bacon, Locke, and Condillac, whose methods, he said, were in turn taken up by François Chaussier, by the misguided Pinel (who fortunately had taught them to Bichat), by the "judicious and profound" Destutt de Tracy, and by Cabanis, whose "precious works gave to physiology and medicine the exclusive right to dictate laws to ideology."[225] Broussais's heroes were matched by enemies. He denounced the "Kanto-platonists" who "pretended to certainty in the science of man" yet knew nothing of what medicine had to teach about human nature.[226] But he was most angered by the "eclectics" and so-called psychologists, whose specious claim to have reconciled sensationalism with orthodox theology had lulled the scientific world into a "singular stupor."[227] Broussais scorned those philosophers who purported to say something about human nature by reflecting on their own experience or constructing some metaphysical ideal of "man." To doctors the futility of this superannuated method was obvious since "man is known only by half if he is observed in health alone."[228] Thus for Broussais the true "physical and moral science of man" was rooted in and wholly dependent on the insights of medicine.

This injunction to know human beings in the lack or absence of health was not a simple call to observe the progress of disease. Rather it was an exhortation to study all human life that varied from the "normal and healthy state," in whatever ways. As Broussais did not articulate what the "normal state" was, its meaning must be constructed from his descriptions

223 Ackerknecht, "Forgotten Medical Revolution."
224 Cf. Goldstein, *Console and Classify*, 242–45.   225 Broussais, *De l'irritation*, xi–xiii.
226 *Ibid.*, xxvi–xxvii.   227 *Ibid.*, xix–xx, xxv–xxvi.   228 *Ibid.*, xxvi.

of what was "unhealthy," "defective," "limited," and "incomplete." These latter categories included, for Broussais, fetuses, infants, the young, and the aged; women; "savages" and "barbarians"; monsters; amputees; "idiots"; and the blind and deaf.[229] Only by studying all these types, which were "pathological" since not wholly "normal," could investigators discern the essence, truth, or inner reality of "man." These inquirers must be doctors, moreover, since only they were equipped to observe and analyze pathological phenomena. That the delineation of pathological types rested on an already constituted conception of the "normal" (mature man, in civilized society, who had all his limbs, was not consigned to a madhouse, and so on) was a fact that did not rise to consciousness with Broussais or any other doctor of the period.[230] This should cause no surprise: the admonition to study the sick in order to know the healthy could not have seemed a fruitful course had doctors not felt confident of their own capacity to know the difference between the two. The conviction of physicians that they could recognize "the sick" as no one else could was in fact the single strongest support available for the view that a genuine science of man must be medical in character. Broussais pressed this claim more forcefully than any other doctor of the Restoration, reasserting – against all the compromises worked up by his contemporaries with moralism, theology, and metaphysics – the singularity of medical training, medical methods and procedures, and general medical philosophy.[231]

None of this means that Broussais adopted Cabanisian doctrine wholesale. In his reworking of Cabanis's vitalism, especially in his own rendering of sensibility doctrine, Broussais detached himself from classical sensationalism in a much more concerted fashion than Cabanis ever had and afforded much greater room in the analysis of human psychology to instinct and innate characteristics, a movement that culminated in the 1830s with his embrace of phrenology.[232] Where Cabanis had seen "interior impressions" as resulting from diverse, not clearly motivated internal activities, Broussais attributed such impressions directly to instinctual formations:

229 Broussais disputed the claim of the "psychologists" that all human beings naturally have "elevated ideas," the capacity to comprehend cause-and-effect relations, and a knowledge of God: "I respond [to this]: yes, the adult man, wide awake, in good health, having long exercised his senses, can feel all this. No, the embryo, the fetus, the child, the man deprived of his senses of sight and hearing, do not feel all this. No, the man who is an idiot from birth by reason of the defective development of the anterior part of the brain, he does not feel all this." See *De l'irritation*, 149–50.
230 Cf. Quetelet, who wrote in 1835 that for anomalies to be recognized, norms must be constituted by statistical means; see my earlier discussion.
231 Broussais, *De l'irritation*, xxvi–xxix, 123–28.
232 Braunstein, *Broussais et le matérialisme*, 156–57. Before his full embrace of phrenology, Broussais criticized Gall for exaggerating the influence of the brain and neglecting the role of other organs; cf. the critique of Gall by Moreau de la Sarthe (see Chapter 2, "Commentary on Gall").

When an internal need is pronouncedly felt because of stimuli brought to the brain by the nerves of the viscera, external objects are observed in the interest of this need because the brain is originally destined for the satisfaction of instinctual needs.[233]

Broussais also rejected Cabanis's teaching that all vital functions were differing "modes of action" of the one primordial force of sensibility. Instead Broussais posited two forces – irritability and sensibility – that differed in character and function and whose presence or absence depended on the degree of development of the organism. In Broussais's view it was irritability rather than sensibility that was the common property of all living beings no matter how primitive; sensibility was present only in beings with a nervous system and a brain. Parting company with Barthezian vitalists, including Cabanis, Broussais insisted that sensibility was dependent on the functional integrity of material structures.[234] The brain and nervous system must, moreover, be in a certain state of action or receptivity for sensibility to operate. Again what this "certain state" was Broussais did not elaborate, except in its negativity: it was lacking, for example, in embryos and in apopleptics, who were capable of irritable response to "excitants" but were unable to "feel."[235] In the most highly developed human beings, on the other hand, the material structures that made sensibility possible were fully elaborated. This dependence of sensibility – and, by extension, intellect and intellectual function – on the material apparatus of brain and nerves was something, Broussais maintained, that "metaphysicians" could not bear to contemplate. They were not prepared to accept the "anatomist's" judgment that "[man] is nothing other than the ensemble of the encephalic apparatus."[236]

If we attempt to sort out what greater theoretical purposes this formulation served for Broussais, we are led in several directions. First, it is apparent that Broussais was attempting to effect a juncture between his peculiar brand of medical materialism and the larger currents of the increasingly rigorous and reductionist sciences of life. It is not necessary to picture Broussais as an avid follower of the Académie des sciences proceedings or to represent him as meticulously knowledgeable about developments in bioscience – he was neither of these things – to recognize that he wanted medicine to be not only in the mainstream but at the head of materialist, scientific developments in the study of life. This was only fitting, in Broussais's view, for it was medicine that had developed the *méthode physiologique* for the study of life, and medicine that had broken with the ancients' procedure of treating life as pure abstraction in favor of the study of "living organs."[237] By the 1820s the desire to align medicine with the other life sciences meant, among other things, that Broussais had to be more attuned than Cabanis, Pinel, or Bichat – and certainly the Montpellier doctors – ever were to the comparativist perspective that had encouraged the

233 Broussais, *De l'irritation*, 208.　234 *Ibid.*, 1–3.　235 *Ibid.*, 3.　236 *Ibid.*, 123.
237 *Ibid.*, v.

emergence of biology from the older biomedical domain. In discussing sensibility, for example, Broussais denied that human beings alone possessed it. Thousands of cases proved to the contrary that animals "possess, to a certain point, the faculty of feeling; that they perceive and have perceived different impressions and even that they have the faculty of induction."[238] Though as a doctor Broussais could still consign all animals to the attention of the *art vétérinaire*, he could not build a general doctrine of sensibility from reflections on human psychology alone, as Cabanis had still done in 1800.[239] And though he himself undertook no comparativist or experimental investigations, he attempted to develop a theoretical understanding of life and vitality that included the lowest of the natural orders. Hence his opposition to any unitary doctrine of vital force that explained all activities from simple movement to human intellectual processes, and his insistence on the importance of irritability, which constituted in the animal realm a kind of prefiguring of fully constituted sensibility.

The other chief theoretical end served by Broussais's movement away from sensationalism and his approach to the comparativist perspective of bioscience was his development of typologies based on the innate characteristics of individuals under observation. Like other physicians who put stock in classical temperament theory, Broussais adumbrated types established by age, gender, "level of civilization," and similar factors. But with Broussais the typologizing procedure became central because of the great importance he gave to the role of instinct in human activity – instinct conceived not with Alibert as an innate capacity to recognize moral truth, but with naturalists as an animal, organically founded urge to engage in practices that conserved life of a certain variety.[240] As Braunstein rightly observes of Broussais, nothing gave him greater pleasure than to *épater le bourgeois* by recounting details of human animality or dredging up such Voltairean maxims as the dictum that "the stomach controls the brain."[241] If human beings were much more fully governed by instinct than had so far been allowed, the scope and importance left to the universals of Christian and rationalist discourse on human nature (the moral light, reason) diminished correspondingly. What was left in the wake of this full retreat from universalism was a much-enhanced disposition to seek out and emphasize those characteristics, patterns, and habits that appeared to be given for children, women, savages, and assorted other physiological types.

There are several ironies in the fact that Broussais occupies a pivotal role in this process of leading medicine away from its preoccupation with the discretely human. One is that he wanted at the same time to maintain med-

238 *Ibid.*, 132.   239 *Ibid.*, 2 (reference to "*art vétérinaire*").
240 *Ibid.*, 92–105, 208–9.
241 On the deliberate violence of Broussais's polemics, see Braunstein, *Broussais et le matérialisme*, 183–85.

icine's specificity, a project much more easily reconciled with a perspective such as Lordat's (humans are unique so medicine as the science of the human must be unique) than with Broussais's biologized medicine. A paradox becomes apparent too if one accepts the Canguilhem-Foucault reading of Broussais – that precisely while he was creating distance between human beings by accenting instinctual predispositions, he was diminishing the distance between the "normal" and the "pathological" by arguing that illness was not a qualitatively different state but a quantitative deviation, perhaps slight, from the healthy state.[242] This new "physiological" sense of illness, it is argued, was at the root of Broussais's attack on medical essentialism; fevers were not invading entities but symptoms of deviation from normal function. The logical corollary in doctrines of human nature would seem to have been that savages, for example, were not fixed types but mere deviations from the normal, fully developed human. This kind of thinking about the medical construction of the normal and the pathological has prompted some historians to argue that the full-blown medical anthropology of the 1860s and 1870s – of which the Broussaisian science of man was an important progenitor – had no true doctrine of "race" since only individuals mattered in a medical perspective that saw all difference merely as quantitative variation from a norm.[243]

Logically rigorous, this interpretation nonetheless obscures the effects of Broussais's work on the development of anthropological as opposed to experimental medicine. Canguilhem demonstrates that the "physiological" conception of pathology had manifold ramifications for experimental medicine. Patients were no longer sick; instead organs were, quantifiably, defective. This perspective certainly had great significance for medical physiology in that it encouraged investigators to focus their attention on minute variations in function, a task best accomplished – as Magendie and Bernard convinced everyone – by highly controlled experiment. This was not, however, the only meaning medical physiology had in the era of Broussais, nor was experiment the sole path of investigation opened up by the "physiological" viewpoint. Despite Broussais's attack on nosology and his attempt to undermine any conception of pathology as entity, medical physiology continued to carry within it a propensity to a classificatory enterprise that still treated diseases as entities and diseased creatures as typical representatives of commonly observed, more or less distinct, pathological patterns. The evidence for this in Broussais's own writing is abundant: in his examination of the etiology of madness, for example, Broussais defines madness on the one hand as something that could happen to any in-

242 Canguilhem, *On the Normal and the Pathological*, 13–14, 17–28; Foucault, *Birth of the Clinic*, 184–92.
243 Claude Blanckaert, "Médecine et histoire naturelle de l'homme: l'anthropologie française dans la seconde moitié du XIXe siècle," in *Médecine et philosophie à la fin du XIXe siècle: Journée d'étude* (Créteil, 1981), 101–16.

dividual if the circumstances were right, and on the other as a condition to which certain individuals clearly had an innate "predisposition."[244] In the former view, madness was an affliction that could strike anywhere and that might represent only a minor, partial, or reversible deviation from normal mental function. In the other, madness was the state of being of the "madman" as such, whose tendency to insanity lurked somewhere in the blood of his type. These unfortunate individuals, furthermore, frequently fell victim to a host of other diseases and degenerated into complete dementia or total paralysis.[245] Broussais's "madman" stands in a clear line of development, then, toward the fully articulated "cretin" of later medical anthropological literature. If the simultaneous existence of these conflicting impulses within anthropological medicine (focusing on marginally pathological individuals as opposed to constructing essential pathological types) is not recognized, then much of the subsequent history of the field is incomprehensible. Medical writings of the 1830s to 1860s show an overweening interest in describing and classifying the alcoholic, the cretin, and ultimately, as Robert A. Nye has meticulously demonstrated, the "degenerate." Thus while a certain kind of medical physiology insisted there was no alcoholic "type" but only individuals who consumed too much alcohol and in so doing distorted the function of their liver, medical anthropology insisted – and with much greater force derived from ideological, social, and political circumstances – that there were clear pathological types that, if not wholly fixed, were to only a limited extent malleable or susceptible to any therapy.[246]

Broussais's innatism, which to a large extent was already apparent in the 1820s in his critique of classical sensationalism and in his frequent references to pathological types, culminated in his embrace of phrenology around 1830. This part of his career is examined in the next chapter in connection with the reemergence of the phrenological movement. But already under the Restoration Broussais denied categorically that physiology should be divided from "psychology," study of the body from study of the mind and morals. He summed up the claims of the new psychology ("not a science but a game of the imagination much like poetry") by noting that psychologists sought to arrogate to themselves the whole domain of investigation of the moral. By their account

if naturalists or physiologists want to study the moral [dimension] of man, they must abandon investigations that call on the senses for help, leave behind their scalpels and microscopes, and give themselves over, just as the philosophers do, to meditation, in the absence of any exterior impressions, with an eye to becoming, uniquely, psychologists.[247]

244 Broussais, *De l'irritation*, 340.   245 *Ibid.*, 389–98.
246 Nye, *Crime, Madness, and Politics*, 230–32, 244–47.
247 Broussais, *De l'irritation*, 126.

Such a point of view was wholly unacceptable to Broussais since there could be no mental activity without the physical substratum; the brain and nervous system must be intact and healthy for full mental function to proceed. Furthermore, mental activity at every turn was inextricably tied up with the phenomena of the body. Even the theologians' much-vaunted will was a slave to the viscera, especially to the powerful and inescapable influences of digestion and sex:

The will, equally with perceptions and ideas, is obstructed, forced, vanquished, obscured, and denatured in the strangest manner by the stimulations that the viscera – especially the digestive and genital – when excited in a certain mode, send to the brain.[248]

If the intellectual functions were the province of doctors, all the more so were the passions since all emotions are seated in the organs of the body. The education and direction of the passions were crucial tasks of "medicine and hygiene," which "must know the nature of man in order to guide him in the intellectual and moral exercises required to cure the diseased states of the nervous system."[249] The moralists had but one legitimate task in this whole enterprise, and that was to undertake the "study of instinctive and intellectual phenomena in their relations with the different modes of development of the social state." This essentially historical endeavor Broussais was willing to grant them, but the foundations of the physicomoral science could be established only by medicine.[250]

Whatever the interest of other physicians in closing the gap between "materialism" and "spiritualism," Broussais was determined that the distance between a rigorously "physiological" approach to the science of man and the obscurities of the metaphysicians be marked. His celebrity (and his immense popularity with medical students) no doubt stemmed precisely from his eagerness to engage an ideological battle that other physicians had come to see as intellectually futile or as damaging to the professional and institutional interests of the medical establishment. Yet, for all the vitriol that flowed in response to the appearance of Broussais's "physiological medicine," we may question whether ultimately there was so profound an antagonism between the materialists and the spiritualists as they themselves were inclined to see. Although the rhetorical fields on which they stood were widely separated, there were regions of theoretical affinity – the existence of the physical-moral bond, the ineluctably social character of medicine, the significance of types – that linked all the diverse bearers of the legacy of anthropological medicine. These affinities began to emerge with real clarity once the passions of the Restoration subsided and the era of the political and intellectual *juste milieu* arrived.

248 *Ibid.*, 215.   249 *Ibid.*, 223–26; the quotation is at pp. 225–26.   250 *Ibid.*, 554.

4

Decline and dispersal: The science of man, 1830–1848

The final stage of the history of the medical science of man unfolds under the July Monarchy. During the 1830s and 1840s, for a complex of theoretical, institutional, and socioprofessional reasons, most medical theorists relinquished the vision of a comprehensive medical science of the physical and the moral. Only some extremists at either end of the ideological spectrum – phrenological materialists on the Left and vitalist conservatives on the Right – continued to argue that medicine should constitute an independent science of man because of its unique grasp of the physical-moral relation. Between these extremes, physicians who inherited the legacy of anthropological medicine and wanted to carry it forward sought to effect junctures with related fields of inquiry and thus to blend anthropological medicine into a more general science of man based not only on medicine but also on the developing natural and human sciences. The outcome of such efforts in fields ranging from medical psychiatry to anthropology will be examined in the Epilogue.

The intellectual and political environment in which medical theorists labored was significantly, if not dramatically, altered by the July Revolution. Changes in the press laws abolished censorship and lifted the requirement of prior authorization for printed material, thus widening the spectrum of expressible opinion.[1] In 1832 the government moved to reestablish the long-defunct Académie des sciences morales et politiques, which Bonaparte had closed as part of his campaign against the Ideologues. Although the academy was quickly integrated into the system of rule by "notables," its very existence signified the failure of attempts by conservatives to reassert their intellectual hegemony. The reemergence of Destutt de Tracy, who was named to the academy at the age of seventy-eight, was nicely symbolic of the limited but genuine shift in the intellectual atmosphere.[2] Although no

1 James Smith Allen, *In the Public Eye: A History of Reading in Modern France, 1800–1940* (Princeton: Princeton University Press, 1991), 86–87, 98–99.
2 William Coleman, *Death Is a Social Disease: Public Health and Political Economy in Early Industrial France* (Madison: University of Wisconsin Press, 1982), 7–8.

major changes in the structure or organization of the university were undertaken by the July Monarchy, the feel and texture of university life altered. Under the new king the university had, as Liard observed, "not an instant of anxiety" since no one in Louis-Philippe's entourage advocated any fundamental change in university structure, personnel, or procedures.[3] The freedom of the administration and the faculties to go their own way without fear of harassment or the kind of outright spoliation worked on the medical faculty in 1822 now seemed assured, even if the government did refuse, when pressed by liberals, to repudiate its prerogative to dismiss professors at will.[4]

Greater breathing space opened for medical education and institutions as well. Soon after the Revolution, the government took some steps to please its supporters: the *concours* was reestablished for professorial posts and new chairs were created, including one for Broussais in general pathology and therapeutics.[5] A clear sign that times had changed was the government's decision to allow the founding of a society devoted to phrenology, a move that had been blocked by the Restoration regime. The Ministry of Public Instruction officially authorized the founding of the Société phrénologique de Paris on April 16, 1831, only some ten months after the July Revolution.[6] The government also encouraged the establishment of "free" medical education, that is, courses outside the public educational system. This move allowed for the founding in 1837 of an "auxiliary" medical school where instruction was offered by some of the most celebrated figures of the period – Magendie, Broussais, Geoffroy Saint-Hilaire, and Buchez among them.[7]

Although the government was not interested in any major structural changes in the university, the later 1830s and 1840s saw a great deal of activity within the Ministry of Public Instruction aimed at reorganizing medical training, practice, and institutions. The comte de Salvandy, who was Minister of Public Instruction for two separate periods from 1837–39 and again from 1845–48, was especially active in this regard. He made a number of small changes in the curriculum, the teaching load of professors, the examination system, and other areas by ministerial decree. He then organized two separate ministerial inquiries that investigated the pedagogical, financial, and intellectual well-being of the medical faculties and the secondary

3 Louis Liard, *L'enseignement supérieur en France (1789–1893)*, 2 vols. (Paris: Armand Colin, 1888, 1894), 1:180.
4 Louis Trenard, "Les études médicales sous Louis-Philippe," *Actes du 91ᵉ Congrès national des Sociétés savantes (Section d'histoire moderne et contemporaine)* (Rennes, 1969), 3:167–214, at 210.
5 Jean-François Braunstein, *Broussais et le matérialisme: Médecine et philosophie au XIXᵉ siècle* (Paris: Méridiens Klincksieck, 1986), 19.
6 AN F¹⁷ 3038.
7 François-André Isambert, *Politique, religion et science de l'homme chez Philippe Buchez (1796–1865)* (Paris: Cujas, 1967), 51, n. 77; Trenard, "Etudes médicales," 172–73, 181; see also Pierre Huard, "L'enseignement libre de la médecine à Paris au XIXᵉ siècle," *RHS* 27 (1974): 45–62.

schools of medicine. In 1845 Salvandy appointed a commission to develop a law that would integrally reform the organization and practice of medicine by addressing the much-contested issues of the continued existence of the second-rank *officiers de santé;* the procedures for appointment to faculty posts; the establishment of new, or closing of old, medical faculties and *écoles secondaires;* and the formation of a corps of cantonal physicians. After taking the advice of this commission, the ministry drafted the text of a law that was sent to the Peers for debate, approved by them with modifications, and then stalled in the lower house at the time of the outbreak of the 1848 Revolution.[8]

In this changed climate of the July Monarchy the medical project for a science of man underwent yet another series of permutations. Thanks to a series of developments both theoretical and structural, the phrase "science of man" gradually began to lose currency in the medical vocabulary. The whole construction of medicine as science of man was increasingly irrelevant to a new generation of physicians who believed that only the elaboration of discrete problematics and the application of rigorous scientific methods would lead to certain knowledge of the nature of disease and to an efficacious therapeutics that would convince the world of medicine's utility. In their view the progress of medicine depended not on its self-construction as a science of man but on its embrace of scientific positivity. The new positive medicine, wrote one observer, attempted "to explain life and, in consequence, health and sickness only by the laws of organization."[9] It must adopt severe methods and, most important, limit its purview to the kind of problems a "natural" science could hope to solve.[10]

In many instances the progressive physicians who insisted that medicine must become a natural science like any other articulated their vision of medicine in explicit opposition to vitalism, and thus rejected constructions of the medical science of man that were rooted in vitalist thinking. Increasingly over the period 1830–48 vitalism came to be regarded as a dead letter and its defenders to be seen as individuals whose idea of medicine was frozen in an earlier time. L.-C. Roche's article of 1852 is typical of the antivitalist sentiments current by around 1850:

Vitalism must disappear. Vitalism is disappearing. If we still see it casting a certain light, this is only the last flickering of a lamp whose light is only vacillating and soon to be extinguished, the last sparks from a meteor that grows ever more distant.[11]

8 The commission was founded in part to respond to the proposals of the 1845 medical congress; see Jacques Léonard, *Les médecins de l'Ouest au XIXème siècle,* 3 vols. (Lille: Atelier reproduction des thèses, Université de Lille III, 1978), 2:787–822; Trenard, "Etudes médicales," 73–79, 189–214.

9 L.-C. Roche, "Anatomie et vitalisme," *L'Union médicale* (April 20, 1852), 192.

10 For a résumé of the medical advances caused by "the intervention of the physical sciences" into medicine, see Hippolyte Royer-Collard, "Considérations physiologiques sur la vie et sur l'âme," *MANM* 14 (1849): 251–69.

11 Roche, "Anatomie et vitalisme," 192.

Such statements should not be taken wholly at face value: vitalism continued to have diverse and powerful influence long after medical progressives
had consigned it to the historical dustbin. Nonetheless, it is true that from
the 1830s forward the dominant discourse of medicine came to exclude vitalist concepts and terminology that earlier had been commonplaces.[12]

The effects of this antivitalist movement on the tradition of the science of
man were complex. One consequence was the driving of an even sharper
institutional wedge between the medical faculties of Paris and Montpellier
than had previously existed. In Paris, Montpellier came to be widely regarded as an intellectual backwater. The commission charged with review-
ing Salvandy's medical reform projects in 1845 observed that Montpellier
was devoted to the search for elevated principles and the criticism of diverse
systems, language that did not conceal the increasingly common view of
Paris doctors that Montpellier was sunk in metaphysical murk.[13] In the
1840s some Parisian doctors even began to demand that the Montpellier faculty be abolished, a move that made Montpellier's defenders more obdurate
than ever in insisting on the glories of its ancient traditions and the unalterable verities of the vitalist science of man.[14]

As vitalist conservatives dug in their heels, medical materialists at the
opposite end of the ideological spectrum intensified their rhetoric and
stated emboldened claims. The phrenologists, emerging from their rather
furtive existence under the Restoration, claimed with new assurance that
medical science could discern human peculiarities and capacities with exactitude. Asserting that phrenology was a mature, accomplished science, they
moved to realize the social ambitions of the science of man in therapeutic
and pedagogical endeavors. In one of the real ironies of the period, the
phrenologists' desire to play an important social and therapeutic role forced
them to modify the rigorous determinism that ostensibly divided them
from theorists (including vitalists) who conceived of the physical-moral
relation in terms of reciprocities rather than strict physicalist determinism.
Although materialists and vitalists clung to the old dichotomies of the
science of man, there were a number of theorists who articulated new
versions of the science of man that deliberately avoided doctrinal extremes.
The Parisian physiologist Pierre-Nicolas Gerdy, for example, maintained
the specificity of medical methods and of the problems presented by hu-

12 For one attack on vitalism, see J.-B. Bouillaud's review of *Physiologie médicale et philosophique*, by A. R. J. Lepelletier, *Journal universel et hebdomadaire de médecine* 4 (1831): 27–28,
where Bouillaud nonetheless expresses satisfaction that Lepelletier's vitalism is less extreme
and not so "absurd" as that of "Bérard of Montpellier."
13 Trenard, "Etudes médicales," 201, 175.
14 See M.-H. Kuenholtz, *Le national aristocrate, ou les Facultés de Montpellier et de Paris sous le
point de vue de la centralisation et de la décentralisation* (Montpellier: J. Martel ainé, 1843).
When the question of whether France should have only one medical faculty was posed by
the commission preparing the 1845 medical congress, most of the Montpellier professors
decided to boycott the congress; see Léonard, *Médecins de l'Ouest*, 797.

man physiology yet rejected the vitalist view that life phenomena were refractory to the ordinary laws of nature. A singular approach to transcending rude dichotomies was developed by a circle of physicians that operated initially within the Saint-Simonian movement but later developed a social-Christian vision of medicine. Social-Christian physicians rejected "analysis" in favor of "synthesis" and in other respects too revamped basic principles of the science of man accepted since Cabanis and Bichat. In keeping with their aim of fostering not only intellectual but also social reconciliation, they argued with new urgency that doctors must get about the concrete work of moral and social regeneration the science of man had long envisaged.

The dominant trend of the period, however, was the attempt of physicians who were still powerfully drawn to the problem of the physical and the moral to effect a juncture between the medical science of man and the developing biological and "human" sciences. This was not of course a wholly new development. Already at the turn of the century, doctors had participated in the Société des observateurs de l'homme, the Société philomathique, and other organizations that brought together scholars from diverse fields of inquiry.[15] But the links that began to be forged in the 1830s and 1840s between physicians and investigators in other sciences were of a new and different character, since doctors now had to accommodate not isolated facts or observations but full-blown paradigms, including the comparativist perspective of general biology (the full "science of life" rather than the limited "science of man") and the historicism that lent new power and complexity to the emergent human sciences.[16] Thus doctors in this period moved, on the one hand, toward comparative physiology, natural history, and "philosophical anatomy," and, on the other, toward the emergent disciplines of "ethnology" and "anthropology," both of which had roots in the medical science of man but whose promoters sought to forge links with as broad a range of scientific activity as possible.

The intellectual developments that undercut the idea of an independent medical science of man in the 1830s and 1840s were strongly reinforced by changes in the structure and organization of medicine that took place in these years. As the development of medical specialties gained momentum, the idea that any one doctor could master the range of problems addressed by Cabanis in his Institute lectures came to seem outmoded, even chimer-

15 See Chapter 2.
16 On comparativism in life science, see Edwin Clarke and L. S. Jacyna, *Nineteenth-Century Origins of Neuroscientific Concepts* (Berkeley: University of California Press, 1987), 20–21; William Coleman, *Georges Cuvier, Zoologist: A Study in the History of Evolution Theory* (Cambridge, Mass.: Harvard University Press, 1964), 1, 45–51, 62–65. On historicism and the emergence of the human sciences, see Charles Rearick, *Beyond the Enlightenment: Historians and Folklore in Nineteenth-Century France* (Bloomington: Indiana University Press, 1974).

ical. The two new specialties of mental medicine and hygiene grew up on the landscape of the general science of man, and their bureaucratic and institutional successes helped to realize some of the ambitions of anthropological medicine. Nevertheless, the rhetoric of specialization blended readily with methodological demands that medicine become more rigorous and more clearly focused on discrete problems. Thus it too challenged the very idea of a comprehensive medical science of man. The specializing tendency went hand in hand, moreover, with the developing ethos of "professionalism," and the joint claims that doctors had special expertise and upheld uniquely rigorous professional standards tended to replace the science of man as the basis on which doctors argued for greater social standing and authority.[17]

Finally, the social and economic developments of the period posed new problems for anthropological medicine. The most significant economic trends of the period – the increasing commercialization of small-scale peasant agriculture and the extension of industrial labor – intensified class conflict and brought to high visibility what contemporaries called the "Social Question." In turn the aggressive capitalism of the era provoked the impassioned, often embittered responses of critics now coming to be known as "socialists."[18] In this context the long-standing assertion of anthropological medicine that it would improve the lot of the people by its general contributions to "perfectibility" appeared empty indeed. The medical corps thus found itself under new pressure (mostly internally generated) to give concrete dimensions to their supposed "social mission." Yet efforts to develop for medicine a posture of general social reformism met with many obstacles. Social "engagement" blended ill with physicians' preoccupations with their own professional advancement. And concrete proposals for social action – such as plans to establish a corps of cantonal physicians – sparked vociferous controversy.[19] In these debates the ideological ambiguities and conflicts within the conception of medicine's "social mission" became manifest. Thus in the broad social arena, as in methodological and professional contexts, the rhetoric of the science of man seemed again to have outlived its day.

17 On the processes of specialization and professionalization, see Jan Goldstein, *Console and Classify: The French Psychiatric Profession in the Nineteenth Century* (Cambridge: Cambridge University Press, 1987), 56–63, 148–51, 346–50; Matthew Ramsey, *Professional and Popular Medicine in France, 1770–1830: The Social World of Medical Practice* (Cambridge: Cambridge University Press, 1988), 3–5, 23; George Weisz, "The Politics of Medical Professionalization, 1845–48," *Journal of Social History* 12 (1978): 3–30. There was a real disjuncture between the rhetoric of specialization and the social reality of medical practice. Ramsey observes that "in Paris, as late as 1845, all but about twelve percent of physicians were still general practitioners" (23).
18 Coleman, *Death Is a Social Disease*, 34–56; François-André Isambert, *De la charbonnerie au Saint-Simonisme: Etude sur la jeunesse de Buchez* (Paris: Editions de Minuit, 1966).
19 Léonard, *Les médecins de l'Ouest*, 744–55, 803–4.

The pace, range, and effects of these developments that tended to undermine the medical science of man should not be exaggerated. As the opening sections of this chapter indicate, there were elements of medicine that continued resolutely to argue that medicine was the science of the physical and the moral and to construe it in broad anthropological fashion. More important, crucial features and elements of anthropological medicine survived this era in diverse reconfigurings that would carry its legacy into the years beyond 1848.

THE REEMERGENCE OF PHRENOLOGY

To the extent that medical progressives or modernists continued to argue on behalf of a medical science of man, they did so chiefly under the rubric of phrenology. Although in the era of Cabanis and Bichat there had been marked theoretical divergences between vitalist-influenced medical Ideology and the perspective of organology, there had also been, as noted in Chapter 2, clear affinities between the two. During the Restoration, when phrenology went largely underground, there continued to be among doctors a small group of real disciples of Gall and a larger group who took inspiration from his work.[20] In the emerging fields of neuroanatomy and mental medicine, for example, figures such as Etienne-Jean Georget openly avowed principles derived from Gall. Indeed among alienists, Jan Goldstein observes, the "influence of Gall was pervasive."[21] Thus doctors continued to carry the phrenological lantern until the change in the political climate made possible phrenology's full reemergence. Whereas during the Restoration phrenology remained a marginal endeavor, held at bay by the academic greats and watched by the royal authorities, with the coming of the Orleanist regime phrenology entered, as Georges Lantéri-Laura observes, its "golden age."[22]

The Société phrénologique founded in 1831 had eighty-four founding members, two-thirds of whom were doctors. Most of the society's officers were also physicians: Casimir Broussais, who worked at the military hospital of Gros-Caillou, was elected secretary-general; J.-B. Bouillaud became editor of the society's publications; the alienists Jean-Pierre Falret and

20 On the reception of Gall's work during the Empire and the Restoration, see François Azouvi, "Psychologie et physiologie en France, 1800–1830," *History and Philosophy of the Life Sciences* 6 (1984): 151–70; Georges Lantéri-Laura, *Histoire de la phrénologie: L'homme et son cerveau selon F. J. Gall* (Paris: Presses universitaires de France, 1970), 126–32; Robert Young, *Mind, Brain and Adaptation in the Nineteenth Century* (Oxford: Clarendon Press, 1970), 24–27.
21 Quoted in Goldstein, *Console and Classify*, 256.
22 Lantéri-Laura, *Histoire de la phrénologie*, 145–46. Phrenology was taught in *cours libre* by Joseph Vimont in 1829 and then by P. C. A. Dumoutier in 1832–33; see Huard, "L'enseignement libre," 53–54.

Félix Voisin held other offices as well.[23] The object of the society, expressed in its opening prospectus, was to pursue intensive investigations of the brain, which "of all the viscera of the human body, was the most important because of its mass, the artfulness [*artifice*] of its structure, and the agglomeration of organs that protect it or are dependent on it."[24]

The phrenological society was not exclusively Gallian. Both J.-G. Spurzheim and the English phrenologist George Combe were made honorary members. Indeed there were certain respects in which the phrenologists of the 1830s believed that Spurzheim had clearly improved on the work of Gall. F. J. V. Broussais credited Spurzheim, for example, with advancing beyond Gall in recognizing that the development of the faculties varied with stages of maturation and growth and that certain penchants proper to children persisted into adulthood.[25] Broussais's emphasis on problems associated with aging is but one instance of ways in which Parisian phrenology of the 1830s blended the original Gallian perspective with elements adapted from the indigenous, vitalist-inspired medical science of man. The phrenologists of this era were much more concerned than Gall had been with the general problems of moral and physical hygiene, especially the agents and influences that could aggravate inherent tendencies.[26]

In respect to the fundamentals of the science, however, phrenology of this period differed little from that taught in the classic texts of Gall. Broussais's 1836 lectures, for example, contained much material on the implications and significance of phrenology that was not to be found in the early texts but little that could be regarded as a genuine development of the anatomical or physiological foundations of the science.[27] Nor was Broussais the only phrenologist who was content merely to repeat the organological truisms of yesteryear.[28] In Parisian phrenology generally in these years there was little that was new except the disposition of its advocates to see phrenology as the achieved, accomplished science of man that Gall and so many others had called for, and to urge society to accept its services without further delay.

23 *Journal de la Société phrénologique de Paris* 1 (1832): 21–25.   24 *Ibid.*, 29.
25 F. J. V. Broussais, *Leçons de phrénologie* (Brussels: Société encyclographique des sciences médicales, 1839), 32. On the differences between Gall and Spurzheim, see Clarke and Jacyna, *Nineteenth-Century Origins*, 223–25; for a contemporary account that includes Broussais's system, see Laurent Cerise, *Exposé et examen critique du système phrénologique* (Paris: Trinquart, 1836), 58–64.
26 See, for example, Casimir Broussais, *Hygiène morale ou application de la physiologie à la morale et à l'éducation* (Paris: Baillière, 1837).
27 Broussais, *Leçons*. These lectures were a rhetorical and theatrical smash. At the first session the audience spilled out of the amphitheater and the lecture had to be postponed until a larger room could be found. Broussais wanted to move the course to the Muséum d'histoire naturelle but the professors' assembly there refused his request. At that point, a private subscription was raised and the course reopened in a *salle libre*. The remainder of the course was no less successful than its dramatic opener, and for a time it restored to Broussais the immense popularity he had enjoyed in the 1820s. See Braunstein, *Broussais et le matérialisme*, 154–55.
28 This is the judgment of Lantéri-Laura, *Histoire de la phrénologie*, 151–52.

Yet it was difficult for phrenology to present itself as an interventionist branch of medicine, equipped with a full range of prophylactic and therapeutic techniques, so long as it was saddled with what many saw as the "fatalism" of Gall's science.[29] The Parisian phrenologists were in any event inclined to such a position both by the meliorative tendencies of the indigenous science of man (especially as developed by hygiene) and by their own generally left-leaning politics. The Paris phrenologists were intent on proving that, far from being incompatible with social progress, phrenology was ready to supply a medical solution to seemingly intractable social problems. Society must recognize, they argued, the phrenological truth that "we are born with different organic dispositions that communicate diverse impulsions."[30] Phrenology alone could devise the means to maximize the social benefits of diversity and to struggle against innate dispositions that disrupted social harmony. Broussais held, for example, that phrenological techniques would allow pedagogues readily to separate students according to their given skills, thus making education more realistic in its aims and ultimately encouraging a more efficacious division of labor. As Jean-François Braunstein has aptly observed, "what was a pessimistic affirmation of human inequality with Gall, became in this case an optimistic – if disquieting – belief that the recognition of inequalities was itself a factor conducing to progress."[31] Broussais argued elsewhere that one of the chief merits of phrenology was that as it became known and understood it would supply a reliable guide to the moral penchants of individuals. Since tendencies to murderousness, lust, or thievery would be literally written on the cranium of the individual, "everyone would fix his eyes on his neighbor's head," and act according to what he saw there. In such circumstances individuals would be forced by public sentiment to work against their own antisocial dispositions; there would be no hiding behind facades of goodwill and intention.[32]

In keeping with this reformist spirit, Parisian phrenology concerned itself not so much with the theoretical or empirical basis of phrenological science as with elaborating an interventionist, utilitarian program and with proving that phrenology could perform a range of useful social functions. In 1834 Voisin and Philippe-Nicolas Cheneau (1796–1855) established an "Institut orthophrénique" in Issy-les-Moulineaux whose purpose was to anticipate

29 Gall had defended himself against this charge but to little avail; see F.-J. Gall and J.-G. Spurzheim, *Anatomie et physiologie du système nerveux en général et du cerveau en particulier*, 4 vols. (Paris: F. Schoell, 1810–19), 1:xxxii.

30 Broussais, *Leçons*, 18.

31 Braunstein, *Broussais et le matérialisme*, 171. This phrenological meliorism may be compared to developments in Victorian Britain, where phrenology played a key role in secular reformism and the popularization of science; see Roger Cooter, *The Cultural Meaning of Popular Science: Phrenology and the Organization of Consent in Nineteenth-Century Britain* (Cambridge: Cambridge University Press, 1985).

32 Quoted in Braunstein, *Broussais et le matérialisme*, 170.

and forestall the development of delinquency among the children of miners. This project was commended in the pages of the *Moniteur universel* by the prominent hygienist C. C. H. Marc. Marc observed that the institute was intended to handle "four principal classes" of children: those born with poor intelligence, those born like everyone else but whose early education had taken "a vicious direction," those with extraordinary capacities that could be developed for good or ill, and, finally, those whose parents were afflicted with alienation and who were thus "predisposed to mental alienation or other nervous affections."[33] Noting that Voisin's ideas "rested on the incontestable facts of observation," Marc argued that in the mental and moral constitution of individuals "organization" exercised the most powerful influence, so that it was crucial in education "to know the organic peculiarities of the child."[34]

No one can any longer deny the evidence that nature is unequal in her distributions and that the system of equality, so vigorously affirmed by the philosophers in the last century, can no longer sustain a moment's examination.[35]

Yet Marc ended by sounding a note of optimism, observing that it was only through education such as that offered by Voisin's institute that the talents of exceptional and unusual individuals could be recognized.[36]

The significance of Parisian phrenology of the 1830s and 1840s has been variously interpreted. For a long time historians of science tended readily to accept the judgment of some contemporaries that phrenology was completely discredited in these years by critiques such as that undertaken by Pierre Flourens in his famous *Examen de la phrénologie* (1842). In this work Flourens set out to demolish all versions of phrenology (Gall, Spurzheim, Broussais), using philosophical, moral, and scientific arguments. Against phrenology's primary postulate that distinct faculties were seated in particular regions of the brain, he asserted with Descartes the incontrovertible existence of a unified *moi*: "the unity of the self is a fact [directly] known to the interior sense [*sens intime*], and the interior sense is stronger than all philosophies."[37] Although he acknowledged that Gall was an observer *plein de finesse*, he insisted that Gall had ignored all observations that tended to demonstrate the unity of the self. Arguing next from the pure exigencies of morality, Flourens held that the primary fact of the moral life was the capacity to choose a course of action and that without free will, morality

---

33 [C. C. H.] Marc, "Rapport fait à M. le conseiller-d'Etat, préfet de police, sur l'établissement orthophrénique de MM. Félix Voisin et P. Cheneau, docteurs en médecine, avenue de Vaugirard, à Issy, no. 14," *Moniteur universel*, no. 297 (October 24, 1834), 1986; see also Lantéri-Laura, *Histoire de la phrénologie,* 149–50.
34 Marc, "Rapport." 35 *Ibid.* 36 *Ibid.*
37 Pierre Flourens, *Examen de la phrénologie* (Paris: Paulin, 1842), 28; see also Clarke and Jacyna, *Nineteenth-Century Origins,* 244–56.

was impossible.[38] Finally, Flourens ridiculed Gall's scientific pretensions by observing that he had never even attempted the kinds of specialized anatomical investigations that would be required to prove the faculty-organ correspondence:

> Strange fact! The whole of Gall's doctrine, the whole of phrenology, depends on the *organs of the brain*, for without distinct cerebral organs there are no independent faculties, and without independent faculties there is no phrenology. Yet neither Gall nor any phrenologist after him has said anything of what a *cerebral organ* truly is.[39]

Flourens finished by asserting that Gall's epigones, Spurzheim and Broussais, had made no advances on Gall's original work and that Broussais's *Cours* of 1836 was a "confused melange" of sensationalism and phrenology.[40]

Flourens's attack on phrenology was but one of many, and although recent historiography is disinclined to accept the view that phrenology was wholly discredited by these assaults, it is true that phrenology lost many important adherents in the intellectual climate of the later July Monarchy.[41] Throughout this period phrenology faced two main camps of critics, one philosophical and the other scientific. The philosophers, with Cousin in the lead, rejected phrenology in favor of "psychology," denied the material basis of mental functions, and in so doing excluded doctors from the work of investigating psychic phenomena.[42] The scientists found phrenology wanting in both method and content, and championed instead more strictly defined investigations in neuroanatomy and neurophysiology. Phrenology suffered much more at the hands of its scientific than its philosophical detractors. While the Cousinians were predictable enemies whom doctors could cheerfully deride, the scientific critics of phrenology were not so easily dismissed, especially since they included representatives of official science like Flourens. The July Monarchy was the period when "official science" began clearly to emerge – a scientific establishment that took the path of moderation, deemphasized conflicts between science and religion, and sought support and validation from public authority. In respect to inquiry into psychophysiological relations, this official science had come to settle on laboratory and clinical techniques as the preferred methods of investigation, and on discrete and uncontroversial problems of sensorimotor

---

38 Flourens, *Examen*, 28, 32–33, 42.   39 *Ibid.*, 57.   40 *Ibid.*, 95.

41 For one important instance, see the section on François Leuret later in this chapter; J.-B. Bouillaud distanced himself from Gall's organology, while continuing to champion localization; see Clarke and Jacyna, *Nineteenth-Century Origins*, 262; J.-B. Bouillaud, *Essai sur la philosophie médicale, et sur les généralités de la clinique médicale* (Paris: De Just Rouvier and E. Le Bouvier, 1836), where Bouillaud pays a warm tribute to Gall while recognizing that "immense research" remained to be done (69–71, n. 1).

42 See Chapter 3.

function as privileged subject matter. Phrenology answered to neither of these criteria.[43]

It remains to be asked why, if the critiques of phrenology were so damning, it enjoyed the success it did and, further, what relation there was between phrenology's difficulties and its self-construal as the embracive science of man long prepared for in medical circles. Phrenology was able to prosper to the extent that it did in part simply because the bogey of materialism, though still formidable, lost much of its power in this period. Indeed one of the principal complaints made by critics of the regime was that it was dominated by "Voltaireans" imbued with the spirit of materialism and skepticism.[44] Yet phrenology seems to have enjoyed its greatest acclaim precisely at those points in its program that were the least theoretical and the most utilitarian. It is noteworthy that in Marc's tribute to Voisin he emphasized the services the Institut orthophrénique would perform without ever mentioning the word "phrenology."[45] Like hygiene, which eschewed theory with all its attendant problems and devised a practical program of service to the expanding state apparatus, phrenology gained public support to the extent that it promised concrete services.[46]

Yet, paradoxically, it was precisely phrenology's claim to be ready to deliver practical services that was in large part responsible for the ridicule to which it was subjected. It is in this connection that the importance of phrenology as science of man emerges. Phrenologists could not assert authority on matters of pedagogy, the treatment of criminals, and like matters if they publicly admitted that their science rested on a hypothesis that still needed much work to be demonstrated. The phrenologists tended, therefore, to lodge themselves within the rhetorical field of the science of man so that the accumulated prestige of that tradition would redound to their benefit while allowing them to ignore the theoretical and methodological problems at the heart of the phrenological system. In the opening to his phrenology course in 1836, Broussais chided any among his listeners who might be inclined to think the grand problems of the science of man irrelevant: "No subject is foreign to doctors since everything is relative to man, since society interrogates doctors about everything."[47]

This evocation of the science of man still had real power among doctors. Long after the public mania for phrenology had passed and long after of-

---

43 On Flourens's influence, see Clarke and Jacyna, *Nineteenth-Century Origins*, 279–85; Michael Gross, "The Lessened Locus of Feelings: A Transformation in French Physiology in the Early Nineteenth Century," *JHB* 12, no. 2 (1979): 231–71, esp. 255–58; Young, *Mind, Brain and Adaptation*, chap. 2 and 246–47.
44 Edward Berenson, *Populist Religion and Left-Wing Politics in France, 1830–1852* (Princeton: Princeton University Press, 1984), 38, 45, 51.
45 Marc, "Rapport."   46 On the hygienic movement, see Chapter 3.
47 Broussais, *Leçons*, 15.

ficial biological science had dismissed it, phrenology continued nonetheless to exert strong influence in medical circles. During the authoritarian years of the early Second Empire phrenology again lapsed into silence, only to resurface among the physician-anthropologists of the Broca circle in the 1860s. It reappeared in that context not only because of the appeal exerted by phrenology's specific problematics – the nature and number of the faculties, the localization of brain function, and the psychophysical link – but also because phrenology had played, from Gall forward, a critical role in pressing the claim that medicine must serve as the foundation of the science of man.[48] The phrenologists were crucial in this respect, moreover, because they were virtually the only element within progressive, materialist medicine that continued as late as the 1830s to make such assertions. Medical progressives were required by the logic of their own epistemological and methodological commitments to oppose such extravagances. Even when sympathetic to the tradition of the science of man, they tended to articulate their conception of the physical-moral link in a much more austere register that that of phrenology and to insist on the broadly scientific rather than specifically medical character of their endeavors. This double movement away from phrenology and the rhetoric of the science of man may be traced in the work of medical investigators who, unlike the phrenologists, did undertake close studies of the brain and nervous system.

CHARTING THE BRAIN AND NERVOUS SYSTEM

Although the phrenologists did little in the 1830s and 1840s to strengthen the anatomical and physiological foundations of their system, close study of the brain was being undertaken in other quarters, often by investigators who were determined to overthrow the phrenological system. Ever since Cuvier's pioneering comparative work on the cerebronervous system, the major concern of naturalists had been to extend knowledge of the cerebronervous system of the different animal orders, for which in some cases even the most basic information was still lacking.[49] Throughout the first decade of the Restoration, specialized work on the cerebronervous system of individual animal groups was reported in the publications of the natural history museum and by the mid-1820s a number of syntheses had been attempted.[50]

---

48 See the tribute to Gall by Paul Broca in *BSAP* 2 (1861): 191.
49 On Cuvier's use of the cerebronervous system in classification, see Dorinda Outram, "Uncertain Legislator: Georges Cuvier's Laws of Nature in Their Intellectual Context," *JHB* 19, no. 3 (1986): 323–68, esp. 361–62.
50 See, for example, Louis-Antoine Desmoulins, *Anatomie des systèmes nerveux des animaux à vertèbres, appliquée à la physiologie et à la zoologie*, 2 vols. (Paris: Méquignon-Marvis, 1825); E. R. A. Serres, *Anatomie comparée du cerveau, dans les quatre classes des animaux vertébrés, appliquée à la physiologie et la pathologie du système nerveaux*, 2 vols. (Paris: Gabon, 1824–26).

In medical circles too there was a rash of publications in this period on anomalies or diseases of the brain and the spinal cord, many of them chiefly descriptive and therapeutic in intent. By the mid to late 1820s, however, there was a branch of medically oriented brain science that aimed at resolving some of the great and long-standing problems of cerebral function by applying the new methods of clinicopathological observation. Indeed for a time in the late 1820s and early 1830s physicians had high hopes that, by joining clinical observations with autopsy results, they would not only find the local lesions responsible for psychic and nervous disorders but, in the process, would illuminate the structure and functions of the brain itself.[51] Although Pinel had rejected the view that mental disorders would ultimately be traceable to lesions in the cerebral or nervous apparatus, mental medicine of the 1820s and 1830s was increasingly attuned to the localist perspective of the new pathological anatomy and anticipated finding precise "seats" for mental disease.[52] Some successes were in fact achieved. Bouillaud, who after his early association with phrenology ultimately came to reject it, was responsible for the most notable triumph of clinicopathological brain studies, in his demonstration of a correlation between a motor disturbance of speech and a frontal lobe lesion. Bouillaud's findings were not widely accepted but they were well enough established to sustain interest in cerebral localization despite the opprobrium increasingly attached to phrenology. Bouillaud's results were supported by the work of the physician J. B. M. Parchappe (1800–66) who, arguing from the cases of patients suffering from neurosyphilis, held that the frontal lobes were the seat of both mental and speech function.[53]

The high hopes for the clinicopathological method were, however, for the most part dashed by the mid-1830s. Where pathologists had anticipated that autopsy investigation would corroborate and clarify clinical cases, such evidence often obscured and sometimes flatly contradicted clinical observations. Bouillaud had warned in 1825 that "although we cannot deny that cerebral pathology may be a precious means of elucidating the mysterious functions of the brain, we cannot but at the same time allow that this method of research is surrounded with great difficulties."[54] Within a decade this warning proved apt.

The failure of the clinicopathological approach to elucidate brain function encouraged some medical investigators to turn away from predominantly

51 Clarke and Jacyna, *Nineteenth-Century Origins*, 22–27.
52 Philippe Pinel, *Traité médico-philosophique sur l'aliénation mentale, ou la manie* (Paris: Richard, Caille et Ravier, 1801), 3, 16, 107; see also Goldstein, *Console and Classify*, 250–54.
53 Clarke and Jacyna, *Nineteenth-Century Origins*, 26, 243, 262–63, 266; on the importance of Bouillaud's work in sustaining interest in cerebral localization, see Francis Schiller, *Paul Broca, Founder of French Anthropology, Explorer of the Brain* (Berkeley: University of California Press, 1979), 172–74.
54 Quoted in Clarke and Jacyna, *Nineteenth-Century Origins*, 26.

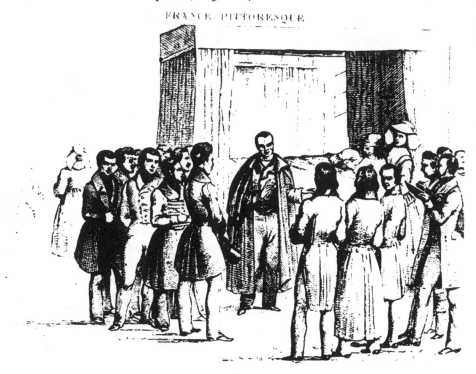

FRANCE PITTORESQUE

Interior view of a hospital ward – bedside teaching, by A. Lacauchie.

medical methods toward the comparativist studies to which naturalists had been dedicated all along. Physicians invariably brought to such investigations much of the baggage of the medical science of man, with its characteristic approaches to the problem of the physical-moral relation. Yet at the same time, medical progressives moved to incorporate the techniques, perspectives, and findings of the natural sciences. Of these works in comparative brain studies undertaken by physicians, one illustrates with particular clarity how progressive neuromedicine of this period simultaneously lingered within and moved beyond the framework of the science of man: the alienist François Leuret's *Anatomie comparative du système nerveux considéré dans ses rapports avec l'intelligence* (1839).[55] Leuret's own contribution to the work of this title was contained in volume one, which synthesized diverse observations on the anatomy and physiology of mollusks, articulates, fish, reptiles, birds, and mammals. Leuret had intended to devote the second volume exclusively to the human brain, but perhaps because he was ab-

---

55 François Leuret and Louis-Pierre Gratiolet, *Anatomie comparée du système nerveux considéré dans ses rapports avec l'intelligence*, 2 vols. (Paris: Baillière, 1839–57). (Subsequent references are to volume 1, by Leuret.)

sorbed in bureaucratic tasks, work with patients, and the composition of more specialized works in his own field of mental medicine, he never did so. The work was formally completed in 1857 by Louis-Pierre Gratiolet, a student of Blainville, and an *aide-naturaliste* at the Muséum d'histoire naturelle, who took the book in a vitalist-spiritualist direction at odds with the tenor of Leuret's original work.[56]

As a student of mental medicine Leuret was originally attracted to phrenology and was for a time very enthusiastic about the clinicopathological search for the local lesions responsible for mental maladies. When the results of such investigations proved disappointing, Leuret initially retreated to the fallback position suggested by Gall himself, that the failure to find a lesion in cases of mental maladies did not prove that there was none. But by 1840 Leuret had become openly skeptical:

> I willingly acknowledge . . . that our means of investigation are often inadequate and that our anatomical knowledge is imperfect on many points. But if, when I see no alteration in the brain, I abstain from concluding that there is, in fact, no alteration in that organ, by the same token I carefully guard against concluding that there is one. When the brain of a lunatic appears healthy to me, I do not affirm . . . that this brain is diseased. I remain in doubt.[57]

In the meantime Leuret had begun seeking illumination of the brain and its functions from the evidence presented by the "lower orders," a technique on which Gall himself of course had often relied.[58] Leuret's 1839 synthesis presented the results of his investigations, which, like those of many physicians turning to natural history in this era, were often not firsthand but collected from the works of specialists in the various branches of animal studies.[59]

Much of Leuret's work was devoted to pointing out the errors of Gall, Spurzheim, Vimont, Broussais, and other phrenologists.[60] Leuret's assault on phrenology rested, not like that of Pierre Flourens, on Cartesian dualism or the demands of Christian morality, but on what he perceived to be a more rigorous naturalism. Leuret's text was in fact as openly materialist as any of the period. He insisted that human beings were fundamentally no different from animals and must be investigated as part of the animal series.

---

56 Ulysse Trélat, "Notice sur François Leuret," in Leuret and Gratiolet, *Anatomie comparée*, xiii–xxx; "Avis de l'éditeur," in *ibid.*, vii.
57 Quoted in Goldstein, *Console and Classify*, 254.
58 Young, *Mind, Brain, and Adaptation*, 33–34.
59 In *Anatomie comparée*, Leuret cited studies undertaken by Cuvier, Lacépède, Soemmering, Blainville, Ehrenburg, Blumenbach, Vicq d'Azyr, Treviranus, Meckel, Gall, Etienne and Isidore Geoffroy Saint-Hilaire, and many other authorities.
60 Leuret also pointed to errors of the phrenologists that the medical anatomist Jean Cruveilhier had accepted uncritically into his celebrated *Anatomie pathologique du corps humain;* see Leuret and Gratiolet, *Anatomie comparée*, 1:365.

Although in other ways critical of the "philosophical anatomy" of Etienne Geoffroy Saint-Hilaire, he praised Geoffroy for demonstrating that all of organized life was subject to natural laws, even the monsters that had long been regarded as proving nature's variability and capriciousness. When he momentarily approached the connection between intellect and soul, Leuret observed that he had nothing to offer on this "metaphysical" subject but insisted that defining "intelligence" as such was a matter properly left to science.[61] Thus in Leuret's materialist critique of phrenology he emerged as more royalist than the king. His specific criticisms of phrenology were all aimed at proving that phrenology was not rigorous enough in its application of the standards of science. He pointed to inaccuracies in the phrenologists' descriptions of animal brains and in their assessments of animal behavior. He was strongly critical of their methods, especially their habit of judging the features of skulls merely by ordinary observation rather than by careful measuring and weighing.[62]

None of this meant, however, that Leuret was antagonistic to the effort to establish the material bases of intelligence. In counterpoint to his critique of the phrenologists' approach, Leuret offered principles of his own. Denying the phrenological claim that the relative size of the brain in relation to body mass increased as the animal series was ascended, Leuret held that although that relation was false, there was an exact correlation between the development of the cerebral ganglia and the development of the mental faculties. Similarly, while he refuted Gall and Spurzheim's contention that throughout the animal series the number of folds in the brain always corresponded to the volume, he nonetheless asserted that in all cases studied the number and complexity of the convolutions did correspond to animal intelligence.[63]

Leuret was also often scornful of the phrenologists' claims about animal "faculties." He regarded as bizarre Gall's faculty of habitativité, which linked the animal drive "to find a domicile on mountains or high in the air with the [human] sentiment of pride."[64] He was equally incredulous at Broussais's contention (in his 1836 Cours) that herbivores demonstrated the faculty of "murderousness" when they "killed" the plants they consumed.[65] In place of what he saw as the phrenologists' fanciful faculties, Leuret relied instead on the more general faculties established in eighteenth-century philosophy and refashioned for modern use by the Ideologues.[66] He had no hesitation in using the omnibus term "intelligence" in his title or in equating it, in his subtitle, with "the instinctive, intellectual, and moral faculties." Similar locutions – "psychic facts," "the works of the intelligence" –

61 Ibid., 100, 69, 88.   62 Ibid., 219, 350.   63 Ibid., 270, 460–61.   64 Ibid., 266.
65 Ibid., 2, 564–66.
66 On the Ideologues' reworking of faculty psychology, see Sergio Moravia, "Philosophie et médecine en France à la fin du XVIIIᵉ siècle," Studies on Voltaire and the Eighteenth Century 89 (1972): 1089–1151, esp. 1107–10.

appear throughout the work. In the sections devoted to the faculties of specific animal groups, the term was used to cover animal activities: eating, swimming, copulating, fighting, and exercising the "senses" as such.[67] Like the Ideologues, Leuret placed particular stress on sociability and language. The reptiles, he observed, exhibited only the "egoistic" faculties and apparently lacked all interest in mutual concourse. Insects and birds, on the other hand, were highly sociable and indeed frequently showed genuine mutual devotion. On the subject of language, Leuret was categorical. Against Buffon and Condillac, he insisted that animals have and use languages appropriate to their conditions.[68] Although as a general rule Leuret asserted that the degree of development of particular faculties depended absolutely on the material development of the corresponding "organs," he made no effort to assign a specific "seat" to the "higher" faculties of sociability and language. These he treated as features of the more general faculty of "intelligence," which he linked to the development of the cerebronervous apparatus.

The most important general argument Leuret developed in respect to human and animal faculties challenged the traditional distinction between instinct and intelligence. Leuret rejected the view that humans enjoyed intelligence while animals had only instinct. He rested his argument in part on Adolphe Quetelet's demonstration of "uniformities" in human actions, which proved human beings were subject to the same kind of unvarying impulses that were usually thought to account for animal behavior. The bulk of his argument aimed, however, to show the "intelligent" character of much animal behavior, from insects' constructions of dwellings to the "choices" made by animal hunters.[69] Yet Leuret was not prepared to say that human beings were wholly determined or utterly lacking in free will. He accepted, if only grudgingly, the molding power of education and training. Having established that even moral behavior was subject to the kind of determining influences revealed in the distribution of crime statistics, Leuret nonetheless observed that "man is free . . . but only rarely, when his passions do not blind him, when, by reason of good training, he submits himself to the moral sense within him."[70]

It is interesting to see the term "passions" in this passage on moral freedom, for the disappearance of the passions was in fact one of the major semantic shifts accomplished by a comparativist approach to the problem of the physical-moral relation such as Leuret adopted in this work. Works positioned within the context of comparativist biology tended to move away from discussions of generalized moral faculties, including the passions, in

67 See, for example, Leuret and Gratiolet, *Anatomie comparée*, 1:90–92 (crustaceans), 204–14 (fish), 248–62 (reptiles), 301–41 (birds).
68 *Ibid.*, 254, 314–15, 100–34, 127.   69 *Ibid.*, 128–33.   70 *Ibid.*, 130.

the direction of the purely intellectual faculties. Where the older vitalist-dominated discourse of Cabanis, Alibert, and even Broussais had encompassed both intellectual and passional life, the new framework privileged the "intelligence."[71] Subtle and gradual, this terminological shift had important implications for the tradition of anthropological medicine that Leuret refrained from exploring in this text, framed as it was as a contribution to natural science. First, it encouraged a departure from the holistic perspective on the physical-moral relation toward the localism that in progressive medicine had become the dominant mode of conceptualizing disease and all other physiological activity. The passions, as conceived in the vitalist-dominated science of man, did not have localized "seats" in the body. They might be concentrated in one of the vital domains, but even in that case they exercised a kind of free-flowing influence throughout the body through sympathies and similar channels. One of the major objections of physicians such as Moreau de la Sarthe to Gall's organology was that it attempted to locate at precise points in the brain passions that were in fact systemic in origin and influence.[72] Eliminating the passions also served to distance medical progressives from the Christian moralizing tradition that had long dominated discourse on the passions, and therefore from conservatives like Alibert, who continued to blend the medical with the archaic, moralizing mode.[73]

Finally, and perhaps most important, deemphasizing the passions helped to deflect ethical problems attached to severely determinist constructions of the physical-moral relation. It was one thing, after all, to claim that human beings had different intellectual capacities, and that these were determined by such organic features as the number and distribution of the cerebral ganglia. Every moral and social orthodoxy was prepared to accept – indeed often insisted on – the existence of intellectual inequalities. It was another thing altogether to hold that human passions – tendencies to love or hate, to honesty or deceit, to moderation or excess – were implacably governed by physical characteristics. Such a contention was, if carried to its rigorous conclusions, universally unacceptable, for it negated both individual moral responsibility and the capacity of human beings (including doctors with their therapeutics) to accomplish anything through striving. Accordingly, the more rigorously determinist the discourse of the physical-moral rela-

71 For the older approach, which included the passions, see, for example, F. J. V. Broussais, *De l'irritation et de la folie, ouvrage dans lequel les rapports du physique et du moral sont établis sur la base de la médecine physiologique* (Paris: Delaunay, 1828), 223–26.
72 On the dominance of localism, see Jacques Léonard, *La médecine entre les pouvoirs et les savoirs: Histoire intellectuelle et politique de la médecine française au XIXe siècle* (Paris: Aubier, 1981), 132–38. On the vitalist conception of the passions, see Chapter 1.
73 Leuret emphasized his differences with the "spiritualists," especially the German alienist Heinroth, in *Du traitement moral de la folie* (Paris: J. B. Baillière, 1840), 147–48.

tion, the more likely it was to excise the passions and to privilege instead "intelligence," "the capacity for progress," and the like. To the extent that works such as Leuret's comparativist treatise continued to attend to the emotional and the passional, they did so by shunting these matters into the domain of instinct. Thus maternal love, sociability, sexual desire, and like tendencies were all treated as natural outcomes of innate "needs," but the multiple permutations and degrees of intensity in the passions gradually lapsed from view.[74]

The passions did not of course altogether disappear: they still had a crucial role to play in the purely therapeutic context of mental medicine. Indeed the difficulties the comparativist perspective presented to physicians such as Leuret, who were eager to embrace the principles of natural science yet still reluctant to apply them to human beings, are fully evident in his own career. There was a sharp dichotomy between Leuret's treatise of 1839 on the comparative structures of the human and animal brain and nervous system and a work he published only the following year on therapeutic techniques in mental medicine, *Du traitement moral de la folie* (1840). In the latter Leuret criticized those among his alienist colleagues who continued to claim all mental disease had a precise organic site and who treated alienation only by traditional physical therapies such as baths, medicines, and purgatives. In this context Leuret reasserted the importance of the passions and abused his colleagues for abandoning Pinel's "moral treatment."[75] Thus the role of the passions in Leuret's practical therapeutics differed starkly from their position in his comparativist discourse of the link between "organic structures" and "faculties." Thus Leuret accepted an uneasy bifurcation between scientific inquiry into the material foundations of the diverse faculties and a therapeutics that bracketed theoretical considerations and was based purely on empirical trial and error. Ultimately Leuret's position earned him few friends. To the alienists who were trying to establish the scientific credentials of mental medicine by emphasizing the need for and efficacy of a physical therapeutics that only doctors could supervise, he was a traitor to a beleaguered cause.[76] To the genuine spiritualists, on the other hand, Leuret's readiness to establish the highest human intellectual faculties at the end of a continuum beginning with the most primitive animal instinct ranked him with the ungodly. By the 1830s and 1840s, this latter position was associated chiefly with the remaining defenders of Montpellier vitalism.

74 For references to instinctual behavior arising from similar "needs" in humans and animals, see Leuret and Gratiolet, *Anatomie comparée*, 1:250–54 (ornamentation, sexual desire), 324–25 (communication through speech), 332–33 (capacity for progress).
75 Leuret, *Du traitement moral*, esp. chaps. 1 and 2. See also Goldstein, *Console and Classify*, 100–1, 177–78, 205, 265.
76 Ian Dowbiggin, *Inheriting Madness: Professionalization and Psychiatric Knowledge in Nineteenth-Century France* (Berkeley: University of California Press, 1991), chap. 2.

MUTATIONS OF VITALISM: MEDICAL CONSERVATIVES AND THE SCIENCE OF MAN

Although vitalism was beginning to come under strong attack by the 1830s many medical doctrines continued to harbor vitalist elements. Sometimes even medical theoreticians who were profoundly hostile to vitalism continued to use vitalist terminology. A case in point is Léon Rostan, the chief theorist of the doctrine called "organicism," who engaged in vigorous polemics against vitalism but nonetheless considered resistance to disease in terms of the "force" manifested by various "constitutions" in struggling against antagonistic external influences.[77] Broussais provides another example. He railed against Montpellier doctrine and vitalism generally and yet himself employed terms and concepts that were recognizably vitalist in origin.[78]

In short, vitalism lived on in the 1830s and 1840s in many forms. In Paris a number of prominent theorists including Frédéric Dubois d'Amiens, François-Joseph Double, and Etienne Pariset continued to defend basic vitalist tenets. In the early years of his career Pariset had translated and edited the *Aphorisms* and other works from the Hippocratic corpus. He later prepared his own edition of Cabanis's *Rapports* and gave public lectures on physiology in courses at the Athénée and the Société des bonnes lettres. Double and Dubois were, as observed earlier, vociferous opponents of medical statistics.[79] Dubois's career illustrates the continuing vitalist tradition in other ways as well. His thesis of 1828 was devoted to the "medical topography" of Saint Petersburg. He later produced a series of works on mental medicine and general medical philosophy in which he argued against materialism from a blended vitalist-spiritualist perspective.[80] His 1833 essay "De l'instinct et des déterminations instinctives dans l'espèce humaine" was ostensibly an attempt to join medical doctrines of instinct with the findings of modern neuroscience and comparative anatomy. Yet Dubois himself had no expertise in comparativist studies and his whole framing of the problem of instinct reflected a grounding in medical vitalism rather than the natural sciences. He argued that doctors must recover for their own science those

---

77 This observation is made in J. B. F. Descuret, *La médecine des passions, ou les passions considérés dans leurs rapports avec les maladies, les lois et la religion* (Paris: Béchet and Labé, 1841), 58, n. 1.

78 Broussais, *De l'irritation et de la folie*, 437–39; on the distinctions between "organic," "metaphysical," and "psychic" vitalism in this period, see Auguste Corlieu, *Le Centenaire de la Faculté de Médecine de Paris (1794–1894)* (Paris: Imprimerie nationale, 1896), 467–71, n. 2.

79 "Etienne Pariset," in *Nouvelle Biographie Générale*, 46 vols. (Paris: Firmin Didot, 1852–77), 39:214–16; on Double and Dubois, see Chapter 3, "The Science of Man at Work."

80 "Frédéric Dubois d'Amiens," *DBF* 11:933; Frédéric Dubois d'Amiens, *Fragments de philosophie médicale: Examen des doctrines de Cabanis, Gall et Broussais* (Paris: H. Cousin, 1842); idem, *Philosophie médicale: Examen des doctrines de Cabanis et de Gall* (Paris: G. Baillière, 1845).

"sensorial acts" that the philosophers had "joined and treated abstractly as . . . *psychology.*" "Everything that belongs to the organism," he wrote, "must henceforth be studied and meditated on by those who would concern themselves with acts of vitality, whatever the mode and source of these acts."[81] In Paris this kind of vitalist formulation was increasingly identified with not only medical but also some variant of social, political, or religious conservatism. This identification was, moreover, powerfully reinforced by the fact that the chief defenders of vitalism were to be found not in Paris but in Montpellier, which was now increasingly regarded as a bastion of both medical and political conservatism.

In Montpellier a number of figures were still attempting to exploit the tradition of the vitalist science of man to the fullest, in the context, by the 1830s, of mounting hostility from Paris and a sometimes desperate sense of institutional decline. During the Restoration many observers had made comparisons between the Paris and Montpellier medical schools that were distinctly unfavorable to Montpellier, but by the 1830s and 1840s these observations had become a chorus of criticism. At the time of Salvandy's inquiries, medical training in Montpellier was found to be deficient in important respects, especially in anatomical education, both classical and pathological; in the "impractical" character of its examinations; and in the botanical garden's stress on exotic rather than useful plants.[82] The Paris medical press was sometimes vociferous in its attacks on Montpellier, and by the early 1840s there were ever more frequent calls for the Montpellier faculty to be dismantled or, at the least, for its prerogatives to be restricted. One proposal, published in the *National* of March 30, 1843, called on the government to limit the medical practice of students with degrees from the provincial faculties to their own region. The article asserted that medical training in Paris was vastly superior to that offered in the provinces and that students who were refused admission in Paris evaded high standards simply by going to Montpellier instead.[83]

This article provoked a bitter response from the Montpellier professor M.-H. Kuehnholtz who denounced "the pretentious and despotic idea of centralization" and asserted that it was thanks only to the efforts of the Montpellier faculty that medicine in France had been saved from the bizarre and rapidly changing doctrinal fashions to which Paris medicine was constantly prey. Commenting on the government's persistent refusal to fund a chair in the history of medicine at the Paris faculty, Kuehnholtz argued that the real reason medical history had languished in Paris was that such a chair

---

81 Frédéric Dubois d'Amiens, "De l'instinct et des déterminations instinctives dans l'espèce humaine," *MARM* 2 (1833): 292–318, at 292.
82 Trenard, "Etudes médicales," 175.
83 H.-K. [M.-H.] Kuehnholtz, *Le national aristocrate, ou les Facultés de Médecine de Montpellier et de Paris considérées sous le point de vue de la centralisation et de la décentralisation* (Montpellier: J. Martel ainé, 1843), 1–4.

would have to be devoted to the "History of [Medical] Revolutions and Doctrinal Variations."[84] Taking advantage of the general repudiation of Broussaisism that set in in the 1830s, Kuehnholtz noted that Montpellier had never fallen victim to Broussais's "so-called physiological medicine, which required no more than twenty-four hours' study to be perfectly comprehended." All the while that the mania for Broussais and his murderous therapeutics had gripped the capital, Kuehnholtz asserted, Montpellier ("the modern Cos") had continued teaching the "Hippocratic and Barthezian doctrine," remaining true to its sacred traditions.[85]

This piece published in the *Echo du Midi* was one of many that Kuehnholtz wrote in the 1830s and 1840s to denounce the pretensions of Paris medicine and to reassert Montpellier's doctrinal purity and steadfastness.[86] The real master of these polemics was not Kuehnholtz himself, however, but his stepfather Jacques Lordat, who had begun defending Montpellier against the Paris materialists during the Restoration.[87] In the 1840s Lordat's campaign on behalf of Montpellier reached a peak of intensity, as the criticism from Paris mounted. Around 1840 a series of exchanges took place between Lordat and the Paris medical publicist Louis Peisse. In 1857 Peisse was to publish a two-volume hagiography of the luminaries of progressive Parisian medicine, but in the 1840s he was already denouncing Montpellier's stagnation the better to demonstrate the brilliance of Paris.[88] The charges Peisse lodged against Montpellier were the same as those made by Montpellier's other detractors: the school neglected the teaching of anatomy and provided its students little opportunity to perform dissections; the curriculum was generally outmoded and the professors hostile to innovation; the vitalist doctrines that still formed the core of Montpellier teaching blocked the progress that resulted when medicine was tied to the natural sciences.[89]

Lordat's response to these charges was both pragmatic and philosophical. On the practical level he answered point by point the criticisms made of Montpellier medical training. He denied that anatomy was poorly taught in Montpellier while acknowledging that anatomical instruction did not occupy the same place in Montpellier pedagogy as it did in Paris. He argued that too much time spent on dissection would prevent students' being trained as "anthropologists, pathologists, therapists." Students elsewhere might know cadavers, he observed, but they did not know pathology, "the

84 *Ibid.*, 12.   85 *Ibid.*, 7.
86 See [M.-] H. Kuehnholtz, *Oeuvres diverses* (a collection of pamphlets and extracts bound by the Wellcome Institute for the History of Medicine).
87 See Chapter 3, "Montpellier as the Bulwark of Orthodoxy."
88 Louis Peisse, *La médecine et les médecins: Philosophie, doctrines, institutions et biographies médicales*, 2 vols. (Paris: Baillière, 1857), esp. 1:238–97.
89 Jacques Lordat, *Réponses à des objections faites contre le principe de la dualité du dynamisme humain* (Montpellier: Martel; Paris: J. B. Baillière, 1854), xlix.

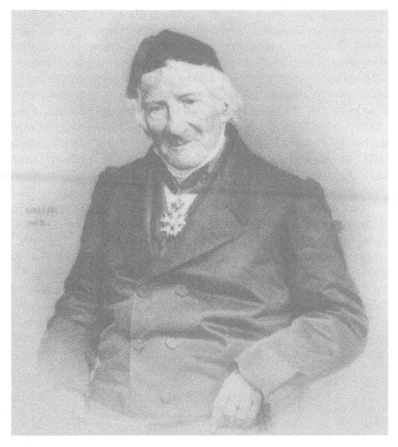

Portrait of Jacques Lordat, by Lafosse.

doctrine of the constitution of man," or the "science of man." Taking up another point of contention, Lordat admitted that Montpellier did not cultivate the new medical specialties but again held that this was a benefit of its teaching, which concentrated instead on "l'homme unitaire, l'homme tout entier." Montpellier's education was, thus, a genuine "intellectual" education, whereas that of other schools was given over to limited, practical matters.[90]

Lordat's defense of Montpellier rested chiefly, however, on the philosophical strengths and historical greatness of Montpellier. As he had in the 1820s, Lordat emphasized Montpellier's ancient traditions and its rooting in Hippocratism. He stressed the uniqueness and fecundity of Barthez's thought, and contrasted Montpellier's theoretical sophistication and solidity

90 *Ibid.*, liii-lv.

to Paris's haphazard empiricism and thirst for novelty. Lordat eventually
came to cast his defense of Montpellier into the form of a new doctrine he
termed "the duality of human dynamism."[91] In this reworking of Montpellier ideas, Lordat broached directly the nature of the relations between
the "thinking soul" and the vital principle, a problem that in the work of
Montpellier's classical eighteenth-century theorists had been kept well in
the background. In all his writings of these years, Lordat insisted upon the
complete orthodoxy of Montpellier teaching, which had always upheld the
unassailable distinction between body and soul. The "vital" and the "intellectual" were the same insofar as each had "an end" and were, unlike brute
matter, characterized by "finality."[92] But this vital principle was never to be
confounded with either the soul or with purely physical forces: "There exists
a cause of life which . . . cannot be either the thinking soul, for which all
was created, nor the ensemble of physical causes that are recognized in inanimate bodies."[93]

This dualist position did not, however, in Lordat's view, alter Montpellier's fundamental commitment to a holistic and unitary approach to man.
Lordat readily disavowed any knowledge or understanding of the "dynamic
nature of the beasts," but he asserted without question that in human beings
the two "powers" of the vital and the intellectual were joined in a "hypo-
static union." This union of the vital and the intellectual was the essence of
human nature and the first principle of any genuine anthropology:

The two dynamic powers of man . . . cooperate in a great number of the functions
of health and of pathology, and the theory of these collaborations forms the anthropological doctrine that we call the doctrine of the alliance.[94]

Lordat separated himself from theorists who insisted that medicine must
link its labors to those of the general life sciences. "Anthropology could
not," he wrote, "be regarded as a part of the general physiology of animals:
it is a physiological science that stands in *isolation*." He denounced all doctrines that controverted this fundamental truth of the uniqueness of human
beings. These included not only the materialist "école Bichato-Cabaniso-
Broussaisienne," which held that the moral and the physical were the same,
but also natural history, whose efforts to invade everything offended "rigorous philosophy, medicine, public decency, and morality."[95]

Such pronouncements did nothing to help Montpellier's reputation or institutional standing, although by the time Lordat wrote these words the
anachronism of such constructions was recognized even in Montpellier.
When Lordat attempted to have a chair established for himself in the study

91 *Ibid.*, xliv, lxi–lxii.   92 *Ibid.*, lx.   93 *Ibid.*, xxiii.   94 *Ibid.*, lxi–lxii.
95 *Ibid.*, lxi, lxv, lxviii.

of "human dynamism," the proposal was rejected.[96] Contrary to the aspersions of the Parisian doctors, there were a number of figures in Montpellier who were as fully committed to modern methods of investigation as medical scientists in the capital.[97] Yet Lordat continued to hold his chair in physiology up to 1860 and throughout these long years always wielded considerable influence in the Montpellier faculty. In 1860 he was promoted to commander in the Legion of Honor on the recommendation of the minister of public instruction Rouland, who reported to Napoleon III that at the age of eighty-seven Lordat was "the most authoritative representative of a school whose doctrines he personifies and of which he is the glory."[98] This being the case, it was all the more imperative that theorists who strove for a distinctly medical yet still scientifically current science of man avoid identification with Montpellier's archaism.

SEEKING MIDDLE GROUND: MEDICAL PHYSIOLOGY AND RACE THEORY IN PARIS

Although conservative notions such as Lordat's that the "natural history of man" constituted an affront to human decency were regarded in Paris as patently absurd, there were diverse medical figures in the capital who sought at one and the same time to embrace medical modernity and yet continue to conceive of medicine as a broad-gauge science of the physical and the moral. The tensions and difficulties involved in finding such middle ground are well exemplified in the career and thought of Pierre-Nicolas Gerdy, who held a chair at the Faculty of Medicine in external pathology but devoted his greatest efforts to work in physiology.

From the point of view of the new experimental science, the medical faculty was the bastion of traditionalist approaches to the problems of life and function. This view was based on the work of such faculty luminaries as P.-H. Bérard, who held the chair in physiology from 1831 to 1858 and who, although not hostile to experimentalism, undertook few experimental investigations of his own until the late 1850s.[99] In the late 1830s and 1840s the

---

96 Louis Dulieu, *La médecine à Montpellier*, vol. 4, *De la première à la troisième république, première partie* (Avignon: Les presses universelles, 1988), 331–33.

97 Antoine Dugès did extensive comparativist work in the 1830s; Claude-François Lallemand uses the techniques of pathological anatomy to explore problems of cerebral localization; see Antoine Dugès, *Traité de physiologie comparée de l'homme et des animaux*, 3 vols. (Montpellier: L. Castel, 1838–39); Claude-François Lallemand, *Recherches anatomo-pathologiques sur l'encéphale et ses dépendances*, 3 vols. (Paris: Béchet jeune, 1830–34). There are biographical sketches of both men in Dulieu, *La médecine à Montpellier*, 4:739–44 (Dugès), 4:825–29 (Lallemand). See also Louis Dulieu, "Claude-François Lallemand," *RHS* 28 (1975): 125–38.

98 Georges Kuehnholtz-Lordat and Henri-F. Peuchot, "Petite histoire de quelques décorations," *Monspeliensis Hippocrates* 4, no. 14 (Winter 1961): 24–28, at 26.

99 Corlieu, *Centenaire de la Faculté de Médecine*, 263–66.

most visible and articulate representative of the older medical physiology was in any event not the chairholder Bérard but Gerdy. Gerdy was for a long time excluded from the faculty; by the time he took up the pathology chair in 1833 he had competed in twelve *concours*.[100] Once appointed to the faculty Gerdy devoted himself for a time to work on osteology, surgery, the dressing of wounds, and similar topics appropriate to his post. But physiology was always the subject Gerdy was the most interested in and preferred to teach. He had offered a *cours libre* in anatomy and physiology at the Charité from 1815 to 1821 and published his first major work in physiology, "Essai de classification naturelle et d'analyse des phenomènes de la vie," in 1821 in the *Journal complémentaire du Dictionaire des sciences médicales.* This work was, in the words of his eulogist Paul Broca, a *coup de maître*.[101] In it, Gerdy attempted to reconcile vitalism in the tradition of Bichat with experimentalism as practiced by Magendie. Gerdy argued that both sides in this conflict had staked out exaggerated, dogmatic positions, the Bichatian physiologist denying that there were "laws of life" and attributing everything to "that great phrase devoid of meaning: the vital principle," and the Magendie-style experimentalist giving far too little significance to "the intervention of life."[102] Gerdy claimed to stand in the middle, recognizing, on the one hand, the importance of purely "physical" functions yet, on the other, categorizing those that could not be explained by physical principles as "vital phenomena" falling into eighteen distinct analytical groups. This, he held, was "*la méthode naturelle* substituted for that of systems."[103]

This work of 1821 outlined in brief the position Gerdy held throughout his whole career. In a discussion at the Académie de médecine in January 1839 he himself referred his listeners back to his 1821 article where he set out views that had remained the same ever since.[104] Gerdy elaborated the principles set forth in that essay in a series of further writings on physiology published from the 1820s to the 1840s, the most substantial of which were *Physiologie médicale, didactique et critique* (1832–33) and *Physiologie philosophique des sensations et de l'intelligence* (1846).[105] In addition, Gerdy spoke at the Académie de médecine, of which he was a member, on the nature of intelligence, the senses and sensory perception, language and speech, the nature of the "understanding," the organization of the brain, and like matters. Many of these presentations were later published in a collection enti-

100 Paul Broca, *Eloge historique de M. P.-N. Gerdy, lu à la Société de Chirurgie le 2 juillet 1856* (Paris, 1856) [extract from *Moniteur des Hôpitaux*], 39.
101 *Ibid.*, 40–41, 34, 7, 20.   102 *Ibid.*, 21.   103 *Ibid.*, 22.
104 P.-N. Gerdy, "Discours sur le système nerveux et la méthode expérimentale," [1839] in *Mélanges d'anatomie, de physiologie et de chirurgie*, ed. Paul Broca and E. Beaugrand, 2 vols. (Paris: P. Asselin, 1875), 1:408.
105 P.-N. Gerdy, *Physiologie médicale, didactique et critique* (Paris: Crochard, 1832–33); *idem, Physiologie philosophique des sensations et de l'intelligence* (Paris: Labé, 1846).

tled *Mélanges d'anatomie, de physiologie et de chirurgie* (1875), edited by Broca and E. Beaugrand, who characterized the work as a tribute to Gerdy's memory and "a genuine service to science."[106]

In his physiological writings Gerdy pressed the argument that medicine was both allied to and separate from the experimental sciences. He praised Magendie for the amazing results he had achieved in the laboratory, yet at the same time regretted the dominance of experimental procedures over others available to physiologists. Those who used only their "hands" and not their "minds" were necessarily hindered from making the most important and privileged observations accessible to physicians ("the more active the hands, the less rational the mind").[107] Experiment was in some cases appropriate but since experimental results were often "deceptive and misleading," clinical observation, reflection, and analysis were generally far superior.[108] To achieve its best results, Gerdy argued, physiology must be closely attuned to the broad concerns of medicine.[109]

It is hard not to feel that Gerdy's concessions to experimentation were the measured words of a man barely concealing his chagrin at the public and official success of procedures that he in fact deplored. His plaudits to experiment were general; no specific gains or advances were ever mentioned. In any event his hostility to experimentation was evident in his description of the laboratory:

> The site of these researches resembles less the study of a meditative man than a place of murder and carnage where there incessantly resound the pleas and cries of animals expiring in the course of frightful tortures. Deaf to their suffering, physiology readily – laughingly – contemplates the horror of their movements and the anguish of their suffering.[110]

Gerdy was, furthermore, one with those physicians who thought it impossible to transfer the results of animal experimentation to the study of human beings. What could be more absurd, he declared to the Académie de médecine in 1839, than "confidently applying to man experimental observations made on animals who are so far removed from him in organization and faculties."[111] Yet his objection to laboratory experimentation was grounded not only in this perceived "distance" between man and animals but also in the long-accepted, specifically medical truth that nature must not

106 "Avertissement," in Gerdy, *Mélanges*, 1:vi.
107 Gerdy, *Physiologie médicale*, "Préface," ix. (References thus cited are to the independently bound "Préface" catalogued at the Bibliothèque nationale under the number 8° Tb⁷.125 and dated 1830.)
108 Gerdy, "Essai de classification naturelle et d'analyse des phénomènes de la vie," in *Mélanges*, 1:161.
109 Gerdy, *Physiologie médicale*,"Préface," ix.
110 *Ibid.*; Gerdy was strongly criticized for this statement by J.-B. Bouillaud who was nonetheless in some ways sympathetic to Gerdy's championing of the science of man; see Bouillaud, *Essai sur la philosophie médicale*, 133–34, n.1.
111 Gerdy, "Discours sur le système nerveux," 1:407.

be "interrogated" but listened to. "To observe is to listen to nature when she speaks spontaneously of herself"; to experiment is to "force nature to speak when one is ready to listen."[112] By their very nature, then, experiments controverted the proper order of inquiry.

These remarks are of special interest in light of Gerdy's attack on the vitalists who, he claimed, explained all phenomena with obscure phrases like the "vital principle" and who stood united against science as their common enemy.[113] Gerdy upbraided vitalists for refusing to accept the determinacy and lawlike behavior of vital phenomena. Although he himself was hostile to experiment, to the laboratory, and to the privileging of hand over mind, he was nonetheless firmly committed to a naturalistic perspective that rejected outmoded dualism, excessively abstract language, and metaphysical obscurity.[114] His antidotes to such unhealthy tendencies within medicine were the standard remedies of his true intellectual forebears – the eighteenth-century sensationalists and, more important than any other, the Ideologues. Indeed Gerdy's works of the 1820s through the 1840s are throwbacks to Condillac, Cabanis, Pinel, and medical Ideology generally. His emphasis on observation, analysis, and classification placed him squarely with what had been modern physiology around 1800. His Hippocratism, clearly revealed in his remarks on the need to listen to nature, reverted to the ritual injunctions of the "Hippocratists" of the revolutionary era.[115]

Medical physiology of Gerdy's sort was thus uneasily poised between the old vitalism, with its recognition of the spontaneity, indeterminacy, and variability of vital phenomena and the modern life sciences; with their insistence on the determinate and fixed character of physiological processes. Gerdy was unwilling to recognize that the internal logic of the expectant-Hippocratic tradition was lost once physicians accepted the lawlike character of vital phenomena. The whole notion that the physician waited patiently for nature to speak had been grounded in the affirmation of the spontaneity and high variability of vital phenomena. The vitalists had taught that one did not interrogate nature because nature spoke in its own way and in its own time, not in response to the inflexible laws of physicochemical reality. Thus although Gerdy accepted the fact of determinacy in the interests of rendering medicine genuinely positive, he was not prepared to accept as one of the consequences of determinacy that the deliberate "interrogation" of vital phenomena was legitimate.

Gerdy's position betwixt and between is perhaps clearest in his treatment of the problem of sensibility, which, as Michael Gross has pointed

112 *Ibid.*   113 Broca, *Eloge historique*, 21.
114 For a denunciation of *esprit de système*, see Gerdy, "Discours sur le système nerveux," 433–36.
115 On the methods of observation, analysis, and classification, see Gerdy, "Science," in *Mélanges*, 1:660–66; and *Physiologie médicale*, "Préface," vii–xi, lxxi–lxxii.

out, supplies a kind of index to the "old" and the "new" physiology in France around 1830.[116] In the tradition of the Montpellier vitalists and the medical Ideologues, Gerdy argued that sensibility was diffused throughout the body, that the individual organs did not merely transmit sensation to the brain but experienced sensation in themselves and reacted to influences or agents both outside and within the body.[117] This issue was a crucial one in anthropological medicine because the argument that sensations – whether external or internal, to use Cabanis's language – were experienced differently by different physiological types depended wholly on viewing sensibility as itself immediately active and determinative in life processes. In the 1830s this point of view was of course in the process of being overthrown by experimental physiology, which regarded sensibility as localized in the neuromuscular system, dependent on the integrity of specific material structures, and not therefore – as the vitalists taught – linked to larger systemic distributions of vital force.[118]

Medical physiologists like Gerdy flatly rejected the experimentalists' reworking of the integral concept of sensibility. When J.-B. Bouillaud argued on behalf of localized, nerve-bound sensibility before the Académie de médecine in 1839, Gerdy responded by reaffirming the

incontestable truths that the sensible parts feel by themselves, as the epithet *sensible* indicates; that the nerves transmit the received sensation and that the brain *does not feel;* that the word sensation can logically be used only for the phenomena that take place in the sensible parts, and perception for the consciousness or sensation that takes place in the brain.[119]

Gerdy opposed the theory of localized sensibility in part simply because it was an argument based on animal experimentation, which he did not trust, but also because to his mind it was actively contradicted by clinical observations such as the well-known fact that lesions suffered in the posterior columns of the spinal cord did not always damage sensation.[120]

Still more important was the fact that if sensibility was confined to the neuromotor system, the entire analytic structure of temperament – and with it much of the larger anthropological imperative of medicine – would be undermined. Anthropological medicine had always taught that sensibility varied with the complex states and dispositions of the solids and humors, and that there was a close correspondence between the character of sensibility and the varied psychophysiological attributes of individual temperaments. If these claims were abandoned, medicine lost the chief tool

116 Gross, "Lessened Locus of Feelings," 232.
117 See esp. Gerdy, "Discours sur le système nerveux," 427–36, where Gerdy mobilizes clinical cases to argue against the view that sensation was dependent on the full integrity of the spinal cord.
118 Gross, "The Lessened Locus of Feelings," 239–46.
119 Gerdy, "Discours sur le système nerveux," 428 (italics in the original).
120 *Ibid.,* 436.

with which it gauged the interrelation of the physical and the moral, and it was precisely the study of the physical and the moral faculties that Gerdy believed should be the "essential object of the physician."[121] That physiology's specific contribution to study of the physical and the moral would be immeasurably weakened if sensibility was reduced to a localized process dependent on a specifically defined apparatus had in fact already been made clear in François Magendie's *Précis élémentaire de physiologie* (1816). In that work the visceral passions of Cabanisian-Bichatian physiology were leveled into so many "judgments" on passion made by the feeling and perceiving brain.[122] In such a rendering there could be no primordial physiological types – brain dominant in the cerebral, feeling in the sensual, movement in the locomotor – because all sensations were ultimately of the same type once moved through the clearinghouse of the central nervous system and the brain. In Magendie's construct emotions were transformed into ideas and, in psychological terms, the clock was set back to the purely externalist sensationalism of Condillac, now buttressed by increasingly detailed knowledge of the workings of the neuranatomical apparatus upon which the transmission of sensation depended.[123] To physiologists like Gerdy – for whom physiology's principal advances lay in its march toward understanding, classifying, and treating variant physical-moral types – the redefinition of sensibility in light of laboratory method was a giant step backward.

Although Gerdy was hostile to experimentalism and determined to retain physiology's focus on human as opposed to animal organization, he nonetheless favored a thoroughly naturalistic approach to physiological investigation and advocated the forging of ever stronger ties between medicine and the other sciences. If in his view the experimental sciences offered little to human physiology, there were nevertheless other fields within the constantly expanding biological sciences with which medical physiology must join its efforts. Since the eighteenth century, investigations of natural historians had markedly advanced the study of human anatomy, to which, in his view, physiology must always be closely allied, and, more significant, had provided a general scientific approach to the study of human beings when considered in relation to organized life in general.

This larger frame of reference was not one to which medical theorists came easily; the absolute uniqueness of the human was both a principle deeply ingrained in medical philosophy and a pragmatic perspective enjoined by the conditions of medical labor. At some level the focus of med-

---

121 Gerdy, "Recherches, discussions et propositions d'anatomie, de physiologie, de pathologie, etc." in *Mélanges*, 1:74.
122 See François Magendie, *Précis élémentaire de physiologie* 2 vols. (Paris: Méquignon-Marvis, 1816), esp. 172–76, where Magendie concluded that "it is principally in our manner of sensing relations or in making judgments that men differ from one another" (1:176).
123 Gross, "The Lessened Locus of Feelings," 246–47.

icine was always on the sick individual and, even where it had developed a perspective that looked beyond individuals to groups and types, such thinking generally remained within the domain of the human. Medical typologizing established human types distributed according to age, sex, climate, and the like; it did not extend to extrahuman comparison. Within the medical framework of "influences," the only concept that provided linkage to the larger world of organized creation was the concept of race, which established a normative, hierarchizing principle permitting conceptualization of the stages or degrees of variability ("inferior races") leading out of the strictly human into the sphere of the animal. Still, although race had been drawn into medical discourse from natural history in the late eighteenth century by figures such as Barthez and Cabanis, its potential for serving as a comparativist instrument had not been much developed in medical discourse since that time.[124] Race tended simply to be added to the list of the long-established influences accounting for intrahuman variability. By the 1830s and 1840s, however, conditions were such that race became an increasingly prominent concept in medical discourse, especially for figures like Gerdy who sought to connect medical inquiry into physical and moral types to larger developments in the natural sciences.

The desire to link the medical science of man more closely to natural history was not of course the only source of the growing importance of race theory in medicine. The new prominence of race in medical thinking resulted from a complex of political, intellectual, and institutional developments that affected all the sciences and indeed the culture at large. As a broad cultural phenomenon, the preoccupation with race resulted from a concatenation of political and ideological imperatives of which the most important was probably the resurgence of extra-European imperialism. For the French this meant especially the conquest of Algeria and the gradual expansion into Africa. Among scholars, the Algerian experience was to a large extent fitted into the preexisting framework of "orientalism," but France's encroachment on black Africa provoked a new conceptualization of what were seen as the profound physical and moral differences separating the "civilized" from the "noncivilized."[125] This larger political and ideological context for the intensified interest in race was reinforced within medicine by local institutional and theoretical developments. The immense

124 Paul-Joseph Barthez, *Nouveaux éléments de la science de l'homme*, 2 vols., 2d ed. (Paris: Goujon, 1806), 2:275; P. J. G. Cabanis, "Rapports du physique et du moral de l'homme," in *Oeuvres philosophiques de Cabanis*, ed. Claude Lehec and Jean Cazeneuve (Paris: Presses universitaires de France, 1956), 1: 468–71.
125 Edward Said, *Orientalism* (New York: Random House, 1978); on the shift in racial thinking that accompanied the French movement into black Africa, see William B. Cohen, *The French Encounter with Africans: White Response to Blacks 1530–1880* (Bloomington: Indiana University Press, 1980).

prestige of the comparativist method exemplified by Cuvier made increasingly dubious any science that purported to examine the differentiation of types without a grounding in comparativist inquiry. Some comparativist instruction had been offered within the medical curriculum from 1802, when a chair in comparative anatomy was created for Cuvier's protégé A. M. C. Duméril.[126] The medical students of the 1820s and 1830s were the first to feel the influence of this institutional innovation and to begin in their own work to acknowledge (if only formally, as in Dubois's essay on instinct) the importance of comparativism. From this period, then, a new framework for medically based race theory, which drew on both the tradition of medical typologizing and on natural history, began to develop. Its outlines may be examined in the work of Gerdy's student Pierre-Paul Broc.[127]

For a short time in the late 1830s Broc was a somewhat notorious figure in Paris medical circles. In 1837 he competed in a hotly contested *concours* for the anatomy chair at the faculty, a contest that became the occasion for one of the most violent student protests of the period. Broc was not the typical *concours* candidate. Although he had received his medical training in Paris, fortune carried him off to a long sojourn in Colombia, where, among other activities, he had operated a school for boys. On his return to Paris, he had offered a *cours libre* in anatomy and gained a considerable reputation for his teaching. He was apparently an impassioned orator and, as a confirmed Rousseauan who condemned schoolmasters as jailers and education as the source of all human misery, he had a fervent student following.[128] The 1835 *concours* for the anatomy chair took place when its previous holder Jean Cruveilhier moved to the new chair in pathological anatomy. This appointment had already caused consternation among student and faculty liberals since the conservative Cruveilhier had been a particular favorite of the Restoration government.[129] Cruveilhier's appointment was, however, a fait

126 Toby Appel, *The Cuvier-Geoffroy Debate: French Biology in the Decades before Darwin* (New York: Oxford University Press, 1987), 61, 65.

127 Gerdy himself did considerable work in racial classification, as did the Faculty of Medicine chairholder in physiology, P.-H. Bérard; see Gerdy, *Physiologie médicale, didactique et critique*, vol. 1; Bérard, *Cours de physiologie fait à la Faculté de Médecine de Paris* (Paris: Labé, 1848), 1: Lessons 21 and 27. Their polygenist constructions helped to form the racial doctrines of Paul Broca; see Claude Blanckaert, " 'L'anthropologie personnifiée': Paul Broca et la biologie du genre humain," Preface to *Paul Broca: Mémoires d'Anthropologie* (Paris: Jean Michel Place, 1989), ix.

128 "Pierre-Paul Broc," *DBF* 7:381; for references to his life in Colombia, see Pierre-Paul Broc, *Essai sur les races humaines considérées sous les rapports anatomique et philosophique* (Paris: Just Ranvier and E. Le Bouvier, 1836), 158–60. Broc's Rousseauism may be traced in *Races humaines*, esp. 121–35, 152–61. His student following is discussed in Corlieu, *Centenaire de la Faculté de Médecine*, 253, and Huard, "L'enseignement libre," 50.

129 In 1824 Cruveilhier was imposed on the Montpellier faculty by the Restoration government; see Dulieu, *La médecine à Montpellier*, 4:277. The new chair in pathological anatomy at the Paris faculty to which he was appointed in 1835 was established on a bequest by Dupuytren; see Russell C. Maulitz, *Morbid Appearances: The Anatomy of Pathology in the Early Nineteenth Century* (Cambridge: Cambridge University Press, 1987), 75.

accompli and so the students apparently set their hopes on the appointment of a kindred spirit to the anatomy chair.

Broc reportedly acquitted himself well in all stages of the contest, which included a written examination on fibrous tissue, an oral on membranes of the brain, a public dissection, and, in the final phase of the competition, the presentation of a synopsis of Broc's soon-to-be-published book on the human races. Despite his fine performances, however, Broc lost out in the voting and the chair went instead to Gilbert Breschet, whose *agrégé* status gave him an edge over Broc. When the decision to appoint Breschet was announced, a riot broke out, the army was called in, and arrests were made. The *concours* was much written about in the medical press, and one critic who denounced the dean, Matthieu Orfila, for the outcome, was fined by the courts.[130]

Broc was, then, a figure much respected by the faculty liberals and, though his anatomical instruction was in many ways traditional in approach, he was nonetheless resolute in urging that medicine incorporate into its own inquiry problems and perspectives current in larger biological science. Much of his slim (161-page) treatise on the human races was devoted to a synopsis of classificatory systems devised by both doctors and naturalists – Cuvier, Gerdy, Linnaeus, Blumenbach, Duméril, J.-J. Virey, J.-B. Bory de Saint-Vincent, and Antoine Desmoulins – as well as the geographer Conrad Malte-Brun.[131] Mobilizing his anatomical expertise, Broc offered a summary of the characters used by taxonomists to differentiate the races, but he also drew attention to general biohistorical problems including the origin of the races, their modifiability, and the best means of defining such terms as "race," "variety," and "species."

Yet despite Broc's efforts to lodge his discussion of race within a broad scientific framework, his own way of defining humans as a distinct species indicates how thoroughly he continued to function within the medical universe. His discussion was ostensibly based on a comparison between humans and the orangoutang:

Like all animals, [the orangoutang] lacks entirely the faculty of comparing things, which makes possible the movement from effect to cause. Hence his incapacity to improve or perfect himself or to make a series of discoveries that can serve as the basis of a science. Unable to articulate sounds, he will never invent the signs of an artificial language. There is nothing to indicate that he forms abstract ideas, that he generalizes . . . that he looks into the future, or that he has any sense of a being who is superior to all others, the creator of the universe.[132]

The characteristics of actual orangoutangs make no appearance here: the orangoutang simply functions as a representative of all animality. The passage

130 Corlieu, *Centenaire de la Faculté de Médecine,* 253–55.   131 Broc, *Races humaines,* 23.
132 *Ibid.,* 5.

in fact reflects not so much the naturalist's interest in actual, living animals as it does the preoccupations of the medical Ideologues with the distinctly human capacities for comparison, analysis, language, generalization, abstraction, and general perfectibility. That the human was the sole focus of this ostensible "comparison" was indicated when, later in the work, Broc declined to offer a description of human moral and intellectual features and simply referred his readers to the characters that "earlier I denied to the orangoutang."[133]

In other ways too it was apparent that Broc did not feel at home with issues raised in natural history and biology. He sometimes merely stated a problem, offering no opinion or resolution of his own. In discussing whether interfertility was the best guide to the demarcation of species, for example, Broc noted that some "zoologists" regarded the capacity for interbreeding as the clearest mark of a distinct species, but he observed with equal interest that others believed "this manner of determining or defining the species" was inexact since animals existed that could produce offspring despite "the great differences separating them."[134] Similarly, on the monogenist-polygenist question that was much disputed among naturalists, Broc merely stated that "it was impossible to respond to this question, at least if one insists on taking it up in a strictly philosophical manner."[135]

No such reticence was apparent in Broc's purely descriptive treatment of the major races (white, yellow, and black), in which he presented physical, moral, and intellectual characters interchangeably. As in many classificatory exercises of the period, Broc did not attempt to develop strictly symmetrical descriptions for each racial stock or group. In one instance he accented geography, in another temperament, in yet others religious practices or phrenological features. The authorities on whom he based these descriptions were, by turn, physicians (Galen, Soemmering, Gerdy), naturalists (Cuvier, Buffon, Isidore Geoffroy Saint-Hilaire), geographers (Malte-Brun, Adrien Balbi), and unspecified "voyagers." And although he incorporated much information from nonmedical sources, Broc's summaries are notable chiefly for assuming as wholly proven many of the standard assumptions of medical typologizing: the virtually inextricable interrelations between the moral and the physical, the limited-energy principle which decreed that sensory acuity necessarily meant diminished intellectual capacity, and the view that external influences such as climate could engender fundamental changes in "organization" if exerted over a long period of time.[136]

The last quarter of Broc's book was lodged, moreover, squarely within the problematic of the physical and the moral. Entitled "Influence de l'état

133 *Ibid.*, 18.   134 *Ibid.*, 3 and n.1.   135 *Ibid.*, 18.   136 *Ibid.*, esp. 14–15, 75, 115–20.

sauvage, de l'état social, du gouvernement, de la religion et de l'éducation," this section presented a long reverie on the primeval human condition of isolation, the awakening to moral and intellectual growth by social interchange, the bitter struggle reason must wage to establish dominance over brute passion, the conquest of nature, and similar topics. Here Broc cited no authorities at all, the better perhaps to emphasize his own originality or to avoid identification with particular philosophical schools. Rousseau's imprint is frequently evident. Yet the opening image of savage, isolated man led Broc not only to the Rousseauan theme of the beneficent effects of sociability but also to a defense of sensationalism in which he held that all knowledge is gained through a sequence of sensations although the sequence is often not remembered.[137]

Like many physicians who worked within the tradition of the science of man, Broc was less interested in the problem of the physical determination of psychic or moral faculties than the reverse. He accepted the general validity of phrenology, even though he noted that in Colombia he had encountered many "good and honest" Indians whose skulls would have condemned them to the gallows according to the phrenologists. He asserted that whites were superior to blacks because of their general "organization" but rejected as unproven assertions that blacks were "brothers" to the monkeys.[138] The problem that really interested Broc, however – and here his thinking is permeated with the spirit of medical moralism and the therapeutic impulse – was the influence that the moral could exert on the physical. In a sentiment reminiscent of Frédéric Bérard (see Chapter 3), he lamented the fact that so little attention was paid to the effects achieved by "the faculties characterized by liberty." It was these faculties that "extended and ennobled existence . . . these faculties that preside over the intellectual and moral life and maintain man in the most perfect harmony with his fellows."[139] To prove his point, Broc recounted in rhapsodic language the successes he had achieved in Colombia educating boys of all races, using not the hateful techniques of the schoolmaster-jailer but the "games and promenades" by which children learn naturally. Here one could see true equality – "the uniform color of intelligence" – as well as the genuine "unity of the species." The effects of education, when undertaken in the true philosophical spirit, could be seen not only in the soul and spirit but on the body itself: the forehead became more commanding, the face took on the rounded form of joy and laughter, and all the traits were altered by "thought and sentiment."[140]

That the students at the Faculty of Medicine should have been moved to tears and blows by Broc's rhetoric is unsurprising when one reads the per-

---

137 *Ibid.*, 126.   138 *Ibid.*, 142, 74–75.   139 *Ibid.*, 135.   140 *Ibid.*, 160.

oration to *Races humaines:* "Ah, that true philosophy had the power to draw from all eternity the centuries it needed [for its work] and that it had command over all education. It would metamorphose all the races and regenerate the human genus!"[141] This text of Broc's is wonderfully revealing of the ramifying ambiguities and rhetorical potentialities of the medical science of man. It shows that even medical figures who sought to put their inquiry into the physical and the moral on a sound footing in the natural sciences might yet cling to their medicomoral, therapeutic framework, with its emphasis on reciprocities, over the strict determinism that was coming to be seen as the only legitimate approach to studies of the animal world. Although Broc accepted that the conformation of the skull and general organization were crucial in establishing moral and intellectual characters, he felt no need to constrain his own thinking on race within a wholly determinist framework. He continued instead to mine the therapeutic vein of anthropological medicine, retrieving for current use the vocabulary of perfectibility, education, and moral-temperamental-psychical molding that had characterized medical Ideology at its more sanguine moments. In this sense, medically grounded race theory provided not so much a bridge between the medical science of man and the natural sciences, with their insistence on the law-bound phenomena of organized creation, as a halfway house occupied before human beings too were brought within the sway of the full-blown naturalism that ultimately would dominate medical discourse as well.

Nor is the fact that Broc's hymn to education and moral-physical regeneration was accompanied by observations typical of the vicious racism of nineteenth-century medical and biological science surprising. Anthropological medicine moved restlessly between the poles of materialism and spiritualism, optimism and pessimism, therapeutic hope and therapeutic nihilism. It supplied, by turns, grounds for insisting on the fixed character of human attributes, and on their malleability; the primacy of the physical over the moral, and of the moral over the physical; of the supreme importance of types, and the essentially variable and nominalist character of all medical observations, including those on racial features. What it always insisted upon was the intricate intermeshing of the physical and the moral, the special capacity of physicians to decipher those relations, and the urgent need for society to note medical counsel on the perils and opportunities presented by the individual and typological permutations of the physical-moral relation. In this respect physicians like Gerdy and Broc who sought to find some methodological and ideological middle ground for the science of man were one with its self-conscious proselytizers on either side of the materialist-vitalist divide. In all cases, the fundamental importance of the

141 *Ibid.,* 161.

physical-moral relation remained and with it the claim that medicine had a special capacity to pierce the obscurities of that relation.

SOCIAL-CHRISTIAN MEDICINE

If physicians such as Gerdy and Broc sought to overcome the dichotomies between materialist and vitalist, progressive and traditionalist, there were other physicians of the period who were concerned not only to transcend theoretical and methodological divisions within medicine but also to direct the science of man toward the task of achieving social reconciliation in a society embittered and divided by its revolutionary past. This was of course one of the stated goals of the "eclectics," both philosophical and medical, who enjoyed great influence in the cultural world of the July Monarchy. Yet philosophical eclecticism, with its aim of reconciling Catholic royalism with liberalism, offered nothing to those whose politics were shaped by the increasingly sharp class divisions caused by the rapid commercial and industrial developments of the era. Medical eclecticism was also increasingly irrelevant as a bridge over the materialist-spiritualist divisions of the past, since the medical eclectics tended increasingly to argue their middle-of-the-road position on the basis of neutral scientism rather than Cousinian or any other philosophical principles.[142] Yet scientistic aloofness was wholly unacceptable to those physicians who believed medicine must engage social problems directly. Thus, if there were to be reconciliation in the changing conditions of the era – both economic and in conceptions of the purpose and goals of science – its themes would have to come from elements that, unlike the eclectics, were attuned to new realities. This was the function that a coterie of physicians dedicated to what may be called "social-Christian" medicine sought to perform.

Developed first in the context of left-wing politics, social-Christian medicine fairly rapidly came to construe the eighteenth-century heritage claimed by much of the Left as one of the principal causes of the divisive spirit of the times. Instead of encouraging social or ideological conflict as a way of achieving progress (in the fashion of Broussais, for example), social-Christian medicine privileged "synthesis" over "analysis," the "organic" spirit over the "critical." It sought to ground medical science in spiritual certainties and to blend its own therapeutics with the healing promised by traditional religiosity. In seeking to accomplish these disparate ends, the social-Christian doctors made creative use not only of the Saint-Simonian and Comtean strains that are evident in such formulations but also of the

142 The economic changes of the era are summarized in Coleman, *Death Is a Social Disease*, 34–56; for a discussion that seeks to displace the medical eclectics' *juste milieu* in favor of the "methods of the physicists and chemists," see Bouillaud, *Essai sur la philosophie médicale*, v–vii.

ambiguities and competing impulses within anthropological medicine.[143] Their reworking of the science of man established social meliorism as its primary goal. The social-Christian doctors were determined to see medicine shoulder the social burdens it had long purportedly sought to assume and devote itself to the general betterment of the lives of the people.

Social-Christian medicine had its roots in the work and thought of Philippe Buchez, who first functioned politically within the Carbonarist movement but then gravitated toward Saint-Simonism. After breaking with the Saint-Simonians in 1829, Buchez went on to develop principles of social action based on his peculiar conception of the science of man. Buchez had many medical associates who either took his lead or developed in their own vein the social-Christian rendering of the science of man. Over the years these included Ulysse Trélat, L. V. F. Amard, Laurent Cerise, Henry Belfield-Lefèvre, Henri Hollard, Louis Cruveilhier, Alphonse Sanson, and other physicians associated with the journals *L'art médical, Journal des progrès des sciences et institutions médicales,* and *Annales médico-psychologiques.*[144] This does not mean, of course, that these doctors endorsed all of Buchez's principles. It does mean that the general conception of medicine he outlined, which reconciled religion and science and sought to realize medicine's longstanding ambition and obligation to "elevate the people," had considerable appeal in the medical world of the July Monarchy.

Born in 1796, Buchez was among that generation of French medical students who in the 1820s began to realize the great benefits of the educational and institutional restructuring of the revolutionary and Napoleonic years. He followed the ordinary course of study at the Faculty of Medicine but also got extensive practical training in dissection at the Ecole pratique and followed courses at the Muséum d'histoire naturelle. Soon after taking his medical degree in 1824 (a process that was slowed down by his involvement with the Carbonari and the Masonic lodge "Les amis de la vérité"), Buchez undertook to write a popular handbook of hygiene in company with the physician and republican activist Ulysse Trélat.[145] This work, *Précis élémentaire d'hygiène,* was intended to overcome the increasingly wide barrier between professional doctors and the people by summarizing hygienic knowledge and diffusing its practical teachings. The authors argued that the only way to improve general health and morality was to "enlighten [the

143 On these strains in Saint-Simonian and Comtean thought, see Henri Gouhier, *La jeunesse d'Auguste Comte et la formation du positivisme,* 3 vols. (Paris: J. Vrin, 1933–41); Frank Manuel, *The New World of Henri Saint-Simon* (Cambridge, Mass.: Harvard University Press, 1956), esp. 118–38.

144 On Buchez's Carbonarist period, see François-André Isambert, *De la charbonnerie au Saint-Simonisme: Etude sur la jeunesse de Buchez* (Paris: Editions de Minuit, 1966), 85–117; the break with Saint-Simonism, and Buchez's medical associates, are covered in François-André Isambert, *Politique, religion et science de l'homme chez Philippe Buchez (1796–1865)* (Paris: Cujas, 1967), 27–40, 49–54, 61–70.

145 Isambert, *De la charbonnerie au Saint-Simonisme,* 34–44.

people], or rather to let them enlighten themselves rather than keeping them in a childish state."[146]

This early book of Buchez's indicates that he was thoroughly grounded in the vitalist-inspired science of man. The work opened with a summary of the vitalist principles on which hygiene was based – the holistic integration of the body economy, the Bichatian division of life-functions into the animal and the vegetative, the crucial importance to health of the "things that surround [us]" and their multiple effects. The authors then offered the standard survey of the "influences" governing health or sickness – temperament, age, sex, and an omnibus category called "circumstances," which included habits, illnesses, "idiosyncrasies," and heredity.[147] As in all hygienic manuals, the chief recommendation made in this work was moderation in all things. Excess was always perilous: drunkenness caused illnesses of all kinds, overeating led "prematurely to the tomb," sexual excess caused frightful maladies (although continence too was dangerous, engendering "a multitude of cerebral and other affections").[148] Reiterating a principle to which Barthez had drawn particular attention, the authors observed that the ill effects of excess were registered in different ways by varying constitutions: the weakest organ in the body economy was always the "most sensitive" and the most likely to fail if habitual abuse destroyed the harmony of the integrated organism.[149]

The chief point of this work by two young, socially engaged physicians was that doctors could help the people best by convincing them to take their health in their own hands and by providing them with the tools to do so. This injunction to "enlighten" the people was uncomplicated enough, but Buchez was simultaneously struggling to achieve an elaborated sense of what else physicians and indeed all men of science must do to heal the grave social wounds of French society. Like many of his contemporaries, Buchez was dissatisfied with what he perceived to be the failure of science to deliver solutions to the problems and conflicts of the social world. In an article on the general character of physiology written for the Saint-Simonian journal *Le Producteur*, Buchez described what he saw as the excessively critical spirit of science, its failure to devise some sense of purpose or direction linking its minute investigations:

Most of the philosophical minds of our era hesitate between two contradictory sentiments. If it is a matter of the fate of civilization, they trust to the progress of the sciences. But if it is a matter of the work actually being undertaken in their own domain, they see nothing but desperate disorder, horrifying chaos![150]

146 Philippe Buchez and Ulysse Trélat, *Précis élémentaire d'hygiène* (Paris: Raymond, 1825), 219–20.
147 *Ibid.*, ii–iii, 5–30, 272.   148 *Ibid.*, 171, 201, 224–25.   149 *Ibid.*, 268–69, n. 2.
150 Philippe Buchez, "De la physiologie," *Le Producteur* 3 (1826): 122–23, 264–80, 459–78, at 460.

Yet in fact, he argued, this chaos was more apparent than real. There was direction and order in the growth of knowledge, an order that was discernible if the full historical development of the sciences was taken into view and their ultimate destination recognized. This destination was the science of man.[151]

In the mid-1820s Buchez gravitated toward the Saint-Simonian movement, in which an idea of the science of man was developed that owed much of its fundamental inspiration to physiology and to the medical science of man and yet that mutated and moved in new directions under the influence of Henri de Saint-Simon's peculiar genius. Saint-Simon had himself produced a key text in the science of man, the *Mémoire sur la science de l'homme* of 1813.[152] This essay, which opened with a tribute to Vicq d'Azyr and was sprinkled with references to Cabanis and Bichat, indicates the extent to which Saint-Simon's social theory was rooted in physiology. It makes clear that Saint-Simon's plan for the reorganization and regeneration of society rested on the view, derived principally from Bichat, that human "capacities" fell into the three domains of intellect, sensation, and physical movement.[153] Indeed all subsequent Saint-Simonian literature showed traces of this original tripartite scheme. The Saint-Simonian newspaper *Le Producteur*, for example, was subtitled "Journal philosophique de l'industrie, des sciences et des beaux-arts," domains of social action that corresponded roughly to Bichat's framework of locomotor, intellectual, and sensory function. In later phases of Saint-Simonism, religion was to replace the *beaux-arts* as the activity best channeling "sentiment" and the "clergy" would supplant the artist in the leadership troika of industrialists, savants, and artists originally envisioned by Saint-Simon. But the original "physiological" conception of the triadic division of human capacities always endured.[154]

In Buchez's Saint-Simonian phase he seems to have conceived of "physiology" and the "science of man" as essentially equivalent. He paid tribute to those scientists who were engaged in comparative anatomy and physiology, but he seemed to see as the true purpose and interest of their work the illumination of the highest development of animal functions, which of course took place in human beings. In any event he argued (more or less following Saint-Simon's historical reveries) that the whole development of the sciences had led to the point where science could elucidate the interre-

---

151 *Ibid.*, 463–64.
152 Henri de Saint-Simon, "Mémoire sur la science de l'homme," in *Oeuvres de Claude-Henri de Saint-Simon* (Paris: Editions Anthropos, 1966), vol. 5.
153 Both Cabanis and Bichat attended Saint-Simon's salon in the years around 1800. See Sébastien Charléty, *Histoire du Saint-Simonisme 1825–1864*, 2d ed. (Paris: P. Hartmann, 1931), 6; Manuel, *New World*, 51–73.
154 On the tripartite scheme, see Frank Manuel, "From Equality to Organicism," *Journal of the History of Ideas* 17 (1956): 54–69. It should be noted, however, that Bichat's system was not rooted in a conception of three "faculties," as Manuel observes, but in the vitalist doctrine of the differential distribution of energy to the three vital domains.

lations between the laws of the universe and the laws of human nature.[155] Indeed, he suggested that all the sciences of life and organization had been in a profound muddle until Cabanis devised a synthesis that made sense of their achievements and gave direction to all subsequent scientific labors. "The work of Cabanis on the relations between the physical and the moral," Buchez wrote, "supplies the link between the past centuries and modern times."[156] Buchez acknowledged that there had been important developments in physiology before Cabanis, in the work of Haller, Reil, Soemmering, Bordeu, and Bichat. But it was Cabanis who had drawn these insights together, using the central concept of sensibility to link the study of the natural and the human worlds:

Cabanis benefited from the insights gained before him, and followed the indications he was given. But he did what no savant before him had yet tried, the first work on the science of man that was free of all theological or psychological admixture. He sought to devise a positive classification of intellectual and moral phenomena.[157]

Buchez saw Cabanis's work as suggesting four possible directions for continuing investigations in the science of man: work on sensibility, which was proceeding both in experimental physiology and in comparative anatomy; ideology itself, which had, however, proved sterile after the work of Destutt; studies of instinct, which had been followed principally by Gall and Spurzheim; and, lastly, inquiry into embryonic development, an anatomical method Buchez thought particularly promising.[158]

It may be worthwhile to pause before following Buchez's break with Saint-Simonism to analyze this peculiar construction of the methods, direction, and goals of the science of man. Buchez was following directly in Saint-Simon's footsteps when he credited physiology with achieving a decisive breakthrough to the natural explanation of human intellectual and moral phenomena. Saint-Simon had attributed this historical achievement to physiology and had argued that all future work on human capacities and social organization must take the lead of that science.[159] Physiology had for the first time, he argued, perceived that human behavior was "lawlike" since it was rooted in the unalterable facts of "organization" – sensibility, pleasure-pain, instinct, and the rest. Buchez clearly believed this too, yet he deflected attention from continued labors in physiology toward anatomical investigation, especially embryological work such as that of Friedrich Tiedemann (1781–1861) in Germany and Etienne Serres in France. Serres was, as we will see, a follower of Etienne Geoffroy Saint-Hilaire; he was known chiefly for a two-volume study of the comparative anatomy of the brain in vertebrates that was based on embryological investigations. How

155 Buchez, "De la physiologie," 463.   156 *Ibid.*   157 *Ibid.*, 464.
158 *Ibid.*, 477; see also Isambert, *Politique, religion et science de l'homme*, 205–6.
159 Saint-Simon, "Mémoire sur la science de l'homme," in *Oeuvres*, 5:17, 29.

precisely studies of this sort were to contribute to the advancement of the science of man Buchez did not specify beyond noting that they would greatly facilitate human-animal comparisons.[160]

Buchez's special championing of anatomy, which marked a departure from both Saint-Simon and the tradition of the medical science of man, may be explained in a number of different ways.[161] At one level, it merely reflects the emphasis of his own medical training and interests, which tended toward the anatomical rather than the physiological. At another it probably is linked to the fact that Geoffroy's "philosophical anatomy," with its central concept of the "unity of plan" underlying all organized creation, functioned ideologically as a confirmation of republican principles of fraternity and equality.[162] Most important, however, is the fact that Buchez was struggling to find some way to move beyond what he saw as the individualist focus of physiology to the level of the collective or the aggregate. At this early stage in his thinking, he did so by arguing that the science of man must concentrate not on the individual but on the "species," a shift in perspective that he credited to comparative anatomy. Buchez argued that in contrast to anatomy, physiology had already yielded its principal insights by demonstrating the unchanging needs and drives established by human organization. What was needed now was scientific inquiry into the changes manifest in human history. These, he argued, could not be explained by fundamental organization, which was invariable, but must be sought in variations peculiar to the species as a whole, that is, in society:

While the individual always presents the same instincts, the same passions, [and] the same needs, social organization differs as much as possible and undergoes numerous and marked mutations. In our view this demonstrates that society is not solely the expression of individual tendencies and that the species is subject to particular laws other than those which belong to physiology.[163]

This early and brief emphasis on the gains to be realized for the science of man from the study of comparative anatomy indicates the extent to which Buchez was dissatisfied with physiology as a framework for the investigation of biohistorical problems. In this respect Buchez resembled many advocates of the science of man in the 1830s and 1840s who were inspired by an emergent historicism of which Saint-Simon himself was one of the principal authors and who sought to transcend the traditional focus of anthropological medicine on the individual or, at best, on abstractly conceived, essentially ahistorical physiological types. As will be seen, this struggle to

160 Buchez, "De la physiologie," 477; on Serres, see the subsequent discussion.
161 Buchez's position may be compared with that of Auguste Comte, who, also writing in the pages of *Le Producteur*, continued to argue for the primacy of physiology; see Isambert, *Politique, religion et science de l'homme*, 205.
162 *Ibid.*, 206; on the diverse political uses made of Geoffroy's ideas, see Appel, *The Cuvier-Geoffroy Debate*, 175–201.
163 Buchez, "De la physiologie," 132–33.

historicize the science of man marked both the "ethnology" and "anthropology" of this period as well. Buchez himself eventually abandoned his equation between species characteristics and social organization, and with it his stress on the importance of anatomy. His determination to move beyond individualism led him later to develop a distinction between "individual physiology" and "social physiology," and to argue that the proper focus of the science of man must be the latter. This "social physiology," although based on "individual physiology," would move to a higher level of understanding in seeking "the general laws of the life of humanity."[164]

Although Buchez always remained loyal to the memory of Saint-Simon himself, he broke early on with the Saint-Simonian coterie. Buchez's break with the movement has been examined in detail by François-André Isambert, who shows that of the many disagreements between Buchez and the other Saint-Simonians, their dispute over the essential philosophical problem of how to reconcile spirit and matter was crucial. Buchez's underlying fidelity to Christian principles was already evident in his hostility to Enfantin's "pantheism" and to Eugène Rodrigues's conception of *Dieu-matière*, views that, to his thinking, differed little from genuine materialism in denying the specific nature of the deity and the existence of an independent spiritual principle.[165]

For several years after his break with the Saint-Simonians, Buchez was preoccupied with ordinary politics, especially as hopes for fundamental social and political change mounted at the time of the 1830 Revolution. After the Orleanist triumph, however, Buchez gave up his involvement in day-to-day politics and began developing a political and intellectual following of his own that included other Saint-Simonian schismatics as well as adherents from the workers' movement and from diverse medical and scientific circles. In the 1830s these "Buchezians" pursued a range of activities intended to blend intellectual labor and social action. Soon after the 1830 Revolution they organized the Athénée des ouvriers, for which Buchez himself planned a hygiene course along the lines he and Trélat had sketched out in the mid-1820s. The medical figures in the group established the journal *L'art médical* to propagate their views. Buchezians also participated in the founding of the Institut historique (1833), which contested the historical program of the Société d'histoire de la France organized by the Orleanist luminaries Guizot, Thiers, and Mignet.[166]

Throughout this period Buchez's chief preoccupation was the need to move society toward a condition of "association" or "harmony" modeled on the functional interdependence of the healthy human organism. In his

164 Augustin Ott, "La doctrine de Buchez sur le système nerveux et sur les rapports de l'esprit avec l'organisme," *Annales médico-psychologiques*, 4th ser., 7 (1866): 1–24, at 6.
165 The schism developed over the course of months and finally became formal in December 1829; see Isambert, *Politique, religion et science de l'homme*, 27–40.
166 *Ibid.*, 42–68.

view humanity was prevented from moving toward such a state by ancient antagonisms between the individual and the social, the theoretical and the practical, the material and the spiritual. His determination that these be overcome in one great synthesis of competing principles led Buchez by the end of the decade to a teleological conception of human "activity" in which all thought and action found their unity in a "common end" that derived ultimately from God. Buchez's synthesis was presented in his *Essai d'un traité complet de philosophie* (1838–40), in which he expressed his intensifying hostility toward all "materialisms," from Cabanis's physiology to phrenology to experimental neuroanatomy.[167] More generally, he argued against all philosophical and scientific systems that concentrated exclusively on analyzing thought and the mental faculties. All such conceptions, he argued, were pure abstractions removed from the only domain where knowledge had any real significance – that of social action. In the place of such systems Buchez developed a theory according to which thought itself *was* action. Rejecting the traditional distinction between knowledge and deed, he elaborated a species of dialectic in which thinking necessarily implied a physiological relation to the exterior world and hence ineluctably connected the individual to the realm of action. "An idea," he wrote,

is not in any way or any circumstance either an image or a simple representation of an object existing in the mind. . . . Take for example the idea of a chair or a house or the name of a number or that of an individual in a certain space, say, among other men, you will readily recognize that the first two have reference to a usage or an end, that the third like the fourth refers to a relation of classification. . . . One can thus conclude with assurance . . . that every idea is a relation, and that as a result the operation that constitutes the idea is an act of affirming a relation.[168]

Thus all knowledge was engaged, relational, and pragmatic; there could be no such thing as abstract theory icily distant from the world of action.

This ontological conception was joined to Buchez's idea that all activity – individual and social, physiological and mental – must be directed toward a "common end." This theme, which Isambert calls the "leitmotiv of Buchezian thought," served to unify his diverse prescriptions for the work of social healing.[169] Arguing that a "common end" was essential to give structure and unity to the activities of competing elements, he asserted that this "end" could be known only through science's capacity to discern the ultimate destination of humanity. Scientific knowledge did not, however, gain any special status or privilege by its performance of this crucial task. Since all thought was inherently active and relational, knowledge too must

167 Philippe Buchez, *Essai d'un traité complet de philosophie du point de vue du catholicisme et du progrès*, 3 vols. (Paris: E. Eveillard, 1838–40).
168 Quoted in Isambert, *Politique, religion et science de l'homme*, 231.   169 *Ibid.*, 273.

be judged by the criterion applied to all other endeavors – that is, by how effectively it contributed to advancing the common end that it perceived.[170]

What all this meant for medicine was that doctors should be focused not on theoretical disputation but on labor in the world; the social mission of medicine must be moved to center stage. Yet precisely what the social tasks of doctors were to be remained only vaguely delineated in the Buchezian program. Although for some time Buchez himself worked to promote workers' associations and other concrete forms of organization, he eventually decided that such efforts were premature and that the first task to be accomplished was that of changing the mentality of the poor and the oppressed through physical and moral education.[171] By this means the Buchezians eventually arrived at a construction of medicine's social mission that bore marked similarities to the program of their ideological antagonists among the phrenologists. Both phrenology and social-Christian medicine argued on behalf of the physician's capacity to recognize and develop (or curb) distinctive human capacities and in so doing contribute to the harmonious operation of a functionally interdependent social organism.

The similarities between phrenological and social-Christian constructions of the social mission of medicine are clearest, paradoxically, in the Buchezian critique of phrenology. This critique was developed not by Buchez himself but by his associate Laurent Cerise, who in a series of articles written for *L'Européen* denounced phrenology as "the grossest materialism" and surveyed the many scientific and moral objections others had made to the system.[172] Cerise insisted that any theory focused on intellection and the cerebral apparatus alone was inherently false. He argued instead on behalf of a tripartite anatomophysiological scheme made up of the visceral ganglia, the senses per se, and the "psychocerebral apparatus" that corresponded to the three vital domains of the affective, the sensory, and the intellectual. In a familiar refrain he argued that only by adopting such a perspective could medicine hope to illuminate the relations between human physical and moral constitution.[173]

Cerise's critique of phrenology was rooted in the vitalist conception that the physical-moral relation was systemic in character and not determined solely by the presence or absence of certain cerebral features. Moreau de la Sarthe had argued in the same fashion when he criticized Gall in the pages of *Décade philosophique* in 1804.[174] Unlike Moreau, however, Cerise also argued that phrenology's very disposition to emphasize differences in capac-

---

170 *Ibid.*, 242–46, 248–49, 273.   171 *Ibid.*, 88–89.
172 These articles were published together in Cerise, *Exposé et examen critique.*
173 Laurent Cerise, *Des fonctions et des maladies nerveuses dans leurs rapports avec l'éducation sociale et privée, morale et physique: Essai d'un nouvel système de recherches physiologiques et pathologiques sur les rapports du physique et du moral* (Paris: Germer-Baillière, 1842), xiii-xix.
174 See Chapter 2, "Commentary on Gall."

ities and human inequality was pernicious. His essay of 1836 opened with an epigraph from Saint Paul: "There is great diversity in gifts but only one spirit." Thus he opposed phrenology in the name of the "universal equality and fraternity" taught "by the law of Jesus Christ."[175]

In pure rhetoric it is hard to see how anything could be further from the formulations of the phrenologists, which were often riddled with anticlerical bombast. Yet once Cerise had made this attack on phrenology, he proceeded to acknowledge that there were in fact profound differences in human capacities. These differences were determined, however, not by the relative dominance or weakness of particular phrenological features but by the variable distribution of vital energy among the visceral, sensual, and psychocerebral domains. Moreover, these differences, far from encouraging social divisiveness, existed for the social good:

> The carnal instruments with which man is endowed are of the same nature and have the same end for all men. If the vital energy is greater in some and lesser in the others, this physiological diversity is regulated according to providential ends that require a diversity of functions. But this diversity of functions does not serve to isolate those who accomplish these functions or to establish them in their individuality; [rather] it facilitates cooperation, it contributes in effect to the realization of a shared idea [*pensée commune*]. And it is this [shared] idea that presides over the organization and conservation of societies.[176]

This vision of providential guidance and organic community differed markedly in tone from the recommendations of phrenological pedagogy. But in fact both of them led to similar calls for functionally arranged and pragmatically hierarchical forms of social organization in which the essential tasks of recognizing, differentiating, and administering physiological differences were accomplished by the physician. Indeed Cerise insisted that the views he upheld in company with his "dearest friend" Buchez had infinitely greater social utility than those systems that charted supposedly inherent, fatal tendencies in human physicomoral makeup. He fully recognized the vast disparities in human capacities, which were especially marked in the physical, moral, and mental degradation of savages.[177] Yet he insisted that this degradation was not a physiological given but a result of the social state in which the savage existed:

> There exists a preestablished relation, a determined functional relation between the nervous organism of man and the social tradition that envelops him and penetrates him on all sides, by means of institutions. It is by this marvelous relation that intellectual and affective diversity among the men of different nations and historical epochs is to be explained.[178]

175 Cerise, *Exposé et examen critique*, xx.   176 *Ibid.*, 6.
177 Cerise, *Des fonctions et des maladies nerveuses*, 53. The reference to Buchez is in the book's dedication.
178 *Ibid.*, 56.

Hence the human ability to live in all conditions – since the body changed with society – and society's great power, when properly attuned to providential ends, to mold the physicomoral character of its members. [179]

In this polemic it suited Cerise's purpose to pretend that only his own point of view recognized the importance of external influences – physical, moral, and otherwise – in the shaping of body and spirit, a claim that of course flew directly in the face of phrenological meliorism. The physiologists ignored, Cerise argued, "the study of the relations that exist between the operations of the nervous system and the teachings of tradition," although this was "one of the gravest and most elevated problems of human physiology." [180] Such study must include religion, political customs, legislation, judicial institutions, hygiene, scientific institutions, the *beaux-arts*, penal institutions, education, and manners. Physiology alone, he concluded, could never take all this into account. It must be completed by history in a comprehensive science of man that would supply the knowledge and instruments for physicomoral amelioration. [181]

The place of the social-Christian doctors themselves in history was not, finally, to be a glorious one, at least in respect to their often-claimed political role. Their attempts to reconcile so many competing impulses – religiosity and scientism, workers' rights and Catholic organicism, Christian fraternity and physiological typologizing – led ultimately to a position of political irresolution that put the lie to Buchez's call to action over words. In the 1848 Revolution Buchez was elected representative from the Seine to the National Assembly and then president of the Assembly itself. For a month he had a platform for action such as few ever command but, as one account puts it, he "showed himself to be scarcely brilliant." [182] His leadership of the Assembly was muddled and indecisive and after the upheavals of May 15 he was not reelected to the presidential post. He ended by voting regularly with the moderates – against the right to work, for the expedition to Rome, against the banning of the clubs. He vigorously opposed Louis-Napoleon Bonaparte's admission to the Assembly, and was therefore among those arrested (at Cerise's home) on December 2, 1851. Released after the intervention of a Bonapartist crony, he played no further role in political life before his death in 1865. [183]

Under the aegis of the science of man, social-Christian medicine developed a program of reconciliation and healing that was intended to overcome ideological antagonisms and usher in an era of social harmony. Yet the career of its principal architect foundered amid the renewed and intensified antagonisms of a new revolution. Historians have often interpreted 1848 as

179 *Ibid.,* 56–73.   180 *Ibid.,* 61.   181 *Ibid.,* 62–76.
182 "Philippe Buchez," *DBF* 7:602–03.
183 *Ibid.;* for a more sympathetic account of Buchez's actions in 1848, see Armand Cuvillier, *P.-J.-B. Buchez et les origines du socialisme chrétien* (Paris: Presses universitaires de France, 1948), 61–69.

the moment when grandiose conceptions of the possibilities for social and scientific progress gave way to a new realism, pragmatism, or, as some see it, cynicism.[184] This view accurately captures the fate of Buchez. It also illuminates the history of another construction of the science of man that coexisted with social-Christian medicine and the visions of Saint-Simon. This was the new science of ethnology, which was promoted within a learned society that began with high ambitions but that also collapsed amid the upheavals of 1848.

MEDICINE AND ETHNOLOGY

Many of the same impulses that had encouraged Buchez and his circle to abandon "individual" for "social" physiology – the disposition to historicize human experience, the deepened concern with the cohesiveness of the social order, the desire to apply scientific knowledge to utilitarian ends – may be seen at work in the Société ethnologique de Paris, founded in 1839.[185] In this instance, however, the goal of broadening the science of man to encompass the great sweep of biohistorical development was to be accomplished not by discerning the providential design of the social organism but by the establishment of a new discipline that would merge biological and historical investigations of the influence of race. The ethnological society brought together scholars from many different fields – physiology, medicine, natural history, geography, history, linguistics, and general belles-lettres. It also attracted individuals from commerce and politics, including an important contingent of ex-Saint-Simonians whose ambitions for the society were for the most part practical rather than scholarly. The presence and importance of the nonscholars was to grow as time passed, but the society at least ostensibly always remained true to its originally declared objective to undertake "serious study of the human races that have peopled the earth."[186]

The chief organizer of the new society was William-Frédéric Edwards, a naturalized Frenchman of Jamaican origin who after receiving his medical degree from the Paris Faculty of Medicine went on to acquire a substantial reputation as an experimental physiologist.[187] Edwards's first major work *De l'influence des agens physiques sur la vie* (1824), was a study of the effects

---

184 For the effects of 1848 on medical aspirations, see Léonard, *La médecine entre les pouvoirs et les savoirs,* 224.

185 *Mémoires de la Société ethnologique de Paris* 1:1 (1841): i–ii.

186 *Ibid.,* i; on the membership and work of the society, see Claude Blanckaert, "On the Origins of French Ethnology: William Edwards and the Doctrine of Race" in *Bones, Bodies, and Behavior: Essays on Biological Anthropology,* ed. George W. Stocking, Jr. (Madison: University of Wisconsin Press, 1988), 18–55, esp. 41–44; Elizabeth A. Williams, "The Science of Man: Anthropological Thought and Institutions in Nineteenth-Century France" (Ph.D. diss., Indiana University, 1983), chap. 2.

187 V. Kruta, "W. F. Edwards," *DSB* 4:285–86.

of "external agents" on the structure, functions, and constitution of four classes of vertebrates including "man."[188] Because the physiological principles developed in this work underlay the doctrine of race that Edwards espoused and that was to orient the work of the Société ethnologique, it is worth considering in some detail. Edwards's work was intended to serve several purposes. It was written in part to follow up on discoveries recently made by Lavoisier and others in animal chemistry. It responded also to research problems addressed in Magendie's prestigious journal, the *Journal de physiologie expérimentale et pathologique*. Finally, the book developed a number of lines of inquiry of continuing interest to hygienists and pathologists.[189] The experiments Edwards undertook on physical agents were carried out at the Collège de France, where he was for a time François Magendie's pupil and laboratory assistant.[190] Among the external agents Edwards investigated were air, liquids and vapors, temperature, light and electricity, and season. Many of these were among the classic agents considered by physicians in their attempts to delineate medical "constitutions," and Edwards made explicit his desire to rationalize and enrich that branch of medical study:

Differences in constitutions and the characters by which they may be recognized have from time immemorial challenged the ingenuity [*sagacité*] of physicians. . . . The facts prove that there are different constitutions but questions remain as to how they may be recognized in advance and what constitutes the differences [among them].[191]

Unlike many physicians of his period who denied that animal experiments could yield anything of interest to the study of human beings, Edwards was firmly committed to experimental procedures. Indeed his work on physical agents illustrates as well as any text of the period the tensions between the techniques of the experimentalist and an older medical approach – with its dependence on bedside observation, privileging of individual cases over group phenomena, and resistance to statistical analysis. The first three sections of the work were devoted exclusively to reporting animal experiments, but in the last Edwards shifted his attention to warm-blooded vertebrates, including human beings.[192] In so doing he confronted directly the objection frequently made by physicians to the use of experimental results obtained with animals – that human beings were not subject to the same laws and influences of nature as the lower orders. In respect to

188 William-Frédéric Edwards, *De l'influence des agens physiques sur la vie* (Paris: Crochard, 1824).
189 Edwards, *De l'influence des agens physiques*, v–xvi.
190 In his *Précis élémentaire de physiologie*, Magendie expressed his gratitude to Edwards "who took part in all my experiments, and whose great knowledge and judicious spirit were of great help to me in the preparation of this work" (vi).
191 Edwards, *De l'influence des agens physiques*, 157.
192 *Ibid.*, part IV, "De l'homme et des animaux vertébrés."

the agents studied in his work, Edwards argued, human beings were properly classified with the mammals, whom they resembled in structure and with whom they shared the need to combat the same "mechanical forces" that worked for their destruction. Edwards fully accepted the Bichatian view that "life" – animal and human – necessitated a ceaseless struggle against physicochemical agents whose principles were antithetical to vitality. Humans were engaged in this combat with external forces no less intensely than animals and often with means that were in no way superior to those available to animals. "Man enjoys no privilege of organization," Edwards wrote, "that frees him from the power of physical laws."[193] Vitalists had always argued against this view by pointing to the extreme variability of medical phenomena, which they took as evidence of the rich individuality and particularity of human vital responsivity. While Edwards was prepared to grant such variability, he perceived it in the activities of animals as well as human beings. He held that two planes of analysis – the individual and the species – were required to make sense of clinical and experimental data indicating variable vital responses to the action of external agents:

Man is affected by diverse agents in the measure that is appropriate to his species but in the same manner as other mammals; in this respect each species – indeed I would say more, each individual, and the individual at different stages of life – has his particular measure. But as a species man belongs in the group we studied in the third part of this work [warm-blooded vertebrates] and the general truths that we established there are equally applicable to him.[194]

All the same Edwards was, at least for a time, a practicing physician as well as a laboratory experimenter, and he used clinical observations to check, reinforce, or modify his experimental findings. Working on the problem of body heat, for example, he noted that nothing in this field of study had more astonished investigators than to find, in trials on patients, that body heat was essentially constant throughout extreme changes of climate and weather. He himself had studied temperature readings, taken first on twenty adults and then on a group of newborns made available to him for observation by his friend, the physician Gilbert Breschet. His researches indicated that a temperature range of 35.5 to 37 degrees centigrade was normal for adults and 34 to 35.5 degrees for newborns. He observed that he "would never have drawn any conclusion from so slight a difference [between adults and newborns] if numerous experiments done on warmblooded animals had not already given me the proper interpretation."[195] Animal experiments had also taught him what to expect about the temperature of human fetuses. This he was eager to check on premature infants, and although "the opportunities are rare," a case came to him via the *ac-*

193 *Ibid.*, 230–31.   194 *Ibid.*, 231.   195 *Ibid.*, 235.

coucheur of one of his own patients. The healthy premature baby had a temperature of 32 degrees, a finding in keeping with those obtained in the laboratory.[196] Such results, he concluded, could only be obtained by a blended clinical-experimental approach.

Edwards closed this work of 1824 with tables presenting the numerical results of his many experiments. Such statistics, he insisted, were essential to medical and physiological investigations since without them reports were vague and unverifiable. Commenting on the observations of the Renaissance physician Sanctorius (1571–1636), Edwards regretted the fact that, although Sanctorius ostensibly derived his results from use of the scales, he in fact rested much of his argument solely on "reasoning." Worse yet, he presented few actual "numerical findings." According to Edwards, "publishing tables of results is the sole means by which we can judge the value of general propositions and distinguish between what belongs to fact and what is only the product of the imagination."[197] In all these respects, then, Edwards proved himself a medical progressive. Rejecting the view that human beings exhibited vital reactions that were qualitatively different from those found among animals, he championed all the methods, including vivisection and statistical investigation, that were opposed by physicians who insisted that human vital phenomena were endlessly variable and not subject to determinate laws.

In the years after the publication of *De l'influence des agens physiques*, Edwards undertook diverse research projects, ranging from work on nutrition to the morphology of infusoria to the character of Celtic dialects. He was one of the few scholars of his generation to belong both to the Académie de médecine and to the Académie des sciences morales et politiques. He also made presentations to, and won prizes from, the Académie des sciences and the Académie des inscriptions et belles-lettres.[198] Eclectic in his interests, Edwards was in a prime position to attempt an interdisciplinary synthesis of the problem that gradually came to dominate his thinking: the cause of diversity in human moral and physical constitution. The synthesis he achieved was a doctrine of race that in turn became the focus of the investigations of the Société ethnologique.

As Claude Blanckaert has shown, Edwards' race theory derived chiefly from the work of natural historians, especially the polygenists whose foremost concern was to demonstrate the differential origins and endurance of distinct human species.[199] In his work *Des caractères physiologiques des races humaines considérés dans leurs rapports avec l'histoire* (1829), Edwards supported the polygenist view that the human races were fixed types whose

196 *Ibid.* 197 *Ibid.*, 313. 198 Kruta, "W. F. Edwards."
199 Blanckaert, "On the Origins of French Ethnology"; see also Claude Blanckaert, "Monogénisme et polygénisme en France de Buffon à Paul Broca (1749–1880)" (Ph.D. diss., University of Paris, 1981).

most important features, especially the physical conformation of head and face, were established at their origin and not subject to change.[200] The unique elements of Edwards's own race doctrine were his concentration on the small-scale, localized "races" of European history rather than the great global races of eighteenth-century tradition and, further, his attempt to mobilize the findings of the new romantic historiography in support of his view that races endure despite the vagaries of history.[201] Edwards was primarily interested in the European past and in European peoples. He regretted that "we know the antipodes better than our own neighbors, the savage people better than the people who were the first to be civilized."[202] In keeping with this emphasis, he argued his case for the fixity of fundamental racial characteristics on the basis of the historic European past, especially the ancient and persistent division between "Galls" and "Kimris" in French history itself.[203]

In order to argue for fixed racial characters, Edwards had to dispose of what had always been – in both the medical and the natural history traditions – the strongest argument in favor of the malleability of human types and against the proposition of fixity: the influence of climate. To do so, he drew a distinction between plant and animal life, accepting that plants, and some elementary animals as well, were subject to climatic influences since they were largely powerless to change the environment or to remove themselves from adverse forces. Such was not the case for more complicated animals, and certainly not for human beings who possessed "powerful means" to shield themselves from the effects of climate.[204] Although he was willing to grant that the capacity of peoples to deflect climatic influence might be less among the less civilized peoples, Edwards nonetheless argued that in general "modifications of the social state" had little influence on physiological types. Pointing to the mixing of races that followed historic cases of conquest, he argued that the primordial racial types of both conqueror and conquered could long after be seen distributed throughout the diverse social classes despite differences in behavior and habits. Finally, Edwards found conclusive proof for the fixity of the races in the classic cases of polygenist literature: the European, whose type remained un-

---

200 William-Frédéric Edwards, *Des caractères physiologiques des races humaines considérés dans leurs rapports avec l'histoire: Lettre à M. Amédée Thierry* (Paris: Compère jeune, 1829).
201 Blanckaert, "Origins of French Ethnology," 24–34.
202 Edwards, *Des caractères physiologiques,* 114.   203 *Ibid.,* 63–78.
204 *Ibid.,* 12. On this point Edwards directly refuted the argument made by Cabanis (in the memoir on climate of the *Rapports*) that of all organized creatures human beings were in fact the most susceptible to external influences because of the intense and highly volatile character of human sensibility. See Cabanis, "Rapports," in *Oeuvres:* "The sensibility of man is, compared to that of all known animal species, the most supple and the most mobile, so that all [the agents] that act on other living creatures act, in general, in an even stronger fashion on him" (1:473).

changed in the colonies and the Jews, whose "traits" and "physiognomy" had remained unaltered from those represented on Egyptian tombs.[205]

That Edwards argued for the inalterability of physiological types was in good part a result of his original experimental orientation. Nothing in the experiments of laboratory physiologists indicated that any known influence was powerful enough to alter fundamentally the organization of advanced animals or human beings. Unlike the physiologists of Cabanis's generation – and his own contemporaries like Broc and Cerise, who argued that moral and social influences had the power to remake the body – he was unwilling to give credence to any influence whose effects could not be demonstrated in the laboratory or at the least be documented by actual incidence. Thus Edwards denied that either physical or social agents had exercised significant influence on the races over time. From this point of view the historical experience of the races was irrelevant to the science of race since the races were now what they had always been.[206]

Although Edwards denied that historical influences could alter physiological types just when other physicians were arguing that history must be mobilized to explain the formation of types, it was nonetheless Edwards who promoted a conception of ethnology that called upon historians to play a crucial role. History, it was true, could not explain the formation and development of the races but it did supply the proofs for the view that the races were inalterable physicomoral entities. The most dramatic cases of the persistence of racial types were to be found in the experience of endogamous people such as the Jews, yet even the historical record of Europe included types that endured through endless conquests, migrations, and intermixings. Indeed the very vagaries of history bore out the truth of racial science, for in the qualities and characters of the races lay the key to the destinies of peoples and the outcomes of complex historical struggles.[207]

Yet despite this affirmation of the crucial role of race in human history, and his rejection of the power of those "influences" long regarded as crucial in the medical science of man, Edwards still did not perceive racial science in terms of a rigorous physicalist determinism. His own method for studying race consisted instead of establishing simple "coincidences" between physical and moral characters.[208] Ethnological science, Edwards argued,

205 Edwards, *Des caractères physiologiques*, 36, 14–20.
206 As was standard in polygenist literature, Edwards held that the races could be substantially changed only by interbreeding, and even this was a subject of much dispute since the races were presumed to have an inherent tendency to remain true to type. See Edwards, *Des caractères physiologiques*, 5–6, 22–23, and the discussion in Blanckaert, "Origins of French Ethnology," 37–38.
207 Edwards, *Des caractères physiologiques*, esp. 37–44, 51–78. See also Edwards, "De l'influence réciproque des races sur le caractère national," *Mémoires de la Société ethnologique*, 2:1 (1845): 1–12, where Edwards argued that when two races coexisted, the "character" of "the most variable and feeble would disappear" (6).
208 Blanckaert, "On the Origins of French Ethnology," 40.

was linked to both "physics" and "metaphysics," but the one could not be called upon to explain the other.[209] Thus in his direct statements on the psychophysiological relation, Edwards reverted to a conventional dualism. He praised Buffon, for example, for recognizing that "man is composed of a body and soul, and that to neglect the latter is to ignore the most distinctive character of his being and the one to which he owes his superiority."[210] In this respect Edwards's conception of the physical-moral relation resembled that of other scientific modernists such as Flourens, who, since they were unwilling to subsume mind, soul, or passion within the determinist framework, reverted when they thought it necessary to the dualist perspective of seventeenth- and eighteenth-century mechanism.

Thus although Edwards argued that the physical organization of the races was supremely important in ethnology, he stopped short of arguing that ethnology could provide genuine cause-and-effect explanations of society, morality, or history based on race. Rather, the science of ethnology would simply describe, with new precision and rigor, the physical and moral characters of the human races throughout history and at present. Much work had already been done: the "great varieties" and some of their subcategories had been delineated by naturalists. These achievements would now be extended and enriched by students of civil history, language, geography, and politics. With the combined efforts of such scholars "we can hope that in but a few years we will have the materials required to write with exactitude a general history of the varieties of the human species."[211]

From its inception, then, the ethnology society was devoted not to explaining the nature of the physical-moral link but to charting the coexistence of physical and moral characters among the human varieties that the ethnologists agreed, taking Edwards's lead, to call "races." All the society's members took for granted that the physical and the moral were somehow conjoined, but they argued throughout the whole life of the society about the nature of the physical-moral link and the extent to which either physical or moral characters were determinative. Some members of the society embraced a strict physicalist determinism, explaining the moral "degradation" of Africans, for example, wholly by faults in their "organization."[212] Others insisted, as one member put it, that

the observation of physical characters . . . is impossible so long as it is not facilitated and directed by the prior observation of moral facts. Without the knowledge of such facts, the anatomist and physiologist lack the guiding thread that must direct them in their research and control their observations.[213]

209 William-Frédéric Edwards, "Esquisse de l'état actuel de l'anthropologie ou de l'histoire naturelle de l'homme," *Mémoires de la Société ethnologique* 1:1 (1841): 109–28, at 109.
210 *Ibid.*, 110.   211 *Ibid.*, 115–128; the quotation is at 128.
212 *Bulletin de la Société ethnologique de Paris* 2 (1847): 174, 182–203.
213 *Ibid.*, 107.

There was, then, no agreement on whether ethnology was fundamentally a physical science or an amalgam of historical and literary pursuits. In 1847 the society voted to divide its members into the three classes devoted to "physical study of the races," "history and linguistics," and "*morale* and politics," a decision that reflected its failure to achieve a sense of theoretical unity. This failure caused anxiety to some members, including the ex-Saint-Simonian Gustave d'Eichtal, who attributed ethnology's apparently slow pace of development to its dependence on contributing sciences that had not yet reached full maturity.[214]

In what direction the society might ultimately have developed its conception of race science cannot be known, for the society succumbed in the late 1840s to its own divided sense of purpose and to the institutional pressures that typically weighed on independent learning societies in this period.[215] Chronically short of funds, the society launched a drive in 1847 to attract more members, and those who wanted to see it assume a more active role in public affairs took the occasion to press for the admission of more members from business, law, and other nonscholarly pursuits.[216] The drive succeeded and, as a result, the society was drawn increasingly away from race science toward pragmatic questions of race relations, especially the slave trade. In 1848 the society was buffeted by the ideological winds and, although not formally dissolved until 1862, it survived the Revolution in little more than name.[217]

Theoretically and institutionally, ethnology was at once tied to and divorced from the medical science of man. Edwards's own perspective on physiological types, his definition of race, and his larger conception of ethnology owed much to his training in medicine and physiology. His original formulation of the influence of "external agents" was rooted in Bichat's fundamental conception of life as struggle against hostile elements. His stress on the importance of the head and face in racial classification derived not only from the work of naturalists but also from phrenology and medical studies of the brain and nervous system. Most important is the fact that Edwards first approached the whole problematic of the identifiability and stability of types in the context of medical constitutions.[218]

214 *Ibid.*, 49, 60.
215 On these pressures, see Robert Fox, "The *Savant* Confronts His Peers: Scientific Societies in France, 1815–1914," in *The Organization of Science and Technology in France, 1808–1914*, ed. Robert Fox and George Weisz (Cambridge: Cambridge University Press, 1980), 240–82.
216 *Bulletin de la Société ethnologique de Paris* 2 (1847): 44–45.
217 For a fuller discussion, see Williams, "The Science of Man," chap. 2.
218 Edwards counted Gall among the greatest contributors to the "study of man considered in his general nature" (the others were Buffon, Kant, and Cabanis). Yet he acknowledged that phrenology was not yet accepted because it "lacked scientific proof" and would require long and arduous work to be established since "there is little precision in the nuances of form and disposition." See Edwards, "Esquisse," 110–13.

Ethnology was clearly perceived by Edward's contemporaries as existing in a medical context. A sizable contingent of the original members of the society were civil or military physicians, and doctors continued to be received into the society throughout the 1840s.[219] The list of medical names includes doctors of mental medicine (Achille Foville), clinicians (Armand Trousseau), phrenologists (P. M. A. Dumoutier, Honoré Jacquinot), and medical publicists and bureaucrats (Jules Guérin, Pierre Rayer, Matthieu Orfila). Yet despite this obvious medical presence and interest, the Société ethnologique was markedly unaffected in the long run by medical problems, perspective, or personnel. In the two volumes of proceedings published by the society, few remarks by medical men appear: aside from Edwards himself, most of the officers of the society were historians, geographers, and belles-lettristes. The preoccupations of the society and cast of its discussions were genuinely "ethnological" in the new sense of this word: a science with roots in medicine and natural history but also closely attuned to the emergent historical sciences.[220]

In this setting doctors had no special claim to prominence. Even Edwards himself regarded physical and moral characteristics as equally necessary components of the synthetic racial descriptions ethnology was to provide. If most of the society's members agreed, furthermore, that physical characters were preeminent in racial classification, they nonetheless regarded classification itself as only one element of a descriptive science that no less urgently required the intensive investigations of historians, linguists, and other men of letters. The doctors were not, moreover, able to offer any genuine medical consensus on the precise character of the physical-moral link that alone could have provided a rationale for ethnology beyond the aim of global description. If for decades one strain within anthropological medicine had tended toward the view that "organization" was primary and that all other features of human nature and constitution flowed from it, still this view was far from embodying a uniform medical conception of the physical-moral relation. Edwards himself shied away from a strict physicalist determinism, although his conception of the fixity of the races and his rejection of the modifying influences long accepted in medicine carried obviously determinist implications. Other physicians in the society, furthermore, occasionally spoke on behalf of the contending strain in anthropological

---

219 Exact figures will be available when Claude Blanckaert completes his sociological study of some three hundred of the society's members; see Blanckaert, "Origins of French Ethnology," 44, n. 2.

220 Before the society became completely absorbed in the discussion of race relations, slavery, and the slave trade, the discussions typically focused on individual ethnic, geographical, or racial groups, including the inhabitants of the United States (December 27, 1839), the "Guanches" of the Canary Islands (January 31, 1840), the Kabyles and the van Diemen Islanders (March 27, 1840), the "three races" of Sicily (April 24, 1840), the Fula of West Africa (February 26, 1841), and so on.

medicine, that physical and moral characters were not fixed but rather were subject to a host of variable influences. The navy doctor Arnoux stated this view in 1847:

I believe that in the human species one searches in vain for an organ whose conformation is peculiar to one race and constitutes its generic character, for there is a multitude of individual anatomical differences by reason of age, sex, and country, and exceptional forms are not rare in any race.[221]

This was nonetheless a rare "medical" intervention into the society's debates on race. For the most part the doctors made little effort to apply their own expertise on the physical-moral relation – garnered in clinical, hygienic, and pedagogical settings – to the global and transhistorical science of race that ethnology purported to be.

There is nothing in the archival or published records of the Société ethnologique to indicate why the medical contribution to ethnology was so thoroughly muted. But if the experience of the Société ethnologique is contrasted to that of the Société d'anthropologie de Paris founded twenty years later, the difference between the two that stands out most clearly is the absolute insistence of the anthropologists of the 1860s that anthropology was not just a marriage of convenience of disparate approaches to the study of human beings but a single science whose unity reflected the reality of nature itself. In contrast to the ethnologists, the anthropologists embraced as the dominant framework of their science the clear primacy of the physical over the moral and the absolute subjugation of the moral sciences to the physical. Certainly there was some dissent within the Anthropology Society from this fixist-determinist paradigm. But the anthropologists nonetheless achieved a high-enough degree of consensus on the nature of the physical-moral link to allow them to succeed, where the ethnologists had not, in establishing a unitary race science that achieved both longevity and influence. The emergence of this consensus depended in turn on changes within medicine that by the 1860s effaced the tension between the competing strains of anthropological medicine and ensured that human beings were brought, with the rest of nature, into a determinist framework.[222] The new anthropological synthesis was not achieved without perplexities and difficulties, however, as is apparent in the career and labors of the physician-naturalist E. R. A. Serres.

E. R. A. SERRES AND THE EMERGENCE OF ANTHROPOLOGY

When W.-F. Edwards submitted his work on external agents to the Académie des sciences competition in 1818, he was awarded half the prize, while the other half was taken by the physician and naturalist E. R. A. Serres for

221 *Bulletin de la Société ethnologique de Paris* 2 (1847): 218.   222 See the Epilogue.

his work on osteogeny.[223] In view of subsequent developments in the science of man, this conjunction of prizewinners was apt. Like Edwards, Serres was trained in medicine, drawn to the experimental path of physiology, and ultimately strove to put the science of man on a broadly scientific rather than exclusively medical footing, in his case with a program for a new science of "anthropology."

Serres took his medical degree from the Paris faculty in 1810 with a thesis entitled "Essai sur la certitude et l'incertitude de la médecine."[224] The title of the thesis recalled Cabanis's work on the same theme, and in other ways too reflected the influence of the Cabanisian science of man.[225] Like Cabanis, Serres argued against both the "blind credulity" of those who accepted any and all remedies offered by medicine and the equally dangerous error of "medical pyrrhonism." He inscribed himself under the banner of Hippocratism, repeating the truisms of expectant medicine that "the doctor must be the minister to nature" and the "executor of nature's laws."[226] Against skeptics who held that medicine was changeable and haphazard, he held that the practice of medicine had been essentially the same everywhere and at all times, except for occasional variations caused by differences in "climate, temperament, age, and sex." He asserted that medicine "was a true science" since it had its "own facts and fixed rules" and like all sciences was based strictly on "experience, observation, and reasoning."[227]

Although this essay repeated principles current in the vitalist-dominated pedagogy of Serres's student years, there were already signs that Serres was unsympathetic to the vitalist idea that medicine had its own laws different in kind from those to be found in the natural sciences. The ritual praise of expectancy was balanced by recognition of nature's *écarts,* cases such as difficult births, malign fevers, and poisonings in which the active intervention of doctors was required. The individual doctors Serres applauded for promoting "medicine founded on observation and the execution of the laws of nature" included the great figures of mechanist rather than vitalist tradition.[228]

After completing his medical studies, Serres began doing clinical work at the Hôtel-Dieu and later at the Hôpital de la Pitié, which was transformed at about this time into a specialized center for the study and treatment of nervous disorders. At the Pitié, Serres undertook intensive clinical work (he later noted he had observed two thousand cases) and was named chief physician in 1822.[229] In 1813 Serres published, with M.-A. Petit, a work on

---

223 Edwards, *De l'influence des agens physiques,* xv; Serres, *Anatomie comparée du cerveau,* xv.
224 E. R. A. Serres, *Essai sur la certitude et l'incertitude de la médecine (presenté et soutenu à la Faculté de Médecine de Paris, le 1er juin 1810)* (Paris: Didot jeune, 1810).
225 Cabanis's work was entitled *Du degré de certitude de la médecine* (1788); in *Oeuvres,* 1:33–103.
226 Serres, *Essai,* 6, 13, 15.   227 *Ibid.,* 12, 11.   228 *Ibid.,* 13, 19.
229 Biographical details on Serres are available in Elizabeth Gasking, "Antoine-Etienne-Reynaud-Augustin Serres," *DSB* 12:315–16; references to his work at the Pitié are in Serres, *Anatomie comparée du cerveau,* viii–ix.

"mesoenteric fevers" that anticipated in important ways Broussais's medical "revolution," which was the product of his attack on the doctrine of essential fevers.[230] This work made clear Serres's evolution toward localist pathology, his increasing interest in anatomical rather than physiological problematics, and his hostility to the systemic, holistic vitalism of Pinel. In this period Serres did numerous dissections at the Ecole pratique and followed courses in comparative anatomy offered at the faculty by Duméril and at the Muséum d'histoire naturelle by Cuvier. Then in 1817 the decisive intellectual encounter of Serres's life took place when he was introduced to Etienne Geoffroy Saint-Hilaire; from this point forward Serres became Geoffroy's loyal friend and intellectual ally.[231]

From very early in his career, then, Serres had been interested in moving beyond the human focus of medical studies and adopting the comparativist perspective of the naturalists. Geoffroy's philosophical anatomy provided the framework and theoretical focus for which Serres had been searching, and in the 1820s Serres produced a series of works in which he explored the implications of Geoffroy's primary concept of the "unity of plan" underlying all organized creation. His 1824–26 *Anatomie comparée du cerveau* was a much-celebrated effort to, as he put it, "apply to the science of man the ideas acquired in comparative anatomy."[232] Following Cuvier and Geoffroy, Serres adopted the method of studying anatomical formations in successive embryological stages. Since the focus of his clinical labors was nervous disorders, he had the idea of using such procedures for a comparative study of the vertebrate brain, a task, he noted, that had not been attempted in three thousand years of brain dissection.[233] The chief result of Serres's labors was the establishment of the general laws of "organogenesis," the most important of which was that, in embryological development, the organs of animals higher on the scale passed successively through stages of development representing the adult forms of creatures lower on the scale. This truth, which Geoffroy was in the process of demonstrating for bony forms, was no less valid for the brain itself:

I demonstrate . . . that the transitory forms of the brains of embryos and the permanent forms of the organ among vertebrates are a repetition one of the other and that they derive from the same causes and are rigorously subject to the same connections [*rapports*].[234]

230 Erwin Ackerknecht, "Broussais or a Forgotten Medical Revolution," *BHM* 27 (1953): 320–43; M.-A. Petit and E. R. A. Serres, *Traité de la fièvre entéro-mésentérique* (Paris: Hacquart, 1813). For a discussion of the contribution of Serres and Petit to the "medical revolution," see Bouillaud, *Essai sur la philosophie médicale*, 48, 58–66.
231 Serres, *Anatomie comparée du cerveau*, xi; Appel, *The Cuvier-Geoffroy Debate*, 122.
232 Serres, *Anatomie comparée du cerveau*, viii.   233 *Ibid.*, 24–26, ii.
234 *Ibid.*, xvii. On the meaning of the term *rapports* in Geoffroy Saint-Hilaire's "philosophical," and Serres's "transcendental," anatomy, see E. S. Russell, *Form and Function: A Contribution to the History of Animal Morphology* (Chicago: University of Chicago Press, 1982), esp. 53–64, 70–71, 79–81.

This general law Serres set out to prove in a survey of the chief anatomical features of the brains of fish, reptiles, birds, and mammals.

Serres was the first to admit that he based his belief in the uniformity of organogenesis on a larger philosophical conception of the necessary orderliness of organic creation. All great observers, he noted, recognized that "the organized universe" must have laws or else all would be chaos. But although this general truth had long been recognized, these laws were only now being explored, thanks to Geoffroy's discovery of the law of the "unity of organic composition" and Cuvier's law of the "harmony of parts." Serres's own contributions were of the same order: he had demonstrated the "fundamental laws of the excentric development of animals" as well as the laws of "symmetry" and *conjugaison*, which dictated that all major organs developed by means of paired or double elements that later fused.[235]

Although the principal focus of Serres's work was anatomical, he did hope to gain insights into the pathology of the brain and nervous system, and ultimately to effect a juncture between what he called "natural physiology" (purely observational) and "experimental physiology" (as pursued by Magendie). One day these would form but "one and the same science."[236] Serres asserted that the pathological and physiological potential of "organogenesis" was best indicated by the light it shed on the development of monsters, which like that of normal creatures was "always subject to an invariable rule, that of the connection of parts." Nature was as orderly in the production of these apparently lawless forms as in all other works: "In these productions nature is subject to a constant order, and it is when she seems to diverge the furthest from this order that we see her the most invariably subjected to the same rules."[237]

Throughout the 1820s and 1830s Serres produced a number of works that developed further the central insights of what he came to call "transcendental anatomy."[238] Along with Isidore Geoffroy Saint-Hilaire, he was Etienne's most loyal supporter even through the trials of the famous Cuvier-Geoffroy debate and the subsequent decline in Geoffroy's reputation. Serres's fidelity to Geoffroy cost him the friendship of Cuvier's circle, delayed his entry into the Académie des sciences, and was probably the cause of his being passed over in 1832 for the chair in human anatomy at the Muséum d'histoire naturelle. The chair went instead to Cuvier's protégé Flou-

---

235 Serres, *Anatomie comparée du cerveau*, xxi–xxv.   236 *Ibid.*, lxxxiii.   237 *Ibid.*, cii.
238 See E. R. A. Serres, "Recherches d'anatomie transcendante, sur les lois de l'organogénie appliquées à l'anatomie pathologique," *Annales des sciences naturelles* 11 (1827): 47–70; *Recherches d'anatomie transcendante et pathologique: Théories des formations et des déformations organiques* (Paris: Baillière, 1832), and *Précis d'anatomie transcendante, appliquée à la physiologie* (Paris: C. Gosselin, 1842); on Serres's continued championing of transcendental anatomy against his critics, see Russell, *Form and Function*, 204–6.

rens, and it was not until 1839 that Serres took it up when Flourens moved to the chair in comparative physiology.[239]

It may be worthwhile to consider for a moment the history of the museum's chair in human anatomy, for its evolution from the late eighteenth century to 1839, when Serres moved to it, illustrates the changing conception among naturalists of the proper relation between human-focused investigation and general natural history. The museum's chair in human anatomy dated from the reorganization of the Jardin des plantes by the Convention in the 1790s. In that restructuring of the museum the old general anatomy chair was split into a new chair in comparative anatomy, which went within a few years to Georges Cuvier, and one in human anatomy, which was taken by the physician Antoine Portal. Portal held this post for some three decades, although from 1817 he had his courses taken over by a *suppléant*. When he died in 1832, the museum professors considered abolishing the chair since strictly human anatomy was now thought by some to be appropriate only in medical instruction. In August 1832, however, the professors finally voted to retain the chair, judging human anatomy "the foundation of natural history and the classification of mammals."[240] This reassertion of the centrality of human anatomy was of course by this time a methodologically conservative view, and when Flourens took up the chair he began offering a course that redefined the chair in the direction of general natural history ("Cours d'anatomie et d'histoire naturelle de l'homme"). This redefinition of the scope and focus of the position was institutionalized on Serre's appointment when it was officially redesignated (after the title of Flourens's course) the chair in "anatomy and the natural history of man."[241]

Throughout his years at the museum, Serres continued to attend to the problems posed by transcendental anatomy, modifying only slightly the principles he had set forth in the 1820s.[242] But in keeping with the specific subject matter of his new chair, he undertook extensive studies in human anatomy and the natural history of man. As a museum professor, he was in charge of a set of collections (in his case inherited chiefly from Cuvier's era), and during his tenure he worked to improve the holdings of human anatomical specimens and other materials, including daguerreotypes, illustrating the physical characters of diverse racial types.[243] Materials came to him from many sources, including officially sponsored expeditions. In the

239 Appel, *The Cuvier-Geoffroy Debate*, 124–25.
240 E.-T. Hamy, "La collection anthropologique du Muséum national d'histoire naturelle," *L'anthropologie* 18 (1907): 257–76 (the quotation is at 265); Armand de Quatrefages, *Rapport sur les progrès de l'anthropologie* (Paris: Imprimerie impériale, 1867), 28. Following Quatrefages, Blanckaert attributes the retention of the chair in human anatomy to the influence of Edwards's work on ethnology; see Blanckaert, "On the Origins of French Ethnology," 45.
241 Hamy, "La collection anthropologique," 266.   242 Russell, *Form and Function*, 205–6.
243 Hamy, "La collection anthropologique," 266–69.

mid-1840s he began receiving drawings of the racial types of Algeria from the Commission scientifique d'Algérie which was under the direction of the minister of war. He was later charged with editing the anthropological section of the commission's publications, although this project was aborted in June 1848 because of the "financial situation" of the Republic.[244]

Serres's manuscripts indicate that he read widely in the science he increasingly preferred to call "anthropology," and they include an undated outline of a course he offered entitled "Leçons sur les races humaines."[245] This course opened with a discussion of human fossil remains, a subject on which Serres published an essay in 1854.[246] He next took up the monogenist-polygenist question, arguing in favor of a generally polygenist position. He avoided categorical pronouncements on the subject, however, asserting only that it was "most likely" that the diverse human types had originated as distinct species. Into this discussion Serres integrated an argument derived from his "organogenetic" principles to the effect that the optimal development of the human brain was found in Caucasians, whereas the other major brain types (Negro, Malay, American, and Mongol) represented "arrests in development" that characterized organic forms low on the animal scale.[247] After a brief discussion of the problem of "abnormal races" (giants and dwarfs), Serres went on to consider the best means to distinguish "the physical powers and structural differences" of the major racial groups and, in eleven subsequent lessons, to survey the characters of the various races.[248]

According to a student outline of Serres's course that was published in 1845, Serres devoted considerable attention to the general problem of how to define "race" and other classificatory units and also took up the theme of the "gradation of power and civilization that could be established on [the basis] of [racial] characters."[249] This summary indicates that Serres argued in favor of a fairly rigorous physicalist determinism, holding that "the functions degrade with the organs" and that animal-like features were to be found in all the "inferior races." The effects of race mixing seem also to have been of great concern to Serres.[250] On this subject he worked out a conception of the differential reproductive compatibility between the races

244 Letter from V. Charon, Ministry of War, to Serres dated June 14, 1848, MNHN, MS 172.
245 The materials in MS 172 include sheets headed "Atlas de l'anthropologie," "Histoire naturelle et anthropologie," "Anthropologie et ethnologie," "De la méthode en anthropologie," and "Philosophie anthropologique." A list of works Serres consulted includes the names of Déramond, Froberville, Dumoutier, Pickering, Guyau, Kant, Jacquinot, Pucheran, J. Jeannel, Moquin-Tandon, Morton, and Dumont d'Urville.
246 E. R. A. Serres, "Notes sur la paléontologie humaine," *Comptes-rendus hebdomadaires des séances de l'Académie des sciences* 37 (1853): 518–25.
247 MNHN, MS 153, "Leçons sur les races humaines."   248 *Ibid.*
249 Alphonse Esquiros, "Du mouvement des races humaines: Cours de M. Serres," *Revue des Deux Mondes*, new ser., 10 (1845): 145–86.
250 *Ibid.*, 165–66.

that anticipated the full-blown doctrines of *métissage* of anthropologists of the 1860s.[251]

Serres's career and work seem in many respects to be in an altogether different universe from the medical science of man. In institutional terms Serres was separated from other physicians working within anthropological medicine, at least once he shifted the major focus of his work from the Pitié to the museum. Even before that move, however, Serres had long struggled to identify himself with the scientific rather than the medical establishment, and his patron Etienne Geoffroy Saint-Hilaire had attempted to help Serres along in this ambition. From 1821 onward Serres sought admission to the Académie des sciences, trying sometimes for entry to the medicine and surgery section but alternatively to the anatomy and zoology section. All Serres's major papers of the 1820s and 1830s were published in the *Annales des sciences naturelles*, a journal devoted to broadly biological rather than to medical science.[252]

In his theoretical preoccupations, too, Serres was, at least after his early work on medical certainty and on fevers, scientific rather than medical in orientation. The great contest between Cuvier and Geoffroy in which he took avid interest unfolded on terrain to which doctors-as-doctors scarcely even had access by their training. The problem of whether all living creatures were made on the same plan was not one that failed to interest doctors (Frédéric Bérard's tribute to Geoffroy may be recalled here), but it was one to which medical science had little to contribute that might seem decisive.[253] The conflict between the morphological and functional approaches represented by Geoffroy and Cuvier was fought out largely in reference to investigations of species other than the human, since the whole problematic of the "unity of plan" derived from the comparativist perspective, and historically became possible only once comparativist labors had got seriously under way from the late eighteenth century forward. In this context knowledge of the human was assumed; knowledge of other species was what was regarded as innovative and crucial to the whole endeavor.[254]

In other ways too Serres's approach to the natural history of man was rooted in broadly biological rather than medical traditions. Such problems as the identification and definition of fundamental classificatory units, the origins and histories of the species or races, the characters that were best

---

251 *Ibid.*; see also the reference to Serres's ideas on the effects of race mixing in Paul Broca, *Recherches sur l'hybridité animale en général et sur l'hybridité humaine en particulier* (Paris: Imprimerie de J. Claye, 1860), 621.

252 Appel, *The Cuvier-Geoffroy Debate*, 122.

253 On Bérard, see Chapter 3, "Eclecticism in Montpellier." A typical medical reaction to the work of Etienne Geoffroy Saint-Hilaire was this comment on a presentation he made at the Académie des sciences: "The nature of this presentation does not permit any analysis giving a clearer idea than what is conveyed in the title." *Archives générales de médecine*, 2d ser., 7 (1835): 279.

254 Serres, *Anatomie comparée du cerveau*, ii.

employed in classification, the limits and possibilities of species or race crossing, these were all posed by natural history. When they were addressed within medical discourse at all, they were addressed only derivatively or as by-products of genuinely medical concerns. The appointment of Serres to a chair at the museum – which had been the institutional home of natural history from its inception – was thus wholly appropriate despite Serres's medical origins and early work; his approach to the natural history of man validated the procedures and concerns of the natural history tradition and the specific biological sciences into which that tradition was gradually transmuting.[255]

All this being said, however, there is another dimension to Serres's career and to his construction of the problematics of "anthropology," as the science taught from his chair was to be officially called after 1855.[256] Serres's manuscripts at the museum include not only the notes for his course on the human races with its focus on the monogenist-polygenist problem and similar issues but also materials on diverse subjects whose links were forged not by the natural history tradition but by anthropological medicine. In June 1848, for example, Serres submitted to the minister of public instruction of the revolutionary government a program for a course in "anthropology and public hygiene." This prospectus included lessons on "organized beings," "anthropogeny," the advantageous effects of work on the longevity of life, the physical and moral character of the races, perfectibility, the influence of physical and moral agents on human development, the foundations of human racial fraternity "deduced from Christianity," a comparison of the physicomoral characters of the French and the Algerians, public hygiene, racial hygiene, hygiene and perfectibility, women's hygiene and education, the obligations of the government in respect to the family, and the organization of work in all the professions.[257] These topics belonged not to general biology but to the medical science of man to which Serres, despite the focus of his published work and his teaching, continued to give great credence. The emphasis in this prospectus on hygiene, education, and perfectibility is especially interesting in light of Serres's generally rigorous fixism – his insistence, for example, that the intellectual potential of the races was established in the course of their embryological development when their movement toward the highest level of human capacities was halted by the work of organogenetic laws. Perhaps in submitting this course to the revolutionary government, Serres was merely swept up in the pas-

255 This division between "medical" and "scientific" concerns is made in Appel, *The Cuvier-Geoffroy Debate*, 122.
256 On the change in title of the chair and the appointment of Armand de Quatrefages in 1855, see Hamy, "La collection anthropologique," 270.
257 Letter from Serres to Minister of Public Instruction, dated June 9, 1848, MNHN, Miscellaneous MS of E. R. A. Serres.

sions of the moment; every revolution so far had brought outpourings of meliorist enthusiasm from doctors who, in soberer moments, saw not much hope for human physical and moral progress. Perhaps Serres always worked two antagonistic veins in his thinking on human prospects: it was he, after all, who declared to his physician colleagues in an opening address to the 1845 medical congress that "the dominant objective of the nineteenth century is the perfecting of the physical and moral well-being of man."[258] The explanation for these competing tendencies may be sought in Serres's private intellectual biography, but if the argument pursued throughout this book is correct, there is not, finally, anything very unusual or particularly in need of explaining in Serres's veering between the fixism of a new anthropological science bent on establishing the natural, determined, and law-like character of its phenomena, and a therapeutic meliorism that still privileged the discretely human, the indeterminate, and the variable. Both these possibilities and tendencies were ever present in the medical science of man in which a physician like Serres and indeed his whole idea of anthropology were at some level inescapably rooted.[259]

In the fevered excitement of spring 1848 it seemed, not just to Serres but to other doctors as well, that the moment had at last arrived when medicine would fulfill the ambitions envisioned for it since the age of enlightenment. Writing for the *Gazette médicale de Paris,* Jules Guérin declared that in the "present cataclysm" medicine must assume "a role that ranked among the first, if not the first" of all those required for the work of "universal regeneration." Arguing that medicine was invested with extensive rights and duties because of the "immense services" it delivered to society, he drew attention to "the many facts, . . . questions, and . . . solutions that require the exclusive competence" of doctors.[260] Society could rely only on medicine in striving to improve the "inferior classes" through the moral and physical education of the young and the eradication of vice, to establish "useful and humanitarian relations" by distributing labor according to age and talents, and, most important of all, to "discern the true capacities and natural rights of the diverse classes to national representation."[261] Only the doctor, "the true priest of present-day society," knew the "complexities of society and could chart the way across so many obscurities of faculties, pas-

---

258 Quoted in Léonard, *La médecine entre les pouvoirs et les savoirs,* 150.

259 That Serres conceived of anthropology as a medical science is further borne out by a lesson he delivered at the museum in 1854 entitled *Considérations sur la méthode d'observation expérimentale en anthropologie* (Paris, 1854), in which the history of anthropology is seen as essentially coterminous with the history of medicine.

260 Jules Guérin, *De l'intervention du corps médical dans la situation actuelle: Programme de médecine sociale* (Paris: Au Bureau de la Gazette médicale, 1848) [extract *Gazette médicale de Paris,* March 11, 1848], 3–5.

261 *Ibid.,* 6.

sions, and instincts." Given the supreme importance of this "high mission of medicine," doctors must now forget "their professional and scientific interests" and devote themselves "solely to society."[262]

As with all other attempts to realize what Guérin called "ideal medicine," the reality fell painfully short. In 1848 the doctors exerted much less influence on events than they had desired. Their numbers were small in the revolutionary assemblies. Buchez's leadership faltered. Concrete proposals for the "amelioration of the people" led to endless wrangling and division.[263] After the Revolution medical visionaries like Guérin survived their disappointments and reverted to a more hardheaded professional pragmatism or to the quiet labors of science.[264] There is a sense, however, in which the "ideal medicine" that they, like so many before them, had dreamed of was dealt a finishing blow by the Revolution. After 1848 the occasions on which doctors chose to call themselves the "priests" of society became rarer and rarer. The "professional and scientific interests" that Guérin believed doctors must shelve for the greater good of society came to dominate medicine more and more. The capability of physicians to discern "true capacities" was trumpeted less as a means to achieve social betterment than as a device to root out criminals and degenerates or to prove the inevitability of racial domination. In short, the postrevolutionary age was to spell the end of the medical science of man.[265]

None of this is to say that medicine moved from being optimistic, meliorist, and generous in spirit to being pessimistic, fixist, and selfishly professional. Long before the watershed of 1848 the anthropological medicine from which visions such as Guérin's derived had sheltered these contending possibilities. What it does mean is that 1848 represented a kind of rhetorical climax for the whole medical tradition and that in the sober, often bitter, aftermath of the Revolution, all the grandiose constructions of medicine that it had encouraged came to seem outmoded and irrelevant. In this way the concrete struggles of 1848 confirmed the theoretical and structural developments within medicine itself that had already begun to undermine the science of man. The failure of the social and scientific messianism of 1848

262 *Ibid.*, 7, 11.
263 The Republic inherited the unsolved problems of the 1845 medical congress; see Léonard, *Les médecins de l'Ouest*, chap. 10, esp. 821–22.
264 On Guérin's more conservative posture after the Revolution, see Léonard, *La médecine entre les pouvoirs et les savoirs*, 200. Serres abandoned anthropology in 1855 when he moved to the museum's chair in comparative anatomy; see Hamy, "La collection anthropologique," 270.
265 Léonard, *La médecine entre les pouvoirs et les savoirs*, argues that after 1848 doctors "followed the evolution of the rest of the petty and middle bourgeoisie toward a prudent realism which encouraged them to subordinate their ideas of progress to men of order" (224). Léonard goes on to document, however, the participation of many doctors in Bonapartist programs for public health. The era of Napoleon III mirrored that of the first Napoleon in quashing medical idealism while extending the state apparatus of public health (226–28).

did not mean that the advocates of science, medical and otherwise, stopped claiming high social utility for their pursuits. It meant rather that they shifted into different registers, on the one hand arguing for the immediate, concrete, often technical efficacy of their labors (their industrial, technological, or therapeutic applications), or, on the other, insisting on the inviolate, "pure" quality of their specialized and intensive researches whose utility might not yet be obvious but whose ultimate value was assured by the un–challengeable value of science itself. Both of these arguments would, in the age to follow, be made by the heirs of the medical science of man.

The science of man after 1850:
The power of tradition

By midcentury the medical science of man, already fragmented and dispersed in multiple directions, was in a full process of disintegration. The phrase "science of man" was now seldom used to designate either medicine generally – as it had been from the late eighteenth into the early nineteenth century – or any of the developing medical specialties. To the extent that the term was used at all, it now referred to the emergent discipline of anthropology, which, although drawing in important ways on medical tradition, repudiated the medical science of man and forged links with a broad range of natural and cultural sciences including archaeology, geology, linguistics, and biology. The central problematic of the medical science of man – the relations between the physical and the moral – was becoming discursively archaic. The "physical" term of the dyad persisted and was diversely reconceived in various disciplines. But the rubric of the "moral" – although still used as a handy catchall term – gave way in the research paradigms of the human sciences to varying constructs including strictly "mental" or "intellectual" phenomena, social and cultural *moeurs,* historical "stages of development," racial or national "spirit," and a range of other categories. Nor did the science of man find any place in the professional and institutional developments of the era. General medicine was witness to the gradual rise of specialties, none of which might reasonably take as their purview the great range of subjects and problems covered by anthropological medicine. Many of these subjects, moreover, were now claimed by specialized disciplines outside medicine or tied to it only by tenuous links. Most important of all, anthropological medicine, with its sense of the free-flowing, protean, indeterminate relations of the physical and the moral, now gave way to constructs and approaches tailored to meet the increasingly stringent methodological requirements of positive science, medical and otherwise.

Thus in the latter half of the nineteenth century the medical science of man fell victim to two trends already evident in the 1830s and 1840s: the spread and enhanced force of the positivist ethos and the tendency toward disciplinary and professional specialization within both medicine and all the emergent human sciences.[1] In the later nineteenth century the medical science of man was an anachronism – it was holistic in an era dominated by localist and reductionist methodologies; it postulated reciprocal physical-moral influences where the new sciences of mind sought unambiguously physicalist explanations for psychic and behavioral phenomena; it propelled medicine into society but failed to offer specific techniques and strategies to undergird the medicosocial enterprise; lastly, it offered a concept of diverse human types rooted in Hippocratism and vitalist medicine that now gave way to the more technical systems of classification offered by the emergent disciplines within the human sciences.

None of this is to say that the tradition of anthropological medicine disappeared abruptly from the French cultural landscape after 1850. Indeed it would seem that, as the unitary science of man disappeared from medical discourse, the warnings and proscriptions of anthropological medicine intensified their hold on public consciousness. The pervasive use of medical metaphors, language, and concepts in French public discourse in the later nineteenth century has been amply demonstrated by historians.[2] And, after a fashion, this medicalized discourse continued to privilege the problem of the physical-moral relation. Yet this discourse altered significantly in the later nineteenth century, when its focus shifted from the constitution of the individual to the well-being of the nation. The "medical concept of national decline," as Robert A. Nye has termed it, traced a direct link between the physical and moral maladies of individual French men and women and the waning strength of the nation in an era of intense international competition and heightened internal divisiveness. In this context the dysfunctions that anthropological medicine had charted in the individual body economy were reconceived to diagnose social ills and national debility. The ultimate exemplar of the enfeebled Frenchman was the "degenerate" – weak, perhaps deformed, deficient in vital energy, prey to addictions and perversions. In some quarters hope was held out for the cure or alleviation of degeneracy, but mostly the degenerate was a figure to be feared and guarded against. The existence of widespread social pathologies – degeneracy, alcoholism, drug addiction, infertility, physical and mental debility – was a theme that ramified throughout French culture and society. It came to constitute standard fare not only in medical and scientific circles but also among politicians, journalists, novelists, playwrights, and other observers.[3]

---

1 On these trends in French medicine in the later nineteenth century, see Jacques Léonard, *La médecine entre les pouvoirs et les savoirs: Histoire intellectuelle et politique de la médecine française au XIXe siècle* (Paris: Aubier, 1981).

2 Ruth Harris, *Murders and Madness: Medicine, Law, and Society in the Fin-de-Siècle* (Oxford: Clarendon Press, 1989); Robert A. Nye, *Crime, Madness, and Politics in Modern France: The Medical Concept of National Decline* (Princeton: Princeton University Press, 1984); Daniel Pick, *Faces of Degeneration: A European Disorder, c. 1848–c. 1918* (Cambridge: Cambridge University Press, 1989).

3 Nye, *Crime, Madness, and Politics*, esp. chap. 5; Pick, *Faces of Degeneration*, esp. chaps. 2–3.

This general cultural phenomenon did not represent a vulgarization of anthropological medicine so much as a refraction of continuing developments within the human sciences in which elements of the science of man discourse persisted and indeed took on new significance. In diverse disciplinary contexts including anthropology, psychiatry, criminology, neurology, legal medicine, and human biology, the thematics and on occasion even the seemingly archaic language of anthropological medicine reappeared in new frameworks. Anthropological medicine continued to exert real force despite its apparent demise chiefly because of its singular role in the most important development in the human and life sciences of the later nineteenth century: the emergence of a peculiarly French conception of heredity. This conception was based on the vitalist doctrine of the equilibration of the body economy through adaptation to "milieux" and argued, despite a putatively strict physicalism, for the blended influence of innate constitution and environment on the formation of the human organism and species, the phenomena of health and disease, and the development of human society.[4] Although based on long-standing tradition, this conception of heredity was articulated in a positivist framework and language suited to the cultural climate of the later nineteenth century. Heredity was now trumpeted as the positive foundation for inquiries that previously had lacked a clear sense of physicalist determinism or indeed any understanding of unidirectional cause-and-effect relations. It is not possible to examine here all the domains of the human sciences where the interplay of innovative hereditarian discourse and medical tradition unfolded. Rather, this discussion will focus on specific moments in the history of medical psychiatry, criminology, neurology, and, especially, the new science of anthropology, to suggest the complex and continuing power of the science of man tradition.

The new importance of hereditarian thinking in the second half of the nineteenth century did not mark a complete break with the past. Heredity had long figured as a possible cause of disease and since at least the 1830s and 1840s some medical theorists had emphasized its role in pathology. In 1840 François Leuret, for example, had ridiculed physicians who discounted heredity in the etiology of mental illness.[5] Yet until midcentury physicians generally adhered to a conception of the reciprocal influence of constitution and "circumstance" rather than one-sided determinism. By the second half of the nineteenth century such indeterminacy was regarded as an inadequate foundation for any enterprise that styled itself scientific. As pressures

---

4 Yvette Conry, *L'introduction du darwinisme en France au XIXe siècle* (Paris: J. Vrin, 1974), 319–23, 348–57. The "ensemble de notions classiques au XVIIIe et au début du XIXe siècle" to which Conry refers as the source of this peculiarly French view of heredity derives from the vitalist medicine and physiology traced in this study.

5 This was Leuret's response to the "spiritualist school," typified by Heinroth in Germany, which argued that mental alienation was the result of sin rather than predisposition to disease. See François Leuret, *Du traitement moral de la folie* (Paris: J. B. Baillière, 1840), 147–48.

mounted for all the human sciences to conform to the investigative methods and explanatory modes offered by the natural sciences, unambiguously physicalist explanations of the phenomena of health and disease seemed to be demanded.[6] In medicine these pressures were exerted by a range of intellectual, professional, and broadly social developments: the increasing importance of the sciences in medical education and training, the intensified emphasis on and demand for therapeutic efficacy, the quest of doctors for enhanced professional status, the competition of an increasingly scientized medical establishment in Germany, and related factors.[7] All of these encouraged recourse to explanatory models based on heredity, which appeared to supply a revolutionary framework for exploring strictly physical causation in the etiology of disease and in the formation of physical and mental characteristics.

The tendency to focus on heredity, as opposed to other possible somaticist approaches, may be explained in various ways. Partly it was a response to the increased prominence – and apparent successes – of embryological and developmental studies in French life science. It was also encouraged by larger cultural factors that focused attention on familial, national, and racial lines of heritage. These ranged from the interest in national genealogy stimulated by romantic nationalism and the new historicism, to the preoccupation with race intensified by the resurgence of imperial ambition, to the challenge mounted by socialists to the validity of the traditional family structure.[8] Whatever the effective cause of the mounting interest in heredity, the problem received its first wide-ranging and influential articulation in 1847 by the alienist Prosper Lucas in the opening volume of his *De l'hérédité naturelle*, a work that recounted numerous case studies to prove the role of heredity in the transmission of mental maladies. Then shortly after the publication of Lucas's work came the events of 1848, which added their own, perhaps decisive, charge to the intensifying interest in heredity by encouraging social observers to seek the root cause of France's penchant for revolutionary violence.[9]

The first major contribution after 1848 to the conceptualization of heredity came in 1857 with the publication of B.-A. Morel's influential treatise,

6 For similar impulses in the Anglo-American context, see Charles E. Rosenberg, "Body and Mind in Nineteenth-Century Medicine: Some Clinical Origins of the Neurosis Construct," *BHM* 63 (1989): 185–97, esp. 195–96.

7 Robert Fox and George Weisz, eds. *The Organization of Science and Technology in France, 1808–1914* (Cambridge: Cambridge University Press, 1980).

8 Claude Blanckaert, "On the Origins of French Ethnology: William Edwards and the Doctrine of Race," in *Bones, Bodies, and Behavior: Essays on Biological Anthropology*, ed. George W. Stocking, Jr. (Madison: University of Wisconsin Press, 1988), 18–55, esp. 24; William B. Cohen, *The French Encounter with Africans: White Response to Blacks, 1530–1880* (Bloomington: Indiana University Press, 1980), esp. chap. 9; Nye, *Crime, Madness, and Politics*, 120–23.

9 Prosper Lucas, *Traité philosophique et physiologique de l'hérédité naturelle dans les états de santé et de maladie du système nerveux*, 2 vols. (Paris: J. B. Baillière, 1847–50); on the effect of 1848, see Pick, *Faces of Degeneration*, 48, 56–59.

Traité des dégénérescences. Morel was a friend and protégé of one of the chief figures of anthropological medicine of the 1840s, Philippe Buchez. He was also a member of the learned society established after 1848 by the founders of the *Annales médico-psychologiques.* Morel's work both manifested and further stimulated the new preoccupation with heredity by articulating the threat posed by hereditary "degeneration."[10] Morel took as his point of departure the effects on the individual of a hostile environment – the diverse, noxious "agents" of anthropological medicine. But unlike earlier physicians he was less interested in the immediate effects of a pathological environment on individuals than in the creation over time of what he called "morbid varieties of the human species."[11] Morel postulated that any abnormal condition induced in the individual by adaptation to a pathological environment would be internalized as a latent tendency or condition and then later fully manifested in the individual's own offspring and in successive generations. This view built on well-established physiological concepts of the necessity for the individual to adapt to external conditions of existence – climatic and otherwise – to assure the uninterrupted harmony of the body economy. But it shifted the emphasis away from the sick individual to the long-term and cumulative effects of an initial reaction to pathological circumstances. How precisely such reactions were transformed into constitutional proclivities and predispositions Morel did not say. This reticence about the actual physical mechanisms of heredity was to be a common feature of hereditarian discourse in France, where much greater attention was always given to the effects of heredity – pathological or beneficial – than to the physical processes involved in the transmission of traits.[12]

The new prominence of theories of heredity had manifold consequences throughout the life and human sciences. The traditional focus of the medical science of man, rooted as it was in vitalist theory and in clinical practice, was the individual, in sickness and health, as these conditions developed and altered in the passage of one lifetime. Anthropological medicine was never distinguished by a historical perspective, either progressivist or degenerationist; instead it was focused on problems of adaptation and equilibration of the body economy in the here and now. That characters and tendencies could be acquired by the individual and passed on to progeny was generally assumed by physicians from Barthez to the hygienists of the 1830s and 1840s. But the science of man never stressed this process of accumulation and transmission. After 1850, on the other hand, concern with heredity became not only an important focus of the human sciences but a virtual ob-

10 B.-A. Morel, *Traité des dégénérescences physiques, intellectuelles et morales de l'espèce humaine* (Paris: J. B. Baillière, 1857). See also Ian Dowbiggin, *Inheriting Madness: Professionalization and Psychiatric Knowledge in Nineteenth-Century France* (Berkeley: University of California Press, 1991), 118–19.
11 Quoted in Harris, *Murders and Madness*, 54.
12 See the discussions of Morel in *ibid.*, 51–56, and in Pick, *Faces of Degeneration*, 40–41, 44–54.

session. As Ian Dowbiggin has recently argued, it came to provide the "somatic missing link" in fields of investigation whose claims to positivity had so far been tenuous and uncertain.[13] In so doing heredity theory strongly encouraged the development of independent disciplines that could mobilize discrete and specialized techniques to solve problems that had seemed intractable. This was a peculiarly welcome development in mental medicine, where the general failure of localization studies of the 1830s and 1840s had left the field without any satisfactory material explanation for mental pathology. Armed with hereditarian constructs, psychiatrists began, from the 1860s forward, to denounce the diagnostic errors made by generalists and to argue that general medicine was an inadequate framework for the understanding of hereditary mental illness.[14]

In medical psychiatry the development of hereditarian thinking unfolded principally with the further elaboration of Morel's "degenerate." The key figure in this work was the medical psychiatrist Valentin Magnan, who was appointed to a post at the Paris mental asylum the Hôpital Sainte-Anne in 1867. Magnan was as eager as any physician of the period to break with the unscientific character of the older anthropological medicine. (To students he denounced, for example, the scientific nullity of the monomania concept of the Esquirol circle.)[15] Strongly impressed by Claude Bernard's experimentalism, Magnan set about studying the "external agents" that influenced mental health – chiefly drugs and intoxicants – by means of animal experiments. He also undertook investigations using hypnosis, likewise conceived as an "agent" whose effect could be experimentally induced and reproduced. Magnan's goal was to elaborate a uniform and predictable sequence by which the degeneration "syndrome" advanced and worsened. To do so he developed what Ruth Harris refers to as a "cerebro-spinal topography of mental pathology."[16]

Despite his vigorous repudiation of nonexperimental investigative and therapeutic methods, however, Magnan's schematization of the forces producing the degenerate had clear affinities with the vitalist-inspired constructs of "prepositive" mental medicine. His attempts to localize the origins of sexually linked mental disorders – in which he posited that healthy sexual function required the harmonious interaction of "psychic, sensory, and spinal centers" – reproduced the triadic form of traditional vitalist pathology.[17] In other instances Magnan abandoned localism altogether in favor of a conception of general nervous degradation set in motion by an

13 Dowbiggin, *Inheriting Madness*, 72.
14 *Ibid.*, 116–60. On the criticism of generalists, see Jan Goldstein, *Console and Classify: The French Psychiatric Profession in the Nineteenth Century* (Cambridge: Cambridge University Press, 1987), 332–33.
15 Goldstein, *Console and Classify*, 191–92 and n. 139.
16 Harris, *Murders and Madness*, 46–47, 70–71.   17 The quotation is in *ibid.*, 46.

initial pathological event.[18] Magnan's links to the tradition of anthropological medicine were further revealed in his characterization of degeneration as
a "state of the organism . . . which . . . only realizes in part the biological
conditions of its hereditary struggle for life."[19] This "struggle for life" in
which the degenerate failed so pitifully was not that of Herbert Spencer or
Charles Darwin, but of the vitalist physiologists who, throughout the
whole tradition of the medical science of man, had insisted that the individual could maintain equilibration of the internal forces of the body economy only by successful adaptation to its circumstances of life.

Magnan's perspective was not peculiar to him but general throughout
medical psychiatry. As efforts to chart the precise organic sites of mental
disease yielded often dubious results, heredity was eagerly mobilized to
provide an alternate – although still clearly physicalist and hence thoroughly scientized – conception of the physical-moral link. Ironically, however, this very search for a somaticist, scientifically secure foundation for
the study of mental phenomena led psychiatrists back to a conception of
free-flowing reciprocities closely akin to the "prepositive" approaches of
anthropological medicine that they consciously rejected. Although heredity
was constantly hailed as a determinist construct that embodied rigorous
"laws" of hereditary influence, the idea of heredity that dominated French
science in this era never in fact incorporated any clear distinction between
the roles of heredity and environment such as that demanded by the
twentieth-century dichotomy of nature and nurture. Rather, the regnant
conception of heredity conceived the individual as an always potentially unstable blend of innate constitution and external influences. The primitive
constitution could be altered – in varying degrees and in ways that remained to be fully explained – by the effects of the individual's struggle for
life. These alterations were then passed on as proclivities or "stigmata," as
Magnan termed them, to offspring.[20] Such tendencies then governed the
adaptive (or maladaptive) responsivity of the next generation.

This understanding of heredity did not rest on a strict concept of physical
inheritance but postulated a reciprocal blend of innate constitution and
molding influences. In allowing for the importance of "milieu" – a concept
that encompassed external environment and individual habits – it continued
to hold the individual responsible for controlling important influences to
which he or she was subjected, such as alcohol and sexual practices, and
also left some room for therapeutic intervention. In these respects the hereditarian discourse of the later nineteenth century differed little from the
concept of reciprocal influences that had always formed the core of anthro-

18 Nye, *Crime, Madness, and Politics*, 123–24.
19 Quoted in *ibid.*, 124 (and see Nye's note 79 in reference to this quotation).
20 *Ibid.*; the anticlerical implications of this usage are examined in Goldstein, *Console and Classify*, 369–74.

pological medicine. Yet this concept of heredity enjoyed a success in the cultural world of the later Second Empire and especially the Third Republic that no direct restatement of the principles of anthropological medicine could ever have achieved. Since heredity was fixed in the blood and transmitted through the mechanisms of sex and reproduction, it was a physicalist, determinist, and therefore unquestionably positive construct. That this peculiar sense of fixed characters embodied its antithesis in assuming that the continuing "struggle for life" could yet again alter the product of heredity constituted no anomaly to theorists nurtured on the tradition of anthropological medicine.

The neovitalist concept of heredity developed by medical psychiatrists such as Magnan commanded widespread approbation among administrators and social reformers who sought to apply the principles of the human sciences directly and without delay to problems of social management. It provided a rationale for incessant campaigns against sexual irregularity, alcoholism, the use of tobacco and drugs, and kindred social evils that could, alone or in combination, trigger the manifestation of latent pathological tendencies.[21] Hereditarian discourse of this character was of special importance to the work of criminologists and medical legists, who sought for their specialties the prestige of scientificity yet were troubled by the full-blown determinism and social fatalism of a criminological doctrine such as that of Cesare Lombroso in Italy.[22] French criminologists were in important instances trained in medicine and, thanks to their efforts, the field incorporated a therapeutic tendency as one of its possible approaches to the management of criminality. Like the anthropologists examined later, the criminologists of this era were generally republican, progressive, and reformist in spirit and as such they were unwilling to relinquish all sense that their scientific labors would have an improving effect on French society. Nor could the criminologists have made much headway in local contests with competing professionals in the law and in social administration by mobilizing a doctrine that ascribed criminality to unvarying laws of biological determinism.

That the medical approach to criminality did not mitigate individual responsibility was definitively demonstrated by the manner in which French criminologists of the 1880s, led by the professor of legal medicine Paul Brouardel, adapted the new bacteriology to their ends.[23] As Brouardel and his followers conceived it, even the microbe, an apparently external, invasive cause of pathology, was transformed into an agent dependent for its effect on suitable "terrain" in the host. As Ruth Harris writes, "in such an

---

21 Dowbiggin, *Inheriting Madness*, 136–40.
22 This discussion is based on Nye, *Crime, Madness, and Politics*, 97–131, and Harris, *Murders and Madness*, 80–98.
23 Harris, *Murders and Madness*, 98–105.

analysis, the offender was regarded as the host rather than the microbe, with the aim of the specialist being to isolate those disease agents in his biological and psycho-social constitution which were the 'germs' of disorder."[24] This was precisely the approach to the menaces of filth and contagion that hygienists had adopted in the 1830s and 1840s. Just as it had then, the tradition of reciprocal influences supplied a welcome, indeed ideologically and professionally indispensable, alternative to strictly determinist constructions of the link between heredity and behavior.[25]

This same ambiguity in the conception of heredity and in the valuation and mechanisms of determinist explanation is apparent in the work of the most prominent neurologist of the fin-de-siècle, Jean-Martin Charcot. Like the asylum doctors who first mobilized the concept of degeneration, Charcot was eager to establish the study of mental pathology on a secure scientific footing. In his work on hysteria Charcot flamboyantly broke with medical tradition and sought to establish a view of hysteria that would be as rigorous and unchallengeable as assertions made by natural scientists. Rejecting the ancient Hippocratist view that hysteria was a female malady caused by the "restless womb," Charcot argued that hysteria afflicted all categories of the population and that its chief characteristics (the four "stages" in which the disease unfolded) were "valid for all countries, all times, all races" and were "consequently universal."[26] In keeping with the focus of neurological science of his era, Charcot was hostile to the view that hysteria reflected a generalized disorder caused by upset in one of the "domains" – the reproductive zone – of vitalist medicine. Like all his positivist colleagues, he anticipated that neuroscience would eventually track the precise lesions in the brain or nervous system responsible for mental disease. Mobilizing the degeneration concept for his own purposes, Charcot argued that the hereditary nature of nervous disease was now amply demonstrated and he avidly searched through the family histories of his patients for the pathological conditions – alcoholism, tuberculosis, melancholia, irritability – that might trigger full-blown mental illness in the current generation. In methodological terms, too, Charcot saw himself as breaking with all medicine that was purely episodic and anecdotal in character: his work with patients was experimental in design and he subjected the results he achieved in work with living patients to the rigorous scrutiny of autopsy.[27]

Yet for all Charcot's determination to establish the study of mental illness on a positivistic, localist, and materialist foundation, he too had recourse – increasingly so as time passed – to constructs borrowed from the anthro-

24 *Ibid.*, 101.   25 See Chapter 3, "The Science of Man at Work."
26 Quoted in Goldstein, *Console and Classify*, 327.
27 Ruth Harris, Introduction to *Clinical Lectures on Diseases of the Nervous System*, by Jean-Martin Charcot (London: Tavistock/Routledge, 1991), ix–lxviii, esp. xxii–xxvi. With his colleague Vulpian, Charcot is said to have "performed as many as 800 autopsies in a single year" (xvi).

pological medicine of old. Charcot's interest in sex-based determination of hysteria did not result merely from his keenness to flout the medical tradition that hysteria was exclusively feminine. Instead it was an approach to the disease that was saturated with the sense of gender-specificity that had long characterized the medical science of man. The language in which Charcot described hysteria was charged with references to sexual vitality and capacity. Opening his lectures with summary descriptions of patients, he frequently referred to the "robust" or "virile" character of his male patients, and on one occasion remarked on the alluring dress and appearance that usually characterized female hysterics. Ruth Harris has suggested, moreover, that in denying that hysteria was an exclusively female disease Charcot nonetheless extended the category only to males of certain types – impressionable and nervous men of the upper classes, but mostly only workers or artisans – whose behavior he "effeminized" by conflating it with the "feminine" features of the disease.[28] This was a procedure wholly in keeping with the approach of anthropological medicine, both in its tendency to slip readily from one domain of influence (sex) to another (occupation, class) and in its reference to the generalized loss of energy and vitality occasioned by an ostensibly localized disease.[29]

Charcot's concept of male hysteria was also heavily indebted to the environmental tradition of anthropological medicine, and especially the peculiar form this tradition had assumed among Parisian hygienists. Hygiene in Paris had always given special attention to the problems of the dirty, crowded, noxious urban environment, and Charcot's work inflected this tradition in attending to the city as the source of traumas (crime, accidents) that led seemingly strong and healthy men to fall into a state of hysteria. The accent on the distress of working men was also in keeping with the science of man of the 1830s and 1840s, which took the lower classes as natural objects for scientific investigation while assuming unselfconsciously that individuals of rank and education had the means (or character) to hold themselves free of noxious influences. Charcot was "sympathetic" to the workers and artisans whose traumas he encountered; in cases of "railway shock," for example, he testified for the victims rather than for the railroad companies. But this does not change the fact that, in a fashion long typical of the medical science of man, his investigations assumed as their foundation the variable physiological responses of discrete social types, and specifically the inherently greater weakness and susceptibility to environmental influences of individuals of the lower classes.[30]

In a similar vein, Charcot put heavy emphasis on the effects of bad habits, common among the working classes, in creating the preconditions for hys-

28 Harris, Introduction to *Clinical Lectures*, xxiii–xxxiii, l–li.   29 See Chapter 1.
30 Harris, Introduction to *Clinical Lectures*, xxvi–xxxi. On this theme in the work of the hygienists, see Chapter 3, "The Science of Man at Work."

teria. Charcot did not, as Freud would do, trace a clearly sexual etiology for hysteria, but he did include sufficient references to "debauchery" in the background of his patients to suggest that sexual excess was an important factor conducing to hysteria.[31] This construct played on two venerable traditions in anthropological medicine. One was the molding power of habit, which had been the subject of sustained attention among French vitalists from at least Lacaze forward. The other, the general neurological debility that was caused by sexual excess and that predisposed individuals to hysteria, was a restatement in modern scientific language of the long-standing assumption that the "higher faculties" were sapped when excessive energy was expended in sexual activity. The principle of limited energy thus reappeared, its vitalist coloring replaced by references to "dynamic alterations" of the nervous system. The vitalist origins of Charcot's framework became curiously obvious when, speculating on the sexual etiology of the disease, Charcot observed that in males the affliction might well begin in the groin and then pass to the "epigastric region" and on to the throat. This itinerary for the disease recalled – consciously or not – the tradition that diseases of the throat were associated in the young with sexual passion. With Charcot thus reemerged the triad – youth/ardor/affliction of the throat – that in classic vitalism prefigured or accompanied the descent into nervous disease.[32]

These theoretical affinities between Charcot's neurology and the old science of man were paralleled, moreover, in Charcot's style and self-presentation as a scientist. The science of man gave way to the new sciences of mind and behavior in part because the old medical tradition seemed too lax, too philosophical, too dependent for effect on rhetorical flights and beautiful metaphors.[33] And Charcot in his early career was careful to cultivate the image of the severe scientist. Yet in this respect too Charcot ended as a throwback. Ruth Harris has observed that in the 1880s Charcot drew on old "medical and natural historical traditions" in presenting himself as a man of broad learned culture and his science as one that revalidated ancient truths about the human spirit.[34] In so doing Charcot made a bow to tradition that was perhaps unique among late nineteenth-century luminaries of the human sciences. The norm was certainly better represented by a figure such as the anthropologist Paul Broca, who was also deeply indebted to anthropological medicine but who nurtured a public image of severity and

---

31 Harris, Introduction to *Clinical Lectures*, xxx.
32 *Ibid.*, xl; on this theme in the vitalist tradition, see Chapter 1, "Vitality and Variability," and Chapter 3, "Physiological Medicine of F. J. V. Broussais."
33 In an 1846 obituary the work of J.-J. Virey was dismissed as the work of a mere rhetorician. The obituarist thought this unfortunate tendency in Virey's work typical of the "era of indecision" in medicine created by the influence of Buffon, Bordeu, Barthez, and Bichat. See *AGM*, 4th ser., 11 (1846): 115–17.
34 Harris, Introduction to *Clinical Lectures*, xlv.

rigor wholly at odds with Charcot's flamboyance. It is clear too that Charcot skated close to the edge of scientific respectability and that his reputation rapidly dissipated once the force of his personality was no longer there to sustain it. But the unique case of Charcot is perhaps best perceived as the exception that proves the rule: doctors were the bearers of a venerable tradition concerning the workings of the soul and could, if so inclined, assert the authority of that tradition far beyond the walls of faculty and clinic.[35]

The notoriety of Charcot resulted in part from the theatricality of his famous lectures but also from his high visibility in the intensified anticlerical struggle that absorbed so many energies in the Third Republic from the ascension of Gambetta onward. Charcot and his school contested the remaining authority of the church within mental medicine on many fronts, especially the campaign to laicize the asylum and the effort to "hystericize" cases – both historical and contemporary – of religious exaltation. And Charcot personally embodied all that the orthodox had most feared in respect to the entrenchment of materialist teaching in public education when in 1882 he was appointed, after long hesitations and machinations, to a chair in "nervous diseases" at the Paris medical faculty. In this respect, too, late century neurological and psychiatric science represented a seemingly definitive break with the tradition of anthropological medicine, which had been marked with few exceptions (Broussais the most notable) by attempts at accommodation with orthodoxy rather than direct confrontation. In company with other Gambettist anticlericals, psychiatrists of the fin-de-siècle finally confronted the church and its teachings about the mind-body relation head on, attacking with bitter sarcasm what they saw as the church's encouragement of religious "hysteria" and its efforts to keep the populace in a condition of ignorance and superstition. Thus Charcot merited his place as one of the Third Republic's "heroes" in part for his efforts to secularize French consciousness and society.[36]

Yet again there are curious paradoxes. In an article on the Lourdes cures written toward the end of his life, Charcot, given the opportunity to press his campaign against superstition, wrote instead in a vein of melancholy tolerance. He was prepared to accept that cures were effected at Lourdes, even if the reasons and the means remained mysterious. In a tacit acknowledgment of the therapeutic paucity of his own work, Charcot admitted that something might be learned from the Lourdes cures about those strange regions of the physical-moral relation where the mind seemed to determine the body rather than, as psychiatric science so stolidly argued, the body governed the mind. As Jan Goldstein has observed, this was a late, fleeting,

---

35 *Ibid.*, xliv–li. On Broca, see the subsequent discussion.
36 *Ibid.*, xii–xiv, xvii–xx; Goldstein, *Console and Classify*, 361–73.

but telling recovery of the physical-moral "reciprocities" so crucial to the Ideologues and to medical tradition.[37]

The final instance to be examined of the persistence of anthropological medicine within the human sciences is found in the emergent discipline of anthropology. The struggle of the anthropologists to establish a new "science of man" – one that would build on medicine and its authority yet achieve genuine positivity – illustrates especially well the strong currents encouraging specialization in the human sciences and yet the simultaneous and continuing power of not only discursive but also institutional tradition.

Unlike psychiatry, which naturally fell heir to the institutional legacy of the asylum doctors, and criminology, which had to struggle for institutional endorsement from the law and public administration, the new science of anthropology was in the peculiar position of seeking disciplinary independence from medicine while still seeking its institutional support. This effort to institutionalize anthropology with the aid of the medical establishment began when in 1859 Paul Broca and nineteen other physicians met in facilities attached to the Ecole pratique of the medical faculty to found the Société d'anthropologie de Paris. The idea of establishing such a group belonged originally to Broca, who later recounted that he had decided to organize an anthropology society when the Société de biologie, to which he also belonged, showed itself reluctant to consider his findings on the subject of "human hybridity."[38] The eighteen individuals who joined Broca to found the society represented the fields of mental medicine, medical and experimental physiology, statistics, medical geography, teratology, hygiene, anatomy and surgery, natural history, and general medicine. The anthropology society later drew many adherents from geography, history, linguistics, archaeology, and similar endeavors, but as late as the 1890s more than half its members were still medical doctors.[39]

When first organized, the anthropology society conducted its meetings at the Ecole pratique. Within a few months it moved to private quarters nearby, but some eight years later (1867) it again took space in the Ecole pratique to establish a laboratory and library. An anthropological museum was added to these facilities in 1872. The final step in this process was the

---

37 Goldstein, *Console and Classify*, 380–82.

38 Paul Broca, "Introduction aux *Mémoires sur l'hybridité*," *MAPB*, 5 vols. (Paris: C. Reinwald, 1871–88), 3:321–25.

39 Besides Broca, the founders of the society were Adrien Antelme, Jules Béclard, Adolphe Bertillon, C.-L. Brown-Séquard, Philippe Boileau de Castelnau, Camille Dareste, L. J. F. Delasiauve, L. J. D. Fleury, F. A. E. Follin, Isidore Geoffroy Saint-Hilaire, Ernest Godard, Louis-Pierre Gratiolet, Gabriel Grimaud de Caux, Lemercier, Martin-Magron, Rambaud, Charles Robin, A. A. S. Verneuil; see the membership lists in *BSAP*, 1 (1860): 2, and for the later era, *BSAP*, 4th ser., 1 (1890): 3. See also Léonce Manouvrier, "La Société d'Anthropologie de Paris depuis sa fondation, 1859–1909," *Bulletins et mémoires de la Société d'anthropologie de Paris*, 5th ser., 10 (1909): 305–28.

founding of the Ecole d'anthropologie, which was also housed in quarters provided by the Faculté de médecine. At its opening in 1876 the school had five instructors, three of whom had received their training and degrees at the Paris medical faculty.[40]

Although anthropology enjoyed this institutional alliance with the medical faculty, it was not made an official part of the medical curriculum. Instead the complex of anthropological institutions was made possible by informal cooperation between the society and the faculty administrators. Thus the continued presence of the anthropologists in the faculty quarters was dependent on mutual goodwill rather than a formal institutional relationship. That anthropology fit, even in this way, in the Paris medical school of the 1860s, is to be explained only by the tradition of anthropological medicine, which made it seem natural for doctors to embark on developing a science of humanity considered, as Broca put it, "as a whole, in its details, and in its relations with the rest of nature."[41] There can be no doubt that by the 1860s this anthropological endeavor was regarded as peripheral to the principal work of the medical faculty. The space given the anthropologists was minimal, the funds required for renovations and installations were in large part privately subscribed, the participation of medical students and teachers in the work of the anthropologists was voluntary and informal.[42] All the same, anthropology did find an institutional base in the medical establishment, and this measure of official support helped to give it a degree of standing and legitimacy not achieved for a generation and more by other fields in the human sciences.[43]

The ties between the new anthropology and the old anthropological medicine are further evident in the intellectual biographies of the founders of the anthropology society, which show prior membership in the phrenology or ethnology societies; work in hygiene, mental medicine, or human physiology and anatomy; personal links to Broussais, Gerdy, Leuret, Buchez. In case after case there exists some institutional or personal tie to

40 These institutional details appear in Paul Topinard, *A la mémoire de Broca: La société, l'école, le laboratoire et le musée Broca* (Paris: Chamerot, 1890), 5–10. See also Elizabeth A. Williams, "Anthropological Institutions in Nineteenth-Century France," *Isis* 76 (1985): 331–48, esp. 339–40.
41 Paul Broca, "Anthropologie," *MAPB* 1:1. This article originally appeared in the *Dictionnaire encyclopédique des sciences médicales*, ed. J. Raige-Delorme and A. Dechambre, 100 vols. (Paris: Asselin, Sr. de Labé, V. Masson et fils, 1864–89), vol. 5.
42 Archives de la Faculté de Médecine de Paris, MS. 5454. This dossier includes a series of letters (nos. 2–8) that Broca wrote to the Ministry of Public Instruction in which he outlined the physical deficiencies of the anthropology laboratory and the financial particulars of its upkeep. A letter dated December 15, 1872, indicates that Broca paid the ordinary maintenance costs of the laboratory himself.
43 Terry N. Clark, *Prophets and Patrons: The French University and the Emergence of the Social Sciences* (Cambridge, Mass.: Harvard University Press, 1973); see also Williams, "Anthropological Institutions."

the tradition of the medical science of man.[44] These patterns reveal, at the level of the personal and anecdotal, what was in fact a structural feature of the intellectual landscape, one that accounted for the demise of anthropological medicine yet the simultaneous rise on medical terrain of a new science of man. French medicine carried ineluctably within it a disposition toward a broadly anthropological as opposed to a strictly clinical or therapeutic perspective, and yet this was a tendency that could no longer be actualized within medicine itself. In this sense the anthropology of the 1860s was not an adventitious synthesis achieved in the thought and ambitions of one man (as Broca's biographer suggests), nor was it a simple gathering together of various ways to study "man."[45] Rather it was a structural transmutation – one of the many that occurred – within a long-standing intellectual tradition that had become methodologically, philosophically, and socioprofessionally obsolete but that continued to have power over people educated and trained within it.

Yet if it is true that the medical science of man had evident power over the anthropologists of the 1860s, it sometimes seems that that power derived chiefly from its providing a model to be negated. The new anthropology utterly repudiated the vitalist perspective so crucial to the science of man tradition: the specificity of the human, the holistic framework, the accent on variability, and, most important, the insistence that vital phenomena were refractory to the ordinary laws of nature. In the place of these features and tendencies of anthropological medicine, Brocan anthropology sought to explain mental and behavioral phenomena by highly specific physical structures, embraced techniques of investigation (especially statistics) whose reliability vitalists had often questioned, and assumed as its very foundation

44 These extensive links can only be partially indicated: Antelme did an 1834 thesis on the physiology of thought and worked as an inspector of madhouses and prisons; Béclard was a student of Gerdy and the author of a major treatise on physiology (1855); Bertillon published extensively on the use of statistics in the science of man; Brown-Séquard did important work on the localization of nervous function; Castelnau wrote for both the *Annales d'hygiène publique et de médecine légale* and the *Annales médico-psychologiques;* Dareste was much influenced by Serres in his teratological work; Delasiauve wrote on phrenology and related subjects for the *Annales médico-psychologiques;* Fleury taught hygiene at the Faculty of Medicine; Isidore Geoffroy Saint-Hilaire, though primarily a naturalist, was trained in medicine and in his early work on teratology blended the approaches of medicine and natural history; Ernest Godard took his degree at the medical faculty and did intensive work in both anatomy and physiology; Gratiolet was a student of Leuret's, worked as an intern at the Salpêtrière and the Pitié, and later did work in the comparative anatomy of the nervous system; Grimaud de Caux was the author of a number of works on human physiology and physicomoral education; Martin-Magron was a private professor of physiology; Robin was influenced by Edwards and worked with P.-H. Bérard on his *Cours de physiologie;* see the biographical articles on these figures in the *DBF, DSB, Nouvelle Biographie Générale,* and *La Grande Encyclopédie.*
45 Francis Schiller, *Paul Broca: Founder of French Anthropology, Explorer of the Brain* (Berkeley: University of California Press, 1979), argues that anthropology would not have existed without Broca since it was he who synthesized a "multiplicity of only moderately germane subjects" (136).

the determinate character of human phenomena. Even in respect to the specificity of the human, anthropology was at least overtly hostile to the vitalist point of view for, although anthropology was itself the science of the human, its advocates insisted that human beings must be studied "in relation to the rest of nature."[46]

This determination to study human beings in nature was both cause and effect of the anthropologists' insistence that human phenomena were determined by and subject to the ordinary laws of nature. The single most important element of Brocan anthropology was its doctrine of race, which was its special contribution to the advancement of hereditarian thinking. The race theory of the anthropologists held that physical organization, especially craniological characters, governed the development of psychic capacities.[47] This conception of race was developed in opposition to traditional ideas of racial influence that in the view of anthropologists were not rigorous, systematic, or determinist enough to satisfy the requirements of science. It was not enough for the Brocan équipe to argue, as Cabanis had at the turn of the century, that racial traits were durable, perhaps even irreversible, if the influences forming them were strong, uninterrupted, and longlasting. Nor were the anthropologists satisfied with Edwards's position that there were marked "coincidences" between physical and moral characters. In the paradigm of racial science that dominated the anthropology society, the races had developed, and they exerted their influence over intellectual and moral characteristics, in accordance with established laws. Certainly the exact nature of these laws was not yet known, nor had adequate proofs been compiled to convince all skeptics. This was to be the work of the society. Yet racial science was already fully enough developed to show that the races had been independently formed at the origin of things, that they had not changed substantially since, in either physical or intellectual characters, that their most important and general features were unchanging and unchangeable.[48] Thus when the anthropologists spoke of

46 See Broca, *Ouverture des cours d'anthropologie au siège de la Société d'anthropologie de Paris à l'Ecole pratique de la Faculté de médecine* (Paris: Imprimerie de Cusset, 1876), where he specifically rejected the phrase *science de l'homme* as a synonym for anthropology because it included a great number of sciences that, like medicine, had a "perfectly distinct existence" (7). That humans were to be studied not as unique beings but as natural creatures like any other was stressed in Paul Topinard, *Eléments d'anthropologie* (Paris: A. Delahaye and E. Lecrosnier, 1885): "Anthropology is the cold and impartial study of man as if he were the most indifferent animal; [it is] the full and complete knowledge of man robbed of his prestige and viewed through the lens of reality" (2).

47 On the centrality of craniology to anthropology, see Broca, "Sur le volume et la forme du cerveau suivant les individus et suivant les races," *BSAP* 2 (1861): 139. Craniology was, Broca asserted, the "common terrain" on which the studies of "anatomical characters" and those of "intellectual and moral characters" could meet (139).

48 This was the dominant view of racial science upheld within the society from its founding to around 1880; for a full discussion, see Claude Blanckaert, "Monogénisme et polygénisme en France de Buffon à Paul Broca (1749–1880)" (Ph.D. diss., University of Paris,

invariable racial laws – comparable to the laws of physics or chemistry – they deliberately repudiated the variable, reciprocal, endlessly interchangeable physical and moral *rapports* of the medical science of man in favor of determinist constructs that in their view rested on a genuinely positive basis. It was this very clarity about the meaning and importance of race that gave Brocan anthropology its authority and distinguished it from both its predecessors and its current competitors in France and elsewhere.[49]

The determined naturalism and scientism of the anthropologists cut them off from the tradition of anthropological medicine in other important ways as well. In the early years of its existence the anthropology society rejected categorically the idea that anthropology had a broad social mission to accomplish. On repeated occasions Broca warned the society against involvement in any kind of political or ideological contest. He argued that controversy had undermined both the Société des observateurs de l'homme of the Napoleonic era and the Société ethnologigue in the 1840s. The ethnology society, he wrote, had strayed from "the path of science and given itself up to the most fantastic speculations"; the public "had ended by believing that ethnology . . . was not a science but something intermediary between politics, sociology, and philanthropy."[50] In truth, however, these historical precedents were less central to Broca's opposition to ideological engagement than his conviction that true science must be unswervingly "neutral" on any question likely to rouse ideological passions. This position of nonengagement put clear distance between the new anthropology and the old anthropological medicine, whose standard-bearers had at virtually every turn proclaimed the moral and social lessons to be learned from their inquiry and the benefits that would derive from the fuller extension throughout society of medical authority.[51]

1981); *idem*, " 'L'anthropologie personnifiée': Paul Broca et la biologie du genre humain," Preface to *Paul Broca: Mémoires d'anthropologie* (Paris: Jean Michel-Place, 1989), esp. v–xi; Cohen, *French Encounter with Africans*, chap. 8; Elizabeth A. Williams, "The Science of Man: Anthropological Thought and Institutions in Nineteenth-Century France" (Ph.D. diss., Indiana University, 1983), chap. 3. The minority view within the society, argued most forcefully in the 1860s and 1870s by Armand de Quatrefages, held that the human "varieties" were susceptible to diverse influences and therefore changeable both in physical and moral features; see Quatrefages, *Rapport sur les progrès de l'anthropologie*, esp. 72–171, 207–39.

49 Broca, "Histoire des progrès des études anthropologiques depuis la fondation de la Société," in *MAPB* 2:493–94; on the differences between anthropology and "ethnography," see Blanckaert, "On the Origins of French Ethnology," 48; the English anthropological tradition, which was strongly imbued with Protestant moralism, is examined in George W. Stocking, Jr., *Victorian Anthropology* (New York: Free Press, 1987), esp. chaps. 5 and 6.

50 Broca, "Histoire des progrès des études anthropologiques," *MAPB* 2:490–91, 493–95.

51 This conception of the ideological neutrality of anthropology was written into the society's founding articles; Article 41 stated that "The president will recall to order anyone who transcends the limits of scientific discussion"; see "Règlement Intérieur," *BSAP* 2 (1861);

Such contrasts between the tradition of anthropological medicine and the realized anthropology of the 1860s and 1870s could be developed at length. Anthropology often seemed bent primarily on repudiating long-standing elements of the medical science of man. This was of course an important kind of influence in its own right. For sciences in the making, the act of rejecting tradition is a crucial element of the work of self-definition. Certainly a good measure of Charcot's notoriety derived from his purportedly radical break with ancient trditions of the etiology of mental illness. The anthropologists were equally radical in their break with the past; indeed anthropology achieved its disciplinary identity in good part by not being the medical science of man. In so doing it repeated the process by which physiology had long ago broken with medicine, as well as that by which medicine itself had charted its movement forward by taking the body alone as its object and ceasing to be "the science of man." Yet although the medical science of man often functioned for the anthropologists chiefly as a tradition to be transcended, its influence operated in active, positive fashions as well. In some cases there is direct, acknowledged linkage. In others the shaping influence of anthropological medicine can be traced in marginal or anomalous formulations that belied the dominant discourse of the field.

The most crucial respect in which anthropology showed the mark of anthropological medicine was in its characteristic construction of the problem of the physical and the moral, or, as the anthropologists reconfigured the issue, the influence of race on physical and intellectual capacities. Broca readily acknowledged his debts to the long line of physicians who had grounded inquiry into mental activity in the study of natural structures and processes rather than metaphysics or psychology.[52] Broca's specialized techniques for investigating the "organ–faculties" correspondence, moreover, were all fundamentally medical approaches: clinical observations of cases of aphasia, dementia, or idiocy; postmortem searches for localized lesions; measurements of anatomical and physiological features in nonliving subjects and specimens; compilations from literary sources of historically and geographically distributed "cases" of the physical and mental characteristics of "typical" representatives of racial groups.[53] These techniques enabled Broca and his co-workers to establish the fundamental claims of craniological and general racial science: that there was a "remarkable" relation between the size of the brain and the development of the intelligence in the diverse

see also Broca, "Histoire des progrès des études anthropologiques," 498, where he wrote that "science must take notice only of its own concerns and must never bend before the exigencies of party" (498).

52 On Broca's debts to medical works in cerebral science, see Schiller, *Paul Broca,* chap. 10; see also Broca, *Eloge de François Lallemand* (Paris, Asselin, 1862).

53 The use of these techniques may be traced in the articles on cerebral and craniological topics in *MAPB,* vol. 4.

racial groups, and that all other significant anatomical and physiological features were in direct correspondence with the "level" of a given race on a hierarchy extending from the "superior" races down to those that occupied an intermediary position between full humanity and the upper reaches of animality.[54] These contentions constituted the bedrock of anthropology as developed within the confines of the anthropology society, and the effort to prove them – by means of thousands of measurements of individuals and specimens recorded in the registers held at the society's laboratory, and by the amassing of testimonials and observations by the anthropologists themselves and their scores of "correspondents" throughout the world – established the practical contours of anthropological labor.[55]

Thus to chart the legacy of the medical science of man to Brocan anthropology, it is necessary to analyze what precisely anthropologists made of the long-standing problem of the physical and the moral. Strictly speaking, the anthropologists considered no such problem. Craniological science held not that there was a correlation between features of the brain and "moral" capacities or tendencies but between the brain and an entity usually called "intelligence." (Synonyms included "intellectual faculties," "mental capacities," "the elevated cerebral functions," and the like.)[56] Insofar as the anthropologists stayed with this contention – that the physical conformation of the brain was in direct correspondence with the intellect – they approached the problem of the physical-moral relation in the way first charted by the materialist neuroscience of the 1830s and 1840s. The anatomists and physiologists of that era shifted emphasis away from the general "moral" capacities of the early science of man toward more narrowly defined "intellectual faculties" and in so doing relieved their science of the weight of postulating the somatic determinism of moral behavior.[57]

This move was of crucial importance to the elaboration of a rigorously determinist science of man for it provided an escape route from a position that the anthropologists, like the criminologists and psychiatrists, found it difficult wholly to accept – that morality or immorality resulted not from moral choice or striving but from inherent, fatal characteristics or tendencies. The disentangling of the "intellectual" and the "moral" relieved anthropology of the burden of moral fatalism and, perhaps more important

54 *BSAP* 2 (1861): 187–88, 176; for the view that the human races shade off into animality, see the discussion by Simonot in *BSAP* 6 (1865): 633–48. Simonot's statement is especially interesting because he was one of the anthropologists who argued that humans should be formally classified as standing apart from the animals, yet even he said that the "series" from man to animal was continuous since the "lower" races showed scarcely any evidence of the higher human faculties (648).

55 On the registers of craniological and other measurements compiled in the anthropologists' laboratory, see Denise Férembach, *Le laboratoire d'anthropologie de l'Ecole pratique des hautes etudes (Laboratoire Broca)* (Paris: Laboratoire d'anthropologie biologique, 1980).

56 These different usages appear in *BSAP* 2 (1861): 70–78, 139–97.

57 See Chapter 4, "Charting the Brain and Nervous System."

given its embrace of neutral scientism, of the very appearance of involvement in moral concerns. When charged after one craniological presentation
with embracing a cruel fatalism that condemned the world's "inferior races"
to a life of unrelieved brutality, Broca responded that such a contention be-
trayed a complete misunderstanding of racial science. Far from contending
that the inferior races were immoral or "ferocious," he readily accepted
travelers' reports that the primitive races had "sweet, gentle manners" and
showed devotion to their fellows. These were the results of "natural" moral
sentiments that appeared to be universal throughout humanity. His contention had only been that there were certain races that, because of their fundamental organization, were wholly incapable of moving up the ladder of
civilization, in short that there were races utterly lacking the capacity for
"perfectibility."[58]

Thus the anthropologists shunted the moral aside and yet, by focusing on
"perfectibility," reintroduced for investigation mental, moral, and psychic
phenomena beyond the strictly "intellectual faculties." In the 1840s François
Leuret had taken a similar step in delineating an aptitude he called the "capacity for progress," and Broca's definition of the scope of "descriptive anthropology" recalled this usage in urging inquiry into the "aptitude to
conceive of progress or be receptive to it."[59] The anthropology society
eventually settled on using the terms "perfectibility" and "civilizability" interchangeably in the first long-sustained debate that took place within its
confines. This debate, which dominated the society's arguments throughout 1861 and 1862, indicates clearly the anthropologists' sometimes precar-
ious suspension between the old anthropological medicine and the new
anthropology.

In the view of most of the anthropologists, the capacity of the various
races for "perfectibility" could be determined by the presence or absence,
development or retardation, simplicity or complexity of features of the
cerebral-nervous system. Broca's own contention was that intelligence/per-
fectibility depended on the size of the brain, and his most intensive research
was devoted to measuring "cranial capacity," the volume of the interior of
the skull. This technique presented certain problems that even Broca himself recognized: the study of cranial capacity focused not on the brain itself
but on the skull; more important, it made possible only measurements of
the whole brain rather than any of its specific regions or parts. Broca whole-
heartedly endorsed the localist framework of modern neuroscience, and he
fully anticipated that further work on charting the brain would reveal the
precise organic "seats" of many human capacities. In his view one of the
most incontestable principles so far established by localization studies was
that the "higher" or "intellectual" faculties were located in the frontal lobes
of the brain. Yet this principle presented a clear problem to craniological

58 *BSAP* 1 (1860): 375.   59 Broca, "Anthropologie," *MAPB* 1:6–7.

research for it meant that to be truly accurate measurements should be made not of the whole brain but of the frontal lobes alone. But it was technically impossible to transport brains of representatives of far-flung races to the anthropology society in good enough condition and large enough numbers to demonstrate the relationship between intellectual capacity and the size of the frontal lobes.[60] Yet Broca was resolute that overall the results of studies of cranial capacity were reliable: they were fully in accord with ordinary assessments of the intellectual superiority and inferiority of the races.[61]

The problems surrounding Broca's approach to craniology were in any event largely irrelevant to members of the society who denied that there was any demonstrable correlation between brain weight generally – or the size of the frontal lobes in particular – and "intellectual capacity." The museum naturalist Louis-Pierre Gratiolet argued, for example, that to the extent that the intellectual faculties depended on any specific anatomical feature, this feature seemed to be not the size of the brain but the number and complexity of the cerebral convolutions. Even this was uncertain: ultimately, Gratiolet argued, the higher faculties depended not on static anatomical features at all but on what he called the "harmony and dynamic architecture" of the cerebral-nervous system, in which were expressed or made manifest the "vital forces whose laws are hidden."[62] This recourse to vitalism within the society was swiftly rebuked. Two speakers who followed Gratiolet condemned him for injecting "metaphysics" into what had been a strictly scientific debate and for resorting to explanations based on the "occult forces" of prepositive medicine. "The object of the society," asserted one member, was "to construct a science of man insofar as man is a distinct, observable, and measurable subject."[63]

As these details from the "perfectibility" debate indicate, the anthropology society attempted to hold fast to a localist and materialist framework that both rested upon and reinforced a rigorously determinist approach to the relation between "structures" and "capacities." And yet Gratiolet's falling away from materialist grace was far from being the only instance in which the anthropologists proved themselves unwilling to embrace a perspective on human potentialities that was absolutely fatalist in character. Even Broca recognized along the margins of craniological science problems and peculiarities that threw into question not only his determinism but his localist and reductionist methodology as well. Not only did he eliminate

---

60 On Broca's work in cerebral localization, see Schiller, *Paul Broca,* chap. 8; on the procedures and difficulties involved in transporting brains, see Broca, *Instructions générales pour les recherches et observations anthropologiques (Anatomie et physiologie)* (Paris: E. Martinet, 1865), 379–81 (these *Instructions* were reprinted from *Mémoires de la Société d'anthropologie de Paris* 2 [1863–66]: 69–204).

61 Broca suggested that difficulties could be avoided "by choosing, for the comparison of brains, races whose intellectual inequality was wholly evident"; see *BSAP* 2 (1861): 176.

62 *BSAP* 2 (1861): 250, 258–59.   63 *Ibid.,* 275, 284.

the "natural" moral sentiments from his construal of the physical-moral relation; he also wavered even on the question of the determinate character of the intellectual faculties. Although craniological science was based on the principle that "stable" physical characters determined intelligence, Broca sometimes seemed willing to accept the reverse view that intelligence – conceived physiologically as the "level of activity" of the brain – determined cranial capacity. The latter view, that intellectual activity might determine the size of the brain, derived not from a static anatomical localism but from the long-standing physiological doctrine that organs and faculties could be improved by habitual use. In such a conception the intellectual faculties were latent and came to be developed only when intellectual "exercise" rendered them active. The naturalist Camille Dareste developed this view within the society on one occasion when he argued that Cuvier's genius was to be explained not by the size of his brain but by his intense and unrelenting intellectual activity. Broca responded that he completely agreed with this physiological principle, but he made no attempt to reconcile it with the static view connecting brain size and intelligence that he ordinarily upheld.[64] Similarly Broca's approach to the subject of the intellectual differences between men and women revealed not a strict determinism but again a readiness to accept that intellectual capacities might be molded by "habits." Although Broca argued that women were slightly inferior intellectually to men, he acknowledged that the difference might well result from women's less demanding education rather than from any inherent physical inferiority. He observed further that if women's brains were put to steadier and more exacting use, they might experience marked improvement.[65]

This conception of the influence of sex on intellectual development was indicative of a more general tendency in the craniological literature to accept, sometimes eagerly to embrace, modifications of the supposedly definitive physical-intellectual relation by the "influences" – age, sex, constitution, and the like – that had always been privileged in anthropological medicine. Indeed the introduction of such influences – the standard agents of medical "variability" that modern anthropology ostensibly repudiated – rescued the anthropologists on repeated occasions from anomalies in their data. When the cranial capacity of "geniuses" was shown to vary widely or to be greater among country people than among Parisians, these oddities were treated as epiphenomena caused by "variations" in the age, sex, general constitution, or mode of existence of the subjects in question.[66] Yet al-

64 Dareste's presentation is in *BSAP* 3 (1862): 26–50; Broca's response is at 54.
65 Compare the contrasting formulation in *BSAP* 2 (1861): 153, to the meliorist view in Broca, *MAPB* 5:214.
66 *BSAP* 2 (1861): 150–51, 165–67, where Broca argued against the findings of the German craniologist Rudolph Wagner, who denied the significance of cranial capacity, by pointing to variations caused by age, sex, and sickness. Wagner's "geniuses," he said, were not re-

though such "influences" were mobilized to explain anomalies, they were never regarded as adequate to alter what were in other contexts presented as the iron laws of craniological science.

Or, rather, it is not that such peculiarities were *never* adequate to subvert anthropology's laws; they were adequate only when bending or overthrowing the law was desirable for some reason external to craniological science or required by its implicit premises. To Broca, who was a political progressive and fervent supporter of female education, assessing women's intellectual capacity as improvable was a case where bending the law was desirable.[67] On the other hand, interpreting the craniological evidence in such a fashion as not to controvert the self-evident intellectual superiority of modern Parisians over peasants was required in the very interest of science itself.

In these instances the ostensibly rigorous determinism of the craniological viewpoint was mitigated or softened by a reversion to older principles of anthropological medicine that left room for the view that "capacities" – intellectual and otherwise – could be altered by use or were subject to diverse systemic influences. This point of view was of course the one that had always been called upon to support medical intervention in education, the life of the family, and other social enterprises. The anthropologists' concept of race denied this soft construction of the physical-moral relation and in so doing supplied anthropology's newly "positive" foundation. Yet at the same time the anthropologists' own hard line excluded meliorist possibilities and led in certain cases to conclusions that were, to the anthropologists themselves, morally, politically, or ideologically unpalatable.

Still, it is important to observe the contexts in which reversions to the meliorist option within anthropological medicine took place. In the "perfectibility" debate, Broca and most of his colleagues agreed that certain races were, by reason of their fundamental "organization," completely incapable of rising to civilization from savagery. Worse yet, some races were not even capable of surviving contact with people of superior organization and were doomed to extinction from the first meeting with Europeans. Thus races like the Tasmanians were lost to history. No adjustments on their part nor any external intervention could have averted their fate.[68] In such cases the desperate conclusions of anthropological science could not be

ally equally intelligent and varied too much in age for comparison; for "country people," see *MAPB* 5:214, where Broca explained their larger cranial capacity as a result of their varied activities (as opposed to the monotony of city life).

67 On Broca's politics, see Schiller, *Paul Broca*, 24–25, 50–51, 54–56, 273–75; on his support for girls' secondary education, see 285–86.

68 *BSAP* 1 (1860): 337–42, 375, 421, 433–37; on the Tasmanians, see *ibid.*, 1 (1860): 255–62; Paul Broca, *Recherches sur l'hybridité animale en général et sur l'hybridité humaine en particulier* (Paris: Imprimerie de J. Claye, 1860), 640–52.

avoided. And yet when anthropology's focus shifted to Europeans and especially to elements of the French population, the anthropologists were usually unwilling to accept such fatalism and became once again, in their general outlook, therapists, meliorists, and reformers. French women could be better educated and aided in leaving their narrow domestic sphere. Criminals, alcoholics, even "degenerates" could be altered through moral and physical education or, at the very least, held responsible for actions they could have controlled if they had tried hard enough. Certainly not all anthropologists availed themselves of this option to revert to the meliorist possibilities of anthropological medicine – criminal anthropologists were often more interested in detecting than in reforming criminals – but the option was definitely there.[69] Determinist anthropology was suitable, then, for those races which approached animality and were, like animals, fatally governed by organization. But the old science of man reasserted its claims when the anthropologists sought to explain the physicomoral link among the races removed from animality by civilization and among whom effort, practice, and habits produced positive results in intellectual, physical, and moral formation.

That the principles of anthropological medicine were only selectively applied was demonstrated when Dareste followed up his challenge to Broca's static craniology by urging that, although in some cases use of the brain could improve both organ and function, in the case of "savages" such capacity for improvement was clearly limited. The intelligence of savages, Dareste held, could improve with use only in the early years of life. At puberty their sexual instinct and urge to physical activity became dominant and blocked further development of the intellectual powers.[70] This was a literal transcription, from the vitalist doctrine of the three domains of force or activity, of the principle that vital energy was limited and could not fuel development in all domains simultaneously. Vitalist constructs of this kind did not commonly appear in the society's deliberations but they were available all the same and formed a kind of sediment – a bedrock of physiological truisms – to which recourse could be had when the localist, static, and reductionist formulations of modern anthropology seemed to falter.

If recalling the medical science of man were only a way to explain the anomalies and inconsistencies of scientific constructs – degeneracy, the "microbial" explanation of criminality, Charcot's hysteria, craniology – whose legitimacy was challenged even within their original disciplines by

69 On the criminal anthropologists' links to police science, see Alphonse Bertillon, *Alphonse Bertillon's Instructions for Taking Descriptions for the Identification of Criminals and Others,* trans. Gallus Muller (New York: AMS Press, 1977); see also Léonce Manouvrier, *L'anthropologie et le droit* (Paris: V. Giard and E. Brière, 1894), 20–27.
70 *BSAP* 3 (1862): 49.

around 1900, then there would be little interest in these intellectual surviv-
als from another age. But in fact the fluid, reciprocal, free-flowing construction of the physical-moral relation that the human sciences inherited
from the old science of man definitively established their larger sociocultural posture in late nineteenth-century France. In the case of anthropology,
this became evident as the anthropologists gradually abandoned their claim
to be interested only in neutral, rigorous science and not in the social applications or utility of their work. Broca preached this principle up to his
death in 1880 and tried to hold the society to it as well. Yet even he was not
beyond all notion of "engagement" and sometimes – as in the case of female education – used the society as a forum to argue for ideological principles or political causes to which he, as a republican, an anticlerical, and a
freethinker, subscribed. Then after the clear triumph of republicanism in
the late 1870s, others within the society became increasingly eager to demonstrate anthropology's immediate and diverse utility. Broca's disciple Paul
Topinard, who both from personal ambitions and fears for anthropology's
future sought to take on Broca's scientistic mantle, observed that even before Broca's death in 1880 the society was bitterly divided between those
who wanted anthropology to be purely scientific and those who wanted it
to function as a standard-bearer for progressive principles in French
society.[71] After Broca's death the whole tenor of the society changed and it
became one of the most visible and controversial forums in French scholarly
life for the advancement of radical republican causes. Like the Charcot circle, the anthropologists became closely identified with Parisian municipal
regimes of the 1880s that concocted diverse schemes to improve the moral,
social, and physical level of the people by applying the insights of the human
sciences. In the last two decades of the nineteenth century, anthropologists
joined with psychiatrists, hygienists, criminologists, and diverse other
"practitioners" in campaigns to eradicate degeneracy, underpopulation, alcoholism, criminality, prostitution, and a host of other maladies using techniques and principles that were now unabashedly mobilized on behalf of
social progress.[72] In so doing none of these sciences abandoned their ostensibly determinist foundations, which undergirded their claims to positivity;
instead they blended, at will and as the changing contexts of their social
"applications" demanded, the fixist/determinist impulse and the meliora-

71 Topinard, *A la mémoire de Broca*, 17–18. Ironically, Topinard, once "liberated" (as he put it)
   from the tradition of Broca, turned to the "social, political, and religious questions" he had
   earlier avoided; see Paul Topinard, *Science et foi: L'anthropologie et la science sociale* (Paris:
   Masson, 1900), v.
72 Topinard, *A la mémoire de Broca*, 13–40; Michael Hammond, "Anthropology as a Weapon
   of Social Combat in Late-Nineteenth-Century France," *Journal of the History of the Behavioral Sciences* 16 (1980): 118–32. On the links between the Charcot circle and the Paris Municipal Council, see Goldstein, *Console and Classify*, 362–64; see also Harris, Introduction to
   Clinical Lectures, xix.

tive/therapeutic impulse that had both long been sheltered by the tradition of anthropological medicine.[73]

In one of the most decisive and significant developments in late nineteenth-century social and human science, the revalorization of the therapeutic impulse of the older anthropological medicine coincided with, reinforced, and even to some extent made possible the neo-Lamarckian revival that began in France after the introduction of Darwinism. The interaction of the medical heritage and neo-Lamarckism in the human sciences was a complex process whose outlines can only be hinted at here, but it is a crucial dimension of the long-term importance of the medical science of man. That Darwinism was even introduced in France owed a good deal to the tendency of the anthropology society, despite its ostensibly strict scientism, to take up questions that to many seemed to border on the metaphysical. The biology society might have seemed a more likely forum for the discussion of Darwin's theory, but just as the society had refused to discuss Broca's arguments on "human hybridity," so it was equally indisposed to examine Darwin's views. Like the Société d'anthropologie, the Société de biologie was made up of doctors who had hived off from medicine proper to effect a juncture with the natural sciences. It too was determined to exclude from its discussions those elements of medicine that seemed archaic and unscientific, and indeed any theory, including that of species transformation, that appeared to rest on speculation or pure hypothesis.[74]

Given the anthropologists' resolutely positivist self-presentation, a similar response to Darwinism might have been expected from the anthropology society. But the anthropologists were committed to the exploration of a range of problematics that was necessarily grand in sweep and that transcended the positivist framework embraced by the biologists. Perfectibility, the monogenist-polygenist thematic, the differences between humans and animals, these were all problems that were only partially susceptible to investigation by the methods and procedures of the laboratory and the autopsy table. Anthropology was forced by its very nature to be open to the sweeping hypothesis and to validate – if against its own positivist grain –

73 See, for example, Manouvrier, *L'anthropologie et le droit*, where in discussing criminality, he embraced both determinism and reformism: "In the psychological and the sociological order, as in the purely biological order, the facts obey a rigorous determinism the knowledge of which may lead to the equally compelling possibility of directing events" (27).

74 On the founding of the Société de biologie in 1848, see E. Gley, "Histoire des Sciences: La Société de Biologie," 4th ser., no. 13 (January 6, 1900): 1–11, and no. 16 (April 21, 1900): 481–91, at 3-4. On the positivism embraced by the society, see V. Genty, *Un grand biologiste Charles Robin, 1821–1885: Sa vie, ses amitiés philosophiques et littéraires* (Lyon: Société anonyme de l'imprimerie A. Rey, 1931), 23–26, 51; see also Charles Robin, "Sur la direction que se sont proposée en se réunissant les membres fondateurs de la Société de biologie pour répondre au titre qu'ils ont choisi," *Comptes-rendus des séances et mémoires de la Société de biologie* 1 (1850): i–x. On the biologists' "positivist" rejection of Darwinism, see Conry, *L'introduction du darwinisme*, 415. This was Broca's initial reaction to Darwin as well; see Blanckaert, "L'anthropologie personnifiée," xiii–xxi.

the kind of grandiose problems that had rested at the heart of anthropological medicine. Thus anthropology could give a hearing to Darwinism where biology could not. As Yvette Conry has demonstrated, the anthropologists were among the few scientists in France even to attempt serious consideration of a theory that not only controverted positivist ideas of "true science" but in its particulars fit ill with hallowed precepts of the French biomedical sciences.[75]

Even among the anthropologists, however, Darwinism soon proved clearly incompatible with regnant doctrines, and this incommensurability rapidly sparked a return to the indigenous transformism of Lamarck, which since the 1820s had had dubious standing in the life sciences. The recovery of Lamarck was pursued nowhere with greater ardor and intensity than among the anthropologists. After early efforts to wrestle with Darwinism as such, the anthropology society moved with alacrity to the more familiar and comprehensible terrain of Lamarckism. By 1875 the anthropologist Clémence Royer, who in her 1862 translation of *Origins* had argued for the originality of Darwin's theory, had assimilated Darwinism to natively French transformism and begun referring to Darwin himself as a continuer of the work of Lamarck. In 1882 the anthropology society established a "Conférence transformiste" that was to sponsor discussions not merely of Darwinism but of all varieties of transformism including that of its original "founder," Lamarck; Darwin's theory was to be treated "as a complement to, not a replacement for," Lamarck's work.[76] The anthropologists were thus instrumental in the Lamarckian revival that soon spread throughout the French life and social sciences.

Although it would require an extended investigation to prove this point, I would suggest that one reason anthropologists, criminologists, psychiatrists, and other human scientists so readily and contentedly incorporated a Lamarckian construction of transformism into their vision of both research and therapeutic possibilities was that the tradition of anthropological medicine had nurtured and carried within it language and concepts that had intimate affinities with Lamarck's thought. It has not fallen within the bounds of this study to develop an extensive comparison between the principles of anthropological medicine and Lamarck's conceptualization of the molding power of external "influences" on the body economy, the adaptive response of creatures motivated by an inner conserving force, the power of habit to remake general constitution, the fluid boundaries between instinc-

75 Conry, *L'introduction du darwinisme*, 31, 52–89. Cf. Joy Harvey, "Evolution Transformed: Positivists and Materialists in the *Société d'Anthropologie de Paris* from Second Empire to Third Republic," in *The Wider Domain of Evolutionary Thought*, ed. D. Oldroyd and I. Langham (Dordrecht: Reidel, 1983), 289–310.

76 On Broca's critique of Darwin, see Conry, *L'introduction du darwinisme*, 52–62, and on Royer's translations, *ibid.*, 19, 41; on the "Conférence transformiste," see Manouvrier, "La Société d'anthropologie de Paris," 311.

tual and intellective response to felt "needs," and the like. And on a few occasions fundamental differences have appeared between the Lamarckian perspective and the conception of the harmony and repose of the body economy that underlay the vitalist conception of health.[77] And yet there are obvious linkages – linguistic and conceptual – between Lamarckism and the medical science of man, especially in their mutual emphasis on the transformative power of habit and usage. When it is recalled that Lamarck had institutional, ideological, and conceptual ties to the medical Ideologues, this conflation of language and principles makes good historical sense.[78] In any event the affinities between Lamarckism and anthropological medicine seem clearly to have encouraged the eager embrace and fostering of the neo-Lamarckian synthesis within the human sciences in the years after 1870. It was no accident that one of the earliest and most influential advocates of the utility of Lamarckism in improving the moral and physical health of the French after the disaster of 1870–71 was the physician Jules Guérin, who amid the passions of 1848 had argued that physicians must take the lead in the work of "universal regeneration."[79]

All of this would seem to leave us at an end point where the human sciences finally settled on one side – the interventionist, therapeutic side – of the meliorist/fixist divide that anthropological medicine had endlessly crossed and recrossed depending on the political, broadly ideological, or socioprofessional pressures of the moment. And yet it would be wholly wrong to convey the impression that under the influence of the progressive spirit of the early Third Republic the human sciences definitively embraced the meliorist "option" within the tradition of anthropological medicine. It is essential as a last word to reaffirm that the human sciences of the late nineteenth century, no less than the medical science of man before them, chose according to their own ambitions and logic the places and moments when they envisaged perfectibility and when they did not. Despite repeated criticisms of the vagueness, inconsistency, and empirical nullity of the concept of hereditary degeneration, the figure of the degenerate disappeared from the cultural landscape only amid the nationalist revival of 1905. Nor did those suffering from Charcot's hereditary and incurable hysteria fade from the pages of psychiatric textbooks until World War I, and even then only to be transformed, in good numbers, into the hereditarily predisposed victims of "shellshock." Throughout the period from the 1890s to World War II, finally, French anthropology was willing and ready, when circumstances seemed to warrant it, to reassert its command of primordial racial

77 See Chapter 1, "Vitality and Variability."
78 For a comparison of Lamarckism with themes of medical Ideology, see Georges Gusdorf, *Les sciences humaines et la pensée occidentale*, vol. 8, *La conscience révolutionnaire: Les Idéologues* (Paris: Payot, 1978), 429–50; see also François Picavet, *Les Idéologues* (Paris: Alcan, 1896), 438–44.
79 Conry, *L'introduction du darwinisme*, 310–11, see also Chapter 4.

laws. When the claims or hopes of black colonials or Jews did not meet favor with the anthropologists, the rhetoric of biohistorical meliorism was once again suppressed and the fatal laws of "organization" resurrected.[80] The science of man could be a science of hope and human betterment, or not. The choice was always there.

80 Dowbiggin, *Inheriting Madness,* 165; Harris, *Murders and Madness,* li; Pick, *Faces of Degeneration,* 231–37. On the Société d'anthropologie de Paris in the twentieth century, see Louis Marin, "Organisation du savoir en France: Les études portant sur l'homme et l'Ecole d'Anthropologie de 1926 à 1956," *Revue anthropologique* (1956): 169–79; the anthropologists Georges Montandon and René Martial offered support to the anti-Semitic laws of the Vichy regime; see Blanckaert, "Origins of French Ethnology," 50–51.

INDEX

continued